HEALTHY CALENDAR
diabetic cooking

SECOND EDITION

Lara Rondinelli-Hamilton, RD, LDN, CDE, and
Chef Jennifer Bucko Lamplough

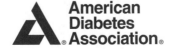

American Diabetes Association.

Director, Book Publishing, Abe Ogden; *Managing Editor,* Greg Guthrie; *Acquisitions Editor,* Victor Van Beuren; *Editor,* Greg Guthrie; *Production Manager,* Melissa Sprott; *Composition,* Circle Graphics; *Cover Design,* Jody Billert; *Photographer,* Renee Comet; *Printer,* Marquis Imprimeur.

Printed in Canada

1 3 5 7 9 10 8 6 4 2

ADA titles may be purchased for business or promotional use or for special sales. To purchase more than 50 copies of this book at a discount, or for custom editions of this book with your logo, contact the American Diabetes Association at the address below, at booksales@diabetes.org, or by calling 703-299-2046.

American Diabetes Association
1701 North Beauregard Street
Alexandria, Virginia 22311

DOI: 10.2337/9781580404624

Library of Congress Cataloging-in-Publication Data
Rondinelli, Lara M., 1974-
 Healthy calendar diabetic cooking / Lara Hamilton, RD, LDN, CDE, and Chef Jennifer Lamplough. -- 2nd edition.
   pages cm
 Summary: "The recipes in this cookbook are not ONLY intended for the person with diabetes, but for the entire family and anyone looking to eat quick, healthy and delicious food!"-- Provided by publisher.
 Includes bibliographical references and index.
 ISBN 978-1-58040-462-4 (pbk.)
 1. Diabetes--Diet therapy--Recipes. 2. Seasonal cooking. I. Lamplough, Jennifer, 1974- II. Title.
 RC662.R65 2012
 641.5'6314--dc23
              2012031878

CONTENTS

PREFACE

Lara Rondinelli-Hamilton

So much has changed since we wrote the first edition of *Healthy Calendar Diabetic Cooking* in 2004. First, nutrition recommendations and products have changed. All Americans are encouraged to increase their fiber intake and make half their grains whole grains, so this means that we have more of these products available to choose from at the grocery store. Lower-carbohydrate versions of many foods are now available, and the good news is that many of these products taste great! We felt these changes needed to be incorporated into this new edition for better nutrition and improved food choices.

My personal life has changed dramatically since 2004. In February 2007, I was biopsy-diagnosed with celiac disease. Celiac disease is an autoimmune disorder that affects the digestive process of the small intestine. When a person with celiac disease eats gluten (a protein found in wheat, rye, and barley), the person's immune system responds by attacking the small intestine (specifically the villi of the intestines) and inhibits the absorption of nutrients into the body. Celiac disease is associated with other autoimmune disorders, such as type 1 diabetes and thyroid disease. An estimated 10% of people with type 1 diabetes also have celiac disease. If celiac disease is undiagnosed and untreated, it can lead to other diseases.

People with celiac disease must avoid gluten. Foods that contain gluten include anything with flour, such as bread, pasta, waffles, cookies, and cakes, but it's also hidden in other foods, such as soy sauce, salad dressings, some canned broth, and many more foods. My life changed with this diagnosis, as I now have to follow a strict gluten-free diet.

Because people with type 1 diabetes have a higher risk of developing celiac disease and it's estimated that 10% of people with type 1 diabetes also have celiac disease, we decided to include some gluten-free tips and recipes in this cookbook too.

In addition to that big change, I have a family now that includes my husband and two children under the age of three. Quick and healthy meals have never been more important to me, since time is limited like never before. I understand that most people don't have a lot of time to get meals on the table. I always encourage the whole family to eat healthy together, so the recipes in this cookbook are not ONLY intended for the person with diabetes, but for the entire family and anyone looking to eat quick, healthy, and delicious food!

Jennifer Bucko Lamplough

We felt it necessary to also incorporate new recipes that focus on updated dietary recommendations and that appeal to a wider audience of people who are not only eating for diabetes but also for general good health. I am actually one of those people. I do not have diabetes but for the last 20 years I have struggled with a weight problem. Being a chef who specializes in cooking and creating recipes for people with diabetes, it has always been a front-and-center issue for me that I needed to focus on my health, too. For the last year or so, I've been on a weight-loss journey, eating healthy (making recipes out of *Healthy Calendar Diabetic Cooking* as well as our other book, *The Healthy Carb Diabetes Cookbook)*, working out, and seeking therapy to deal with my food issues. I've lost 60 pounds and continue to pursue good health and fitness. I have become an avid runner in this process and have received a whole new lease on life.

I'm so thrilled to share my weight-loss journey with you and others who come see us at cooking demonstrations. In the last eight years, I've also gotten married and continue to work as a faculty member teaching futures chefs. I am on a mission to educate them on how to bring healthy options to the public as they pursue their careers in food service.

ACKNOWLEDGMENTS

Thank you to all of you who supported the first edition of *Healthy Calendar Diabetic Cooking*. We were overwhelmed by the positive response to that cookbook and are grateful that so many of you spread the word to your friends and family. The biggest compliment we receive is that people actually use this cookbook and it's not just sitting on the shelf!

Thank you to the efforts of many people at the American Diabetes Association. Big thanks to Abe Ogden, Director of Book Publishing, for allowing us to do this updated edition—you are a true professional and have been great to work with. Thank you to Greg Guthrie for all your time, work, and dedication to this project. Big thanks to Lyn Wheeler for your hours of work on the nutrition analysis (and for taking our calls at any time of night). We were thrilled to work with you again.

Special thanks to my family, including my mom, dad, and sisters, Kari Mender and Jennifer Sebring, who have been wonderful supporters and bought and sold many of the cookbooks. Thank you so much for your love and for sharing in my joy. My closest friends and Dinner Club girls have been wonderful supporters, and I thank you too. A special thanks to Megan Clendening, who has given almost everyone she knows copies of our cookbooks and has been a great help at our book events. Thank you to my fellow certified diabetes educators who recommended the cookbook to their patients. You all have been wonderful and thank you for sharing in my excitement.

I'm forever grateful to my co-author, Jennifer Bucko Lamplough, who isn't only an amazing chef, but also a great writer, my best friend, and one of the smartest and funniest people I know. I'm so glad we've been through it all together—especially this project.

Thank you to my husband, Jared, for your constant love and support and for making so many of my dreams come true. Thanks also for your ability to make me laugh, for your taste-testing skills, and for always giving me your honest feedback. And, to my two little sweeties, Ethan and Penelope, I love you more than you will ever know and I'm so grateful for the joy you have brought into my life.

Finally, thank you to all my patients with diabetes who continue to inspire me every day. I hope this makes your life with diabetes a little easier and healthier.

—Lara Rondinelli-Hamilton, RD, LDN, CDE

This book surely would not have been possible had it not been for my co-author and lifelong best friend, Lara Rondinelli-Hamilton. Lara, your knowledge and experience made this book what it is and continuously inspire me to be healthy, and your unconditional friendship inspires me to be a better person. This book started as a dream and became our reality, and I wouldn't want to share this experience with anyone else.

I want to thank my darling husband, Michael Lamplough, for his unfailing love, support, and encouragement. I feed you healthy food, and you feed my soul. I love you more than any words can say. Thanks for being such an incredible cheerleader, taste tester, and partner.

I want to thank my family for being such great supporters and taste testers, especially my mom, Judy Bucko, for constantly inspiring me to follow my dreams, do what I love, and make a killer pot of soup. Mom, you are the reason I'm the woman I am today. To my entire family: Jill, Rob, Kate, and Erin Kilhefner; Jane, Mike, Gabrielle, and Camille DiMartin; Jackie, Penny, and Ella Burke; Jim, Paula, Lily, and Jackson Bucko; Margaret McKenzie; Joel and Laura Lamplough; and Joel, Josh, Jacob, and Jessica Lamplough; thank you for your constant support, your outstanding recipe ideas, your feedback, and your senses of humor … all of which I couldn't have survived this project without.

Most importantly, to my dad, Jack Bucko, who would have loved this book. Dad, I wish you could have been here to see, experience, and taste all of this.

To all of our friends who acted as our official taste testers and who are always there to support us in whatever we do, especially Draga Beckner, Megan Clendening, and the rest of the Dinner Club girls—Ann Marie Ferguson, Stacey Joyce, Mary Alice Patton, Elizabeth Sheridan, and Heather Johnson—as well as all of my wonderful neighbors and Batavia friends, you have my thanks.

Thank you to everyone at Robert Morris University Institute of Culinary Arts, especially Nancy Rotunno, Amy Keck, Bryan Flower, and all of the incredible faculty, advisors, and students. There is a reason I love my job, and it's all of you.

Thank you to everyone at the American Diabetes Association, especially Abraham Ogden, Director of Book Publishing, for your support and words of wisdom. Thank you to our editor, Greg Guthrie, for all of your hard work, and to Madelyn Wheeler, for your unbelievable dedication in completing the nutrition analysis of the recipes.

I mostly want to thank all of our readers, especially those who come see us every year at the American Diabetes Association Expo in Chicago. Your support and belief in us and our recipes make what we do worth every second of cooking, testing, writing, and reworking to make these recipes happen.

Eat well!

—Chef Jen Bucko Lamplough

KITCHEN TOOLS

Are you confused about which kitchen tools are must-haves and which ones are fads? This list is everything you need to ensure smooth sailing in the kitchen.

A good knife set, including:
- a French or chef's knife
- a paring knife
- a serrated knife
- a honing steel (usually included with knife set) and
- a sharpener

Baking dish (casserole dish), 9 × 13

Baking sheets

Can opener

Colander (small and large)

Garlic press

Immersion blender

Measuring cups (liquid and dry)

Measuring spoons

Meat thermometer

Plastic cutting boards

Potato masher

Prep bowls

Saucepan

Sauté pan (nonstick)

Sauté pan (oven safe)

Skewers and toothpicks

Soup pot

Spatulas, metal and plastic

Spoon, large

Spoon, large, slotted

Sturdy whisk

Tongs

Various sizes of mixing bowls (small to large)

Vegetable peeler

Zester (or microplane)

STOCKING A HEALTHY KITCHEN

Here is a list of healthy kitchen staples that you should always have on hand to prepare quick and tasty meals!

CARBOHYDRATES

Starchy Foods
- Whole-wheat bread with 2 or more grams of fiber per slice or whole-wheat sandwich thins
- Low-carb tortillas
- Oatmeal
- Sweet potatoes
- Canned and dried beans, such as black beans, kidney beans, garbanzo beans, and lentils
- Whole-wheat bread crumbs
- Quinoa
- Barley

Fruits
- Fresh fruit
- Frozen fruit, such as blueberries or strawberries (unsweetened)

Milk and yogurt
- 1% or fat-free milk or unsweetened almond milk
- Plain, fat-free Greek yogurt and/or light yogurt (aim for 15 or fewer grams of carb per serving)

NON-CARBOHYDRATES

Meat and meat substitutes
- Skinless chicken breast
- Lean ground turkey
- Lean beef and pork, round or loin cuts, e.g., sirloin and tenderloin
- Fish, fresh or frozen
- Canned tuna (packed in water)
- Lunch meats, turkey breast, ham, lean beef (reduced sodium)
- Reduced-fat cheese (shredded and slices)
- Low-fat or fat-free cottage cheese
- Eggs and egg substitutes

Vegetables
- Fresh and frozen vegetables
- No-salt-added diced tomatoes and crushed tomatoes

Fats
- Light cream cheese
- Light salad dressings
- Light mayonnaise or Miracle Whip
- Olive or canola oil
- Trans-fat-free margarine, e.g., Smart Balance
- Peanuts, almonds, walnuts, or pecans
- Avocado and olives

Miscellaneous
- Nonstick cooking spray
- Grated Parmesan cheese
- Vinegars: balsamic, apple cider, and red wine
- Chicken broth, fat-free, reduced-sodium
- Dried herbs and spices, such as basil, oregano, paprika, chili powder, garlic powder, cumin, cinnamon, and parsley
- Ketchup
- Dijon mustard
- Lemons or lemon juice
- Limes or lime juice
- Salsa
- Lite soy sauce
- Sugar substitute
- Garlic

MEAL DEALS

HEALTHY BREAKFAST IDEAS

Breakfasts with 30 Grams Total Carbohydrate or Less

Breakfast #1

1 slice whole-wheat toast, served with
    1 tsp sugar-free jam
1 hard-boiled egg
1 cup strawberries

Breakfast #2

1 low-carb tortilla
1 egg or 1/4 cup egg substitute (add veggies
    such as green pepper and onion to egg
    when cooking)
1 ounce reduced-fat cheddar cheese
1 cup mixed berries
*Roll ingredients into a burrito and serve fruit
    on the side.*

Breakfast #3

1 cup almond milk
1 cup unsweetened frozen berries
2 ounces plain Greek yogurt
*Put in a blender and mix for a delicious
    smoothie.*

Breakfast #4

1 whole-wheat English muffin
1 egg or 1/4 cup egg substitute (add veggies
    such as green pepper and onion to egg
    when cooking)
1 ounce reduced-fat cheddar cheese
1 slice Canadian bacon
Serve as a sandwich.

Breakfast #5

1/2 cup egg substitute
1 cup chopped spinach (or vegetables of
    your choice)
1/2 cup diced tomato
2 Tbsp reduced-fat cheddar cheese
1 slice whole-wheat toast
1 slice Canadian bacon
*Prepare omelet with first four ingredients,
    serve with toast and Canadian bacon.*

Breakfast #6

1 slice whole-wheat toast, served with
    2 tsp peanut butter
4 ounces plain, fat-free Greek yogurt
3/4 cup sliced strawberries

Breakfasts with 45 Grams Total Carbohydrate

Breakfast #1
1 cup oatmeal, served with
   cinnamon, to taste, and
   1 Tbsp chopped walnuts
1 cup fat-free milk

Breakfast #2
6 ounces light yogurt
1 cup blueberries
1 Tbsp sliced almonds
1 slice whole-wheat bread, served with
      1 tsp sugar-free jam

Breakfast #3
1/2 cup low-fat cottage cheese
1/2 cup pineapple
1 whole-wheat English muffin, served with
      1 tsp trans-fat-free margarine

Gluten-Free Breakfasts with 30 Grams Total Carbohydrate or Less

Breakfast #1
1 slice gluten-free bread, served with
      1 tsp sugar-free jam
1 hard-boiled egg
1 cup strawberries

Breakfast #2
1/2 cup low-fat cottage cheese
1/2 cup pineapple
1 slice gluten-free bread, served with
      1 tsp trans-fat-free margarine

Breakfast #3
6 ounces plain, fat-free Greek yogurt
1 1/2 cups blueberries
1 Tbsp sliced almonds

Breakfast #4
1 corn tortilla
1 egg or 1/4 cup egg substitute
      add 1 ounce reduced-fat cheese, and
      veggies, such as green pepper and onion,
      to eggs when cooking
1 cup mixed berries
*Combine ingredients in tortilla to make a
   burrito served with berries on the side.*

Breakfast #4
1 cup almond milk
1 cup unsweetened frozen berries
2 ounces plain, fat-free Greek yogurt
*Put in a blender and mix for a delicious
   smoothie.*

Breakfast #5
1/2 cup egg substitute
1 cup chopped spinach (or vegetables of your
   choice)
1/2 cup diced tomato
2 Tbsp reduced-fat cheddar cheese
1 slice gluten-free bread, toasted
1 slice Canadian bacon
*Prepare omelet with first four ingredients, serve
   with toast and Canadian bacon.*

Gluten-Free Breakfasts with 45 Grams Total Carbohydrate

Breakfast #1

1 egg or 1/4 cup egg substitute, cooked with
    1 ounce low-sodium ham, served on
    2 slices gluten-free bread (for lower
      carbs, serve on corn tortillas instead)
1 cup melon
Serve as a sandwich with melon on the side.

Breakfast #2

1/2 cup gluten-free hot cereal (aim for 4 grams
   fiber per serving), served with
   cinnamon
   1 Tbsp chopped walnuts
1 cup fat-free milk

Breakfast #3

1 gluten-free waffle, served with
    2 tsp peanut butter
4 ounces plain, fat-free Greek yogurt
1 cup strawberries

HEALTHY LUNCH IDEAS

Lunches with 30 Grams Total Carbohydrate or Less

Lunch #1 (Turkey or Ham Sandwich)

Whole-wheat sandwich thin, served with
    1 Tbsp hummus spread on light wheat
      bread (15 grams carb for 2 slices)
    lettuce
    tomato
    1 ounce deli-sliced turkey or ham
1 small apple
Small green salad with 1 Tbsp light dressing

Lunch #2 (Chicken Wrap)

1 low-carb tortilla
3 ounces chicken
1/4 avocado, mashed (spread on tortilla)
1/4 cup diced tomatoes
1 small pear
Serve chicken, avocado, and tomatoes wrapped
in the tortilla, serve with pear on the side.

Great Lunch Recipes

Spring Rolls, p. 262

Chicken Caesar Salad, p. 292

Chicken Guacamole Salad, p. 212

Mandarin Orange Chicken Salad, p. 308

Pesto Chicken Pita, p. 366

Toasted Almond Chicken Salad Sandwich, p. 333

Salad Niçoise, p. 303

Taco Salad with Black Beans, p. 231

Mediterranean Shrimp Wrap, p. 136

Tuna Melt, p. 93

Turkey and Artichoke Sandwich, p. 194

Turkey and Avocado Wraps, p. 42

Smokin' Turkey Sandwich, p. 156

Black Bean Soup, p. 328

Hearty Lentil Soup, p. 17

Split Pea Soup, p. 412

Tortilla Soup, p. 151

Lunch #3 (Large Green Salad)
Salad greens
3 ounces sliced chicken breast
1 Tbsp chopped pecans
2 Tbsp lite balsamic vinaigrette dressing
1 cup black bean soup
Serve the soup on the side.

Lunch #4 (Tuna Salad)
3 ounces tuna, packed in water, mixed with
    1 Tbsp light mayonnaise
    celery
    chopped onion, served on
1 whole-wheat sandwich thin
1 cup carrots, cucumbers, and cauliflower,
    served with
    2 Tbsp hummus
1 cup milk or 6 ounces light yogurt
Serve tuna salad on sandwich thin with veggies, hummus, and yogurt on the side.

Lunch #5 (Chicken Salad)
3 ounces cooked chicken, chopped, mixed
    with
    1 Tbsp light mayonnaise
    chopped onion
    1/4 cup grapes, halved
    1 Tbsp slivered almonds
10 whole-wheat crackers (serve salad on
    crackers instead of bread)
1/2 cup cottage cheese
1 cup strawberries
Serve chicken salad on whole-wheat crackers with strawberries and cottage cheese on the side.

Lunch #6 (Egg White Salad)
3 hard-boiled egg whites, mixed with
    1 Tbsp light mayonnaise
    1 tsp Dijon mustard, served on
Mixed greens OR 10 whole-wheat crackers
1 cup fresh fruit
Serve egg salad on salad greens or whole-wheat crackers with fresh fruit on the side.

Lunches with 45 Grams Total Carbohydrate

Lunch #1
1 cup reduced-sodium soup (lentil or beef
    vegetable)
1/2 natural peanut butter and sunflower seed
    sandwich, made with
    1 slice whole-wheat bread
    1 Tbsp peanut butter
    2 tsp sunflower seeds
1 cup strawberries

Lunch #2
3 ounces leftover chicken breast, chopped,
    mixed with
    1/2 cup fat-free refried beans, served
      with
14 baked tortilla chips OR two corn tortillas
    (top with salsa if desired)
Green salad, served with
    2 Tbsp light Ranch dressing
1 medium orange

Gluten-Free Lunches with 30 Grams Total Carbohydrate or Less

Lunch #1 (Chicken Wrap)

1 gluten-free tortilla

3 ounces chicken

1/8 avocado, mashed (spread on tortilla)

1/4 cup diced tomatoes

Serve chicken, avocado, and tomatoes wrapped in the tortilla.

Lunch #2

Large green salad, with

    3 ounces cooked chicken breast

    1 Tbsp chopped pecans

    2 Tbsp balsamic vinaigrette dressing (gluten-free)

1 cup gluten-free black bean soup

Lunch #3 (Chicken Salad)

3 ounces cooked chicken, chopped, mixed with

    1 Tbsp light mayo

    chopped onion

    1/4 cup grapes, halved

    1 Tbsp slivered almonds

10 gluten-free crackers (serve salad on crackers instead of bread)

1/2 cup cottage cheese

1/2 cup strawberries

Serve chicken salad on gluten-free crackers with strawberries and cottage cheese on the side.

Lunch #4 (Egg White Salad)

3 hard-boiled egg whites, mixed with

    1 Tbsp light mayo

    1 tsp Dijon mustard, served on

Mixed greens OR 14 baked corn chips

1 cup fresh fruit

Gluten-Free Lunches with 45 Grams Total Carbohydrate

Lunch #1 (Turkey or Ham Wrap)

1 gluten-free tortilla, with

    1 Tbsp hummus

    lettuce leaves

    tomato slices

1 small apple

Small green salad, with

    1 Tbsp light dressing (gluten-free)

Lunch #2 (Tuna Salad)

3 ounces water-packed tuna, with

    1 Tbsp light mayo

    chopped celery

    chopped onion, served on

2 slices gluten-free bread

1 cup carrots, cucumbers, and cauliflower, served with

    2 Tbsp hummus

1 cup milk or 6 ounces light yogurt

Serve tuna salad on sandwich thin with veggies, hummus, and yogurt on the side.

Lunch #3

1 cup gluten-free canned soup (lentil or black bean)

1/2 natural peanut butter and sunflower seed sandwich, made with
    1 slice gluten-free bread
    1 Tbsp peanut butter
    2 tsp sunflower seeds

1 cup strawberries

Lunch #4

3 ounces leftover chicken breast, chopped, mixed with
    1/2 cup fat-free refried beans, served on

14 baked tortilla chips OR 2 corn tortillas

Green salad, with
    2 Tbsp light ranch dressing (gluten-free)

1 medium orange

LOW-CARB SNACKS

Here are some low-carb snacks with 15–20 grams of carbohydrate:

- 4 whole-wheat crackers with 1 Tbsp natural peanut butter
- 1 small pear and a small handful (12) of almonds
- 3 1/2 ounces flavored Greek yogurt
- 3 cups light microwave or air-popped popcorn with 1 Tbsp butter
- 1/2 cup sugar-free pudding
- 1/2 cup peaches and 1/2 cup low-fat cottage cheese
- 1 small protein bar with around 15 grams carbohydrate
- 1 small apple with 1 Tbsp natural peanut butter
- 1/2 turkey sandwich on whole-wheat bread with light mayonnaise
- 4 baby carrots and 4 celery stalks dipped in 2 Tbsp hummus
- 1 corn tortilla with 1 slice turkey and 1 Tbsp reduced-fat shredded cheese, heated in the microwave

Here are some snacks with even fewer carbs (under 15 grams):

- Small handful (12) of almonds, walnuts, or pecans
- 3 celery stalks with 1 Tbsp natural peanut butter
- String cheese
- Light Laughing Cow Cheese Wedge spread on cucumber slices
- 1/2 cup low-fat cottage cheese
- Hard-boiled egg
- Sugar-free gelatin with whipped topping
- 1 slice of ham spread with 2 tsp light cream cheese, rolled up
- Cucumber rounds topped with 2 Tbsp avocado and 1 tsp sunflower seeds

MORE GLUTEN-FREE TRANSFORMATIONS

Instead of	Try this Gluten-Free Substitute
Canned chicken or beef broth	→ Gluten-free chicken or beef broth
Bread crumbs	→ Gluten-free bread crumbs or gluten-free oats
Flour tortilla	→ Corn or gluten-free tortilla
Soy sauce	→ Gluten-free soy sauce
Pasta	→ Gluten-free quinoa or rice pasta
Couscous	→ Quinoa
Flour	→ Gluten-free flour
Whole-wheat pita	→ Gluten-free tortilla or gluten-free crackers
Hamburger bun	→ Gluten-free bun or lettuce wrap

JANUARY

A Fresh Start

Happy New Year! These three words are followed by another three words—New Year's Resolutions. We all start off the year with good intentions of living a healthier lifestyle. People with diabetes often set goals to practice better diabetes management, including improving their eating habits. This book is designed to help you meet your goals and start the year off right. In the following pages you will find a grocery list for the food items you need to kick off the New Year with healthy recipes. Soon, you'll find that healthy cooking and eating is easier than you thought. And yes, it can taste good, too!

Veggie Pizza (page 48)
You can add almost any veggie you like to this healthy, satisfying pizza, and it will taste delicious! Have a pizza party and let your guests make their own pizzas.

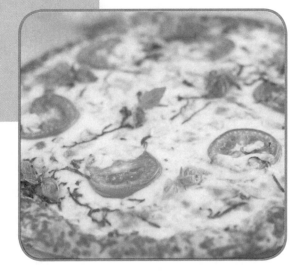

GF gluten-free recipe, but always check ingredients for gluten.

LC these recipes contain 15 grams of carbohydrate or less per serving.

NEW new recipe for the second edition.

JANUARY RECIPES

JANUARY
WEEK 1

GROCERY LIST

Fresh Produce
Basil—1 small bunch
Bell peppers, green—3
Bell pepper, red—1
Cucumber, medium—1
Garlic—1 head
Mushrooms, sliced—1 pint
Onion, red—1 small
Onion, yellow or white—1
Salad greens/mix—8 cups
Spinach—1 large bunch
Tomato, medium—1

Meat, Poultry, & Fish
Beef, ground, 95% lean—
    1 pound
Cod fillets, 4 ounces each—4
Pork tenderloin—1
Turkey sausage, Italian, lean
    or reduced-fat—1 package

Grains, Bread, & Pasta
Hamburger buns, whole-
    wheat—6
Pizza crust, 12-inch, whole-
    wheat, prepackaged—1
Tortellini, cheese, whole-
    wheat—1 package

Dairy & Cheese
Eggs
Mozzarella cheese, part-skim,
    shredded—1/3 cup
Trans-fat-free margarine

Canned Goods & Sauces
Black-eyed peas, 15.5-ounce
    cans—2
Chicken broth, fat-free,
    low-sodium, 14.5-ounce
    cans—3
Preserves, apricot, sugar-
    free—1 jar
Tomato sauce, 8-ounce
    can—1
Tomatoes, diced, no-salt-
    added, 15-ounce cans—2

Frozen Foods
Corn—1 bag

Staples, Seasonings, & Baking Needs
Basil
Cayenne pepper
Crushed red pepper flakes
Flour, all-purpose
Ground black pepper
Mustard, yellow
Nonstick cooking spray
Olive oil
Oregano
Sage
Salt
Thyme
Vinegar, apple cider
Vinegar, balsamic
Worcestershire sauce

Miscellaneous
Peanuts, unsalted—small jar
Wine, red

Sloppy Joes

Makes: 6 servings   *Serving Size: 1 Sloppy Joe*   *Prep Time: 5 minutes*

1 pound 95% lean ground beef
1/2 cup diced onions
2 garlic cloves, minced
8-ounce can tomato sauce
1/2 cup water
1 cup no-salt-added diced tomatoes (fresh or canned; if canned, drain juice)
1 Tbsp yellow mustard
2 Tbsp Worcestershire sauce
1/4 tsp salt (optional)
1/2 tsp ground black pepper
6 whole-wheat hamburger buns

1 In a large skillet, cook ground beef over medium-high heat for about 5 minutes. Drain fat.

2 Add onions and cook 3 minutes or until onions begin to turn clear. Add garlic and cook 1 more minute.

3 Add remaining ingredients except buns and simmer for 10 minutes.

4 Serve on whole-wheat buns.

Resolve to make this your healthiest year yet!

Exchanges/Choices

1 1/2 Starch	1 Vegetable
2 Lean Meat	1/2 Fat

Calories	240
Calories from Fat	55
Total Fat	6.0 g
Saturated Fat	2.2 g
Trans Fat	0.1 g
Cholesterol	45 mg
Sodium	535 mg
Potassium	625 mg
Total Carbohydrate	28 g
Dietary Fiber	5 g
Sugars	7 g
Protein	20 g
Phosphorus	260 mg

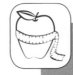

Dietitian's Tip

To reduce this recipe's fat content even further, use lean ground turkey instead of beef.

Corn Salad GF LC

Makes: 7 servings   *Serving Size: 1/2 cup*   *Prep Time: 15 minutes*

2 cups frozen corn
1 cup finely diced green bell pepper
1 cup finely diced red bell pepper
1/2 cup finely diced red onion
1/2 tsp chopped fresh basil
1/4 cup balsamic vinegar
2 tsp olive oil
1/2 tsp salt (optional)
1/4 tsp ground black pepper

1 Place frozen corn in a colander and run under cold water for about 5 minutes to thaw.

2 In a medium bowl, toss together corn, green and red pepper, red onion, and basil.

3 In a small bowl, whisk together remaining ingredients and pour over salad. Toss to coat.

Exchanges/Choices

1/2 Starch	1 Vegetable

Calories 70
  Calories from Fat 15
Total Fat . . . . 1.5 g
  Saturated Fat . . . . 0.3 g
  Trans Fat . . . . 0.0 g
Cholesterol . . . . 0 mg
Sodium . . . . 0 mg
Potassium . . . . 195 mg
Total Carbohydrate . . . . . . 13 g
  Dietary Fiber . . . . 2 g
  Sugars . . . . 4 g
Protein . . . . 2 g
Phosphorus . . . . 40 mg

Chef's Tip

Place a wet paper towel under your cutting board to anchor it while you are dicing vegetables.

Spinach and Mushroom Pizza

Makes: 4 servings   *Serving Size: 2 slices*   *Prep Time: 15 minutes*

4	cups fresh spinach, washed, stemmed, and coarsely chopped
2	cups sliced mushrooms
1 1/2	Tbsp olive oil, divided
1/2	tsp salt (optional)
1/2	tsp ground black pepper
1/2	Tbsp dried basil
1/2	Tbsp dried oregano
1	12-inch whole-wheat prepackaged pizza crust
3	garlic cloves, minced
1/3	cup shredded, part-skim mozzarella cheese

Salad

8	cups salad greens
1	medium tomato, sliced
1	medium cucumber, sliced

1 Preheat oven to 375°F. In a medium nonstick skillet, sauté spinach and mushrooms in 1/2 Tbsp olive oil. Add salt, pepper, basil, and oregano. Sauté until all the moisture is evaporated (about 10 minutes).

2 Rub pizza crust with 1 Tbsp olive oil. Sprinkle minced garlic on top. Spread the spinach and mushroom mixture evenly over the pizza crust.

3 Sprinkle the cheese on top and bake for 15 minutes or until cheese is bubbly and lightly browned.

4 Serve pizza with a side salad.

Exchanges/Choices

3 Starch	1 1/2 Fat
1 Medium-Fat Meat	

Calories	380
Calories from Fat	129
Total Fat	14 g
Saturated Fat	3 g
Cholesterol	8 mg
Sodium	686 mg
Total Carbohydrate	47 g
Dietary Fiber	3 g
Sugars	3 g
Protein	16 g

Dietitian's Tip

If you're looking to lower the carb content in this recipe, eliminate the pizza crust and serve toppings on Portobello mushrooms (using 4 mushrooms).

Tangy Apricot-Glazed Pork Tenderloin GF LC

Makes: 4 servings   *Serving Size: 1/4 recipe*   *Prep Time: 5 minutes*

1	pound pork tenderloin
1/2	cup sugar-free apricot preserves
1/4	cup apple cider vinegar
1/2	Tbsp dried sage
1/2	Tbsp dried basil
1/2	Tbsp dried thyme
2	garlic cloves, minced
1/2	tsp salt (optional)
1/2	tsp ground black pepper

1 Preheat oven to 350°F. Trim tenderloin of all visible fat. Set aside.

2 In small saucepan, combine preserves, vinegar, herbs, and garlic over medium heat. Simmer for 3 minutes to make a glaze.

3 Season all sides of the tenderloin with salt (optional) and pepper. Place tenderloin in a shallow baking dish.

4 Coat tenderloin with apricot glaze and bake for 30 minutes or until pork is done.

Exchanges/Choices
1/2 Carbohydrate
3 Lean Meat

Calories	145
Calories from Fat	25
Total Fat	3.0 g
Saturated Fat	1.0 g
Trans Fat	0.0 g
Cholesterol	60 mg
Sodium	40 mg
Potassium	410 mg
Total Carbohydrate	11 g
Dietary Fiber	0 g
Sugars	0 g
Protein	22 g
Phosphorus	205 mg

Chef's Tip

The tenderloin is a lean cut of any meat. Typically, round or loin cuts are leaner meats.

Lucky Black-Eyed Peas GF

Makes: 7 servings　　　　*Serving Size: 1/2 cup*　　　　*Prep Time: 3 minutes*

2 Tbsp olive oil

1 green bell pepper, cut into 1-inch strips

2 garlic cloves, minced

2 15.5-ounce cans black-eyed peas, rinsed and drained

1/2 tsp crushed red pepper flakes

1 Add oil to a large nonstick skillet over medium-high heat. Add green pepper and sauté for about 10 minutes. Add garlic and sauté 30 seconds.

2 Add black-eyed peas and red pepper flakes and sauté 5–10 more minutes.

Exchanges/Choices
1 Starch　　　　1 Lean Meat
1/2 Fat

Calories 140
　Calories from Fat 40
Total Fat . . . . .4.5 g
　Saturated Fat . . . . .0.7 g
　Trans Fat . . . . .0.0 g
Cholesterol. . . . . 0 mg
Sodium . . . . 140 mg
Potassium. . . . . 280 mg
Total Carbohydrate . . . . . . 19 g
　Dietary Fiber . . . . 6 g
　Sugars . . . . 3 g
Protein . . . . 7 g
Phosphorus . . . . 140 mg

Dietitian's Tip

Black-eyed peas are high in fiber: 6 grams per 1/2 cup. A high-fiber food contains 5 grams of dietary fiber or more per serving.

Peanut-Crusted Cod LC

Makes: 4 servings   *Serving Size: 1 fillet*   *Prep Time: 5 minutes*

1/2   cup all-purpose flour
1/4   tsp cayenne pepper
1/2   cup chopped unsalted peanuts
  4   4-ounce cod fillets
1/2   tsp salt (optional)
1/4   tsp ground black pepper
  2   egg whites, lightly beaten
      nonstick cooking spray
  1   tsp trans-fat-free margarine

1 In a small bowl, combine flour and cayenne pepper. Spread flour mixture on a plate. Spread peanuts on a separate plate.

2 Season fillets with salt and pepper on both sides. Dredge one fillet through flour and shake off excess. Dip floured fillet into egg whites. Press one side of the fillet into chopped peanuts.

3 Coat a large nonstick skillet with cooking spray. Melt trans-fat-free margarine over medium heat. Place fillets peanut side down in skillet and cook for about 3 minutes on each side.

Exchanges/Choices
1 Carbohydrate   3 Lean Meat

Calories 235
  Calories from Fat 80
Total Fat . . . . .9.0 g
  Saturated Fat . . . . .1.4 g
  Trans Fat . . . . .0.0 g
Cholesterol. . . . . 50 mg
Sodium . . . . 105 mg
Potassium. . . . . 355 mg
Total Carbohydrate . . . . . . 11 g
  Dietary Fiber . . . . 2 g
  Sugars . . . . 1 g
Protein . . . . 27 g
Phosphorus . . . . 190 mg

Chef's Tip

You can use tilapia, orange roughy, or perch instead of cod in this recipe.

Tortellini Soup

Makes: 7 servings *Serving Size: 1 cup* *Prep Time: 10 minutes*

nonstick cooking spray

2 cups reduced-fat or lean Italian turkey sausage

1/2 cup finely diced onion

1/4 cup red wine

1/2 Tbsp dried basil

1/2 Tbsp dried oregano

1 15-ounce can no-salt-added diced tomatoes with juice

3 14.5-ounce cans fat-free, low-sodium chicken broth

2 1/2 cups uncooked whole-wheat cheese tortellini

1/2 tsp ground black pepper

1 Coat a large soup pot with cooking spray. Add sausage and onion and cook over medium-high heat for 7 minutes or until sausage begins to brown.

2 Add wine to deglaze pan. Cook for 2 minutes or until wine is almost completely evaporated.

3 Add basil and oregano and cook for 1 more minute. Add tomatoes and broth. Bring to a boil, then reduce heat and simmer for 5 minutes.

4 Add tortellini and pepper. Cook for another 10 minutes.

Exchanges/Choices

1 Starch	1 Vegetable
2 Lean Meat	1 Fat

Calories 220
  Calories from Fat 70
Total Fat . . . . 8.0 g
  Saturated Fat . . . . 2.4 g
  Trans Fat . . . . 0.1 g
Cholesterol . . . . 50 mg
Sodium . . . . 565 mg
Potassium . . . . 415 mg
Total Carbohydrate . . . . . . 21 g
  Dietary Fiber . . . . 3 g
  Sugars . . . . 3 g
Protein . . . . 16 g
Phosphorus . . . . 185 mg

Chef's Tip

If you don't want to use wine in this recipe, you can substitute 1 Tbsp red wine vinegar or balsamic vinegar.

JANUARY
WEEK 2

DAY 1
Blackened Catfish   12

DAY 2
Turkey Chili   13

DAY 3
Chili Mac   14

DAY 4
Pecan Chicken   15
Spaghetti Squash   16

DAY 5
Hearty Lentil Soup   17
Cucumber Onion
    Salad   18

GROCERY LIST

Fresh Produce
Bell pepper, green—1
Carrot—1
Celery—1 head
Cucumbers, large—2
Dill—1 small bunch
Onions, yellow or white,
    medium—3
Squash, spaghetti, medium—1

Meat, Poultry, & Fish
Catfish fillets, 4 ounces
    each—4
Chicken breasts, boneless,
    skinless, 4 ounces each—4
Turkey, ground, lean—
    1 1/4 pounds
Turkey sausage (kielbasa),
    lean, smoked,
    precooked—14 ounces

Grains, Bread, & Pasta
Elbow macaroni, whole-
    wheat—1 box
Cornflakes—1 small box

Dairy & Cheese
Eggs
Parmesan cheese—2 Tbsp
Sour cream, light—1 small
    container
Yogurt, plain, fat-free—
    1 container

Canned Goods & Sauces
Beans, kidney, 15.5-ounce
    cans—2
Broth, chicken, reduced-
    sodium, fat-free,
    14.5-ounce can—1
Tomatoes, diced, no-salt-
    added, 14.5-ounce cans—4

**Staples, Seasonings,
& Baking Needs**
Bay leaves
Black pepper, ground
Cayenne pepper
Chili powder
Cumin
Flour, all-purpose
Garlic powder
Garlic salt
Nonstick cooking spray
Olive oil
Onion salt
Paprika
Salt
Sugar substitute
Vinegar, white wine

Miscellaneous
Chili seasoning packet,
    1.25-ounce—1
Lentils, dried—1 bag
Pecans—1 small can

Blackened Catfish GF LC

Makes: 4 servings   *Serving Size: 1 fillet*   *Prep Time: 5 minutes*

2   Tbsp paprika
1   tsp cayenne pepper
1   Tbsp chili powder
1   tsp cumin
1/2   tsp salt (optional)
1/2   tsp ground black pepper
4   4-ounce catfish fillets
      nonstick cooking spray

1 In a small bowl, combine the first six ingredients and stir well.

2 Rub one side of each fillet well with spice mixture.

3 Coat a large nonstick skillet with cooking spray. Over medium-high heat, place each fillet spice side down and cook for 3 minutes on each side or until fish is done.

Exchanges/Choices
3 Lean Meat   1/2 Fat

Calories 165
  Calories from Fat 70
Total Fat . . . . .8.0 g
  Saturated Fat . . . . .1.8 g
  Trans Fat . . . . .0.1 g
Cholesterol. . . . . 65 mg
Sodium . . . . 145 mg
Potassium. . . . . 500 mg
Total Carbohydrate . . . . 3 g
  Dietary Fiber . . . . 2 g
  Sugars . . . . 1 g
Protein . . . . 20 g
Phosphorus . . . . 270 mg

Chef's Tip

If you prefer this dish less spicy, reduce the cayenne pepper to 1/2–3/4 tsp. Quinoa and broccoli make excellent side dishes for this entrée.

Turkey Chili

Makes: 9 servings   *Serving Size: 1 cup*   *Prep Time: 15 minutes*

1 1/4 pounds lean ground turkey
      nonstick cooking spray
  1   green bell pepper, finely diced
  1   small onion, finely diced
  2   14.5-ounce cans no-salt-added
      diced tomatoes
  2   15.5-ounce cans kidney beans,
      undrained
  1   1.25-ounce chili seasoning
      packet

1 In a large soup pot, cook turkey over medium-high heat until brown. Remove turkey from pot and drain fat.

2 Spray pot with cooking spray and sauté green pepper and onion for 3–4 minutes.

3 Add cooked turkey back to pot with the remaining ingredients. Bring to a boil, cover, and simmer 10 minutes. Reserve 4 cups chili for Chili Mac recipe (see page 14).

Exchanges/Choices
1 Starch   1 Vegetable
2 Lean Meat

Calories 215
　Calories from Fat 55
Total Fat . . . . .6.0 g
　Saturated Fat . . . . .1.6 g
　Trans Fat . . . . .0.1 g
Cholesterol. . . . . 50 mg
Sodium . . . . 580 mg
Potassium. . . . . 605 mg
Total Carbohydrate . . . . . . 22 g
　Dietary Fiber . . . . 7 g
　Sugars . . . . 5 g
Protein . . . . 19 g
Phosphorus . . . . 250 mg

Dietitian's Tip

This recipe not only tastes good, but also has great nutritional value. The meat and beans provide iron, and the vitamin C in the tomatoes helps your body absorb the iron.

Chili Mac

Makes: 4 servings   *Serving Size: 1 cup chili and 1/3 cup pasta*   *Prep Time: 10 minutes*

4 cups Turkey Chili, heated
(see recipe, page 13)

1 1/3 cups cooked whole-wheat
elbow macaroni (about 2/3 cups
uncooked macaroni)

Mix pasta and Turkey Chili and serve.

Exchanges/Choices
1 1/2 Starch   1 Vegetable
2 Lean Meat

Calories 270
   Calories from Fat 65
Total Fat . . . . 7.0 g
   Saturated Fat . . . . 1.6 g
   Trans Fat . . . . 0.1 g
Cholesterol . . . . 50 mg
Sodium . . . . 585 mg
Potassium . . . . 625 mg
Total Carbohydrate . . . . . . 34 g
   Dietary Fiber . . . . 8 g
   Sugars . . . . 5 g
Protein . . . . 21 g
Phosphorus . . . . 290 mg

Dietitian's Tip

If you're looking to lower the carb content of
this recipe, serve the chili over a bed of lettuce
with reduced-fat shredded cheddar cheese for
a quick taco salad.

Pecan Chicken

Makes: 4 servings   *Serving Size: 1 chicken breast*   *Prep Time: 10 minutes*

nonstick cooking spray
1   cup cornflake crumbs
1/2 cup chopped pecans
1/4 tsp garlic powder
1/2 tsp onion salt
1   egg
2   egg whites
2   Tbsp all-purpose flour
4   4-ounce boneless, skinless chicken breasts

1 Preheat oven to 350°F. Coat a shallow baking pan with cooking spray.

2 In a medium bowl, combine cornflake crumbs, pecans, garlic powder, and onion salt. In a separate bowl, lightly beat egg and egg whites. Put the flour in a third bowl.

3 Dip each chicken breast in the flour, then the egg mixture, then in the cornflake and pecan mixture. Coat each side of the chicken breast.

4 Place chicken breasts in the baking pan. Spray chicken lightly with cooking spray and bake 30–35 minutes or until chicken juices run clear.

Exchanges/Choices
1 Starch   4 Lean Meat
1 Fat

Calories 300
 Calories from Fat 110
Total Fat . . . . 12.0 g
 Saturated Fat . . . . 1.8 g
 Trans Fat . . . . 0.0 g
Cholesterol . . . . 105 mg
Sodium . . . . 400 mg
Potassium . . . . 305 mg
Total Carbohydrate . . . . . . 19 g
 Dietary Fiber . . . . 2 g
 Sugars . . . . 2 g
Protein . . . . 30 g
Phosphorus . . . . 245 mg

Dietitian's Tip

Pecans are high in calories but loaded with healthy fat. A small amount provides big flavor!

Spaghetti Squash `GF`

Makes: 5 servings   *Serving Size: 1/2 cup*   *Prep Time: 45 minutes*

1 medium spaghetti squash
  nonstick cooking spray
1 tsp olive oil
2 Tbsp freshly grated Parmesan
  cheese
1/4 tsp salt (optional)
1/4 tsp ground black pepper

1 Preheat oven to 400°F. Cut ends off squash and then cut squash in half lengthwise. Scoop out seeds and wash and dry both sides.

2 Coat a large metal or glass baking dish with cooking spray. Place squash halves face down on baking dish and spray the skins lightly with cooking spray.

3 Bake for 40 minutes.

4 Remove squash meat from rind with fork and place in a medium bowl. Discard rind. Drizzle oil over squash, sprinkle with Parmesan cheese, salt, and pepper, and stir.

Exchanges/Choices
1 Starch

Calories 75
  Calories from Fat 20
Total Fat . . . . .2.0 g
  Saturated Fat . . . . .0.6 g
  Trans Fat . . . . .0.0 g
Cholesterol. . . . . 0 mg
Sodium . . . . 70 mg
Potassium. . . . . 265 mg
Total Carbohydrate . . . . . . 15 g
  Dietary Fiber . . . . 3 g
  Sugars . . . . 6 g
Protein . . . . 2 g
Phosphorus . . . . 45 mg

Chef's Tip

If you've never tried this mild-flavored squash before, you're in for a fun treat.

Hearty Lentil Soup

Makes: 9 servings   *Serving Size: 1 cup*   *Prep Time: 20 minutes*

nonstick cooking spray

14   ounces lean smoked precooked turkey sausage (kielbasa), sliced

1   cup diced celery

1   medium onion, diced

1   carrot, diced

3   cups water

1   14.5-ounce can fat-free, low-sodium chicken broth

2   14.5-ounce cans no-salt-added diced tomatoes

1   cup dried lentils

1/2   tsp salt (optional)

1   tsp ground black pepper

1   bay leaf

1 Coat a large soup pot with cooking spray. Over medium-high heat, sauté sausage until lightly browned. Remove from pan.

2 Add celery, onion, and carrots to pot and sauté over medium-high heat for about 4 minutes.

3 Add the sausage and all remaining ingredients. Bring to a boil; reduce heat and simmer for 1 hour.

4 Remove bay leaf and serve.

Exchanges/Choices

1 Starch   1 Vegetable
1 Lean Meat

Calories	175
Calories from Fat	25
Total Fat	3.0 g
Saturated Fat	1.2 g
Trans Fat	0.0 g
Cholesterol	30 mg
Sodium	605 mg
Potassium	580 mg
Total Carbohydrate	21 g
Dietary Fiber	6 g
Sugars	5 g
Protein	14 g
Phosphorus	215 mg

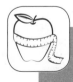

Dietitian's Tip

Lentils, along with all legumes, contain both carbohydrate and protein and are an excellent source of fiber.

Cucumber Onion Salad GF LC

Makes: 5 servings   *Serving Size: 1/5 recipe*   *Prep Time: 5 minutes*

1/2	cup fat-free plain yogurt
1/4	cup light sour cream
1	Tbsp minced fresh dill
1/2	tsp garlic salt
1 1/2	Tbsp white wine vinegar
1/4	tsp ground black pepper
1	packet sugar substitute
2	large cucumbers, peeled and thinly sliced
1	medium onion, thinly sliced

1 In a medium bowl, whisk together all ingredients except cucumber and onion.

2 Add cucumber and onion and toss to coat well. Serve chilled.

Exchanges/Choices
2 Vegetable

Calories	55
Calories from Fat	15
Total Fat	1.5 g
Saturated Fat	0.9 g
Trans Fat	0.0 g
Cholesterol	5 mg
Sodium	160 mg
Potassium	270 mg
Total Carbohydrate	8 g
Dietary Fiber	1 g
Sugars	5 g
Protein	3 g
Phosphorus	85 mg

Chef's Tip

Dill has a distinctive flavor that may be too strong for some people. If you don't care for dill, just leave it out.

JANUARY
WEEK 3

DAY 1
Turkey and Wild Rice
   Soup   20
Spinach Salad with
   Mushrooms   21

DAY 2
Sweet and Sour
   Pork   22

DAY 3
Chicken Breasts
   with Raspberry
   Balsamic Glaze   23
Candied Walnut
   Salad   24

DAY 4
Creamy Macaroni
   and Cheese   25

DAY 5
Stuffed Peppers   26

GROCERY LIST

Fresh Produce
Bell peppers, green—7
Carrots, medium—2
Celery—1 stalk
Salad greens, field, mixed—
   4 cups
Garlic—1 head
Mushrooms—1 pint
Onions, yellow or white—2
Spinach, baby—10-ounce bag

Meat, Poultry, & Fish
Beef, ground, 95% lean—
   1 pound
Chicken breasts, boneless,
   skinless, 4 ounces each—4
Pork chops, center-cut,
   boneless—1 pound
Turkey breast, roasted—
   2 cups

Grains, Bread, & Pasta
Elbow macaroni, whole-
   wheat—1 box (8 ounces)
Quinoa—1 small box or bag
Rice, wild and long-grain—
   1 box or bag

Dairy & Cheese
Cheese, cheddar, 75%
   reduced-fat, shredded—
   1 bag or block
Margarine, trans-fat-free
Milk, fat-free
Milk, fat-free,
   evaporated—1/2 cup

Canned Goods & Sauces
Broth, chicken, fat-free,
   reduced-sodium,
   14.5-ounce cans—4
Hot pepper sauce
Sweet-and-sour sauce—1 jar
Pineapple, chunks, packed in
   juice—1 can
Preserves, raspberry,
   seedless, sugar-free—1 jar
Tomatoes, diced, no-salt-
   added, 14.5-ounce cans—2

**Staples, Seasonings,
& Baking Needs**
Bay leaves
Black pepper, ground
Flour, all-purpose
Mustard, Dijon
Nonstick cooking spray
Oil, canola
Oil, olive
Salt
Splenda Brown Sugar Blend
Thyme
Vinegar, balsamic
Vinegar, red wine

Miscellaneous
Salad dressing, Ranch,
   light—1 bottle
Sunflower seeds—1 small
   package
Walnuts—1 small package

Turkey and Wild Rice Soup

Makes: 7 servings   *Serving Size: 1 cup*   *Prep Time: 15 minutes*

2	tsp trans-fat-free margarine
1	cup finely diced carrot
1	cup finely diced onion
1/2	cup finely diced celery
1	cup sliced mushrooms
1	garlic clove, minced
2	Tbsp all-purpose flour
3	14.5-ounce cans fat-free, low-sodium chicken broth
1/4	tsp dried thyme
1	bay leaf
2	cups roasted turkey breast, chopped
1	cup uncooked wild and long-grain rice
1/2	cup evaporated fat-free milk
1/4	tsp salt (optional)
1/4	tsp ground black pepper

1 Heat margarine in a large soup pot over medium-high heat. Add carrots, onion, celery, and mushrooms and sauté until beginning to brown. Add garlic and sauté for 1 more minute.

2 Add flour, stirring constantly, and cook for 1 minute. Add chicken broth and stir (make sure to scrape the brown bits on the bottom of pan).

3 Add thyme, bay leaf, turkey, and rice; bring to a boil.

4 Reduce heat to a simmer; cover and cook for 25 minutes. Add evaporated milk; bring to a boil for 1 minute. Add salt and pepper. Remove bay leaf before serving.

Exchanges/Choices

1 Starch   1 Vegetable
2 Lean Meat

Calories	175
Calories from Fat	15
Total Fat	1.5 g
Saturated Fat	0.4 g
Trans Fat	0.0 g
Cholesterol	35 mg
Sodium	510 mg
Potassium	490 mg
Total Carbohydrate	22 g
Dietary Fiber	2 g
Sugars	5 g
Protein	18 g
Phosphorus	200 mg

Chef's Tip

Save yourself some prep time and buy pre-sliced mushrooms.

Spinach Salad with Mushrooms GF LC

Makes: 4 servings   *Serving Size: 1 1/2 cups*   *Prep Time: 5 minutes*

10-ounce bag baby spinach
1 cup sliced mushrooms
1/4 cup sunflower seeds
1/3 cup light Ranch dressing

1 In a large salad bowl, toss spinach and mushrooms together.

2 Sprinkle sunflower seeds over the top and drizzle with dressing. Toss well to coat.

Exchanges/Choices
1 Vegetable   2 Fat

Calories 115
  Calories from Fat 80
Total Fat . . . . .9.0 g
  Saturated Fat . . . . .1.1 g
  Trans Fat . . . . .0.0 g
Cholesterol. . . . . 5 mg
Sodium . . . . 240 mg
Potassium. . . . . 465 mg
Total Carbohydrate . . . . . . 7 g
  Dietary Fiber . . . . 2 g
  Sugars . . . . 2 g
Protein . . . . 4 g
Phosphorus . . . . 175 mg

Chef's Tip

Bagged, prewashed spinach will save you time with this recipe.

Sweet and Sour Pork

Makes: 4 servings   *Serving Size: 1/4 recipe*   *Prep Time: 10 minutes*

6 Tbsp jarred sweet-and-sour sauce
3/4 cup fat-free, low-sodium chicken broth
1 pound boneless center-cut pork chops, cubed
1 tsp ground black pepper
1 Tbsp olive oil, divided
1 green bell pepper, diced
1 cup pineapple chunks packed in juice, drained

1 Mix sweet-and-sour sauce with chicken broth and set aside.

2 Sprinkle pork with pepper. In a large nonstick skillet or wok, sauté pork cubes in 1/2 Tbsp olive oil over medium-high heat until cooked through and beginning to brown. Set the cooked pork aside in a bowl.

3 In the same pan, sauté green peppers in 1/2 Tbsp olive oil for 2 minutes. Add the pork and pineapple to the peppers. Pour sauce over pork mixture and simmer for 5 minutes. Serve over brown rice, if desired.

Exchanges/Choices
1 Carbohydrate   3 Lean Meat
1/2 Fat

Calories 255
  Calories from Fat 100
Total Fat . . . . .11.0 g
  Saturated Fat . . . . .3.0 g
  Trans Fat . . . . .0.0 g
Cholesterol. . . . . 60 mg
Sodium . . . . 260 mg
Potassium. . . . . 500 mg
Total Carbohydrate . . . . . . 17 g
  Dietary Fiber . . . . 1 g
  Sugars . . . . 14 g
Protein . . . . 22 g
Phosphorus . . . . 195 mg

Chef's Tip

You can ask your butcher to cube the pork for you, saving yourself a step in this recipe.

Chicken Breasts with Raspberry Balsamic Glaze GF LC

Makes: 4 servings   *Serving Size: 1 chicken breast*   *Prep Time: 10 minutes*

1   tsp canola oil
2   garlic cloves, minced
1/2 cup sugar-free seedless raspberry preserves
1/4 cup balsamic vinegar
1/4 tsp ground black pepper
4   4-ounce boneless, skinless chicken breasts
     nonstick cooking spray

1 Preheat oven to 350°F. In a small saucepan, heat oil, add garlic, and sauté for 30 seconds over medium-high heat.

2 Add raspberry preserves, balsamic vinegar, and pepper and bring to a low boil; simmer 3 minutes or until mixture gets a glaze-like consistency.

3 Reserve half of glaze and set aside. Brush chicken breasts on both sides with remaining glaze.

4 Coat a baking dish with cooking spray. Place chicken breasts in dish and bake 30 minutes. Pour remaining glaze over chicken breasts.

Exchanges/Choices
1 Carbohydrate   3 Lean Meat

Calories 175
  Calories from Fat 35
Total Fat . . . . .4.0 g
  Saturated Fat . . . . .0.9 g
  Trans Fat . . . . .0.0 g
Cholesterol. . . . . 65 mg
Sodium . . . . 60 mg
Potassium. . . . . 250 mg
Total Carbohydrate . . . . . . 13 g
  Dietary Fiber . . . . 0 g
  Sugars . . . . 2 g
Protein . . . . 24 g
Phosphorus . . . . 185 mg

Chef's Tip

Your guests will beg for the recipe for this quick and tasty dish.

Candied Walnut Salad GF LC

Makes: 4 servings   *Serving Size: 1/4 recipe*   *Prep Time: 15 minutes*

2	Tbsp red wine vinegar
1	Tbsp olive oil
1	tsp Dijon mustard
2 1/2	tsp trans-fat-free margarine
1	Tbsp Splenda Brown Sugar Blend
1/4	cup chopped walnuts
4	cups mixed field greens
1/2	cup shredded carrots

1 Preheat oven to 350°F. In a small bowl, whisk together vinegar, oil, and mustard; set aside.

2 In a small bowl, combine trans-fat-free margarine and brown sugar. Microwave on high for 30 seconds to melt margarine, then stir well. Toss walnuts with margarine and sugar and spread on a small baking sheet. Bake for 15–20 minutes or until beginning to brown.

3 In a large salad bowl, toss remaining salad ingredients with the candied nuts. Drizzle dressing over salad and toss to coat.

Exchanges/Choices

1/2 Carbohydrate	2 Fat

Calories	125
Calories from Fat	90
Total Fat	10.0 g
Saturated Fat	1.5 g
Trans Fat	0.0 g
Cholesterol	0 mg
Sodium	70 mg
Potassium	205 mg
Total Carbohydrate	7 g
Dietary Fiber	2 g
Sugars	3 g
Protein	2 g
Phosphorus	45 mg

Chef's Tip

Sweet, crunchy walnuts add great texture to this dish.

Creamy Macaroni and Cheese

Makes: 6 servings   *Serving Size: 1/2 cup*   *Prep Time: 25 minutes*

8 ounces uncooked whole-wheat elbow macaroni
2 tsp trans-fat-free margarine
2 Tbsp all-purpose flour
1 1/2 cups fat-free milk
1 1/4 cups 75% reduced-fat shredded cheddar cheese (reserve 2 Tbsp)
1/2 tsp salt (optional)
1/2 tsp ground black pepper
1/4 tsp hot pepper sauce
   nonstick cooking spray

1 Preheat oven to 350°F. Cook macaroni according to directions on box, omitting salt. Drain.

2 In a small nonstick skillet, heat trans-fat-free margarine over medium heat. Stir in flour and cook for 4–5 minutes to create a roux.

3 In a small saucepan, add milk and bring to a boil; whisk in roux. Reduce to a simmer for 7 minutes.

4 Add cheese (except reserved 2 Tbsp) to pan and whisk while simmering 2 more minutes. Add salt, pepper, and hot pepper sauce.

5 In a large bowl, combine noodles and cheese sauce and mix well.

6 Coat an 8-inch glass baking dish with cooking spray. Spread macaroni mixture in dish. Sprinkle remaining cheese over the top.

7 Bake for 15 minutes.

Exchanges/Choices
2 Starch   1 Lean Meat
1/2 Fat

Calories	220
Calories from Fat	30
Total Fat	3.5 g
Saturated Fat	1.7 g
Trans Fat	0.0 g
Cholesterol	10 mg
Sodium	205 mg
Potassium	175 mg
Total Carbohydrate	33 g
Dietary Fiber	3 g
Sugars	4 g
Protein	15 g
Phosphorus	270 mg

Dietitian's Tip

Increase your veggie intake by mixing in cooked broccoli with this dish.

Stuffed Peppers GF

Makes: 6 servings   *Serving Size: 1 stuffed pepper*   *Prep Time: 20 minutes*

1/2   cup uncooked quinoa
  6   medium green bell peppers
  1   pound 95% lean ground beef
  1   small onion, chopped
  2   14.5-ounce cans no-salt-added diced tomatoes
  2   garlic cloves, minced
1/4   tsp ground black pepper

1 Preheat oven to 350°F. Cook quinoa according to package directions, omitting salt.

2 Fill a large saucepan with water and bring to a boil. Cut the tops off the green peppers and remove the seeds and membranes. Place the peppers in the boiling water and boil for 5 minutes. Remove and drain.

3 In a large skillet, brown ground beef and onion. Drain fat.

4 Add the quinoa and diced tomatoes to the skillet with ground beef and mix well. Add garlic and black pepper.

5 Place peppers right side up in a large baking dish. Fill peppers with beef and quinoa mixture. Bake, covered, for 30 minutes.

Exchanges/Choices
1/2 Starch   3 Vegetable
2 Lean Meat

Basic Nutritional Values:
Calories 215
   Calories from Fat 45
Total Fat . . . . .5.0 g
   Saturated Fat . . . . .2.0 g
   Trans Fat . . . . .0.1 g
Cholesterol. . . . . 45 mg
Sodium . . . . 105 mg
Potassium. . . . . 865 mg
Total Carbohydrate . . . . . . 24 g
   Dietary Fiber . . . . 6 g
   Sugars . . . . 9 g
Protein . . . . 20 g
Phosphorus . . . . 270 mg

Dietitian's Tip

Quinoa provides the highest protein content of any grain and is gluten free!

JANUARY
WEEK 4

DAY 1
Ham and White
    Bean Soup   28
Quick Creamy
    Cornbread   29

DAY 2
Quick Tacos   30

DAY 3
Spinach Pasta
    Shells   31

DAY 4
Tuna with Tomatoes
    and Olives   32
Roasted Asparagus   33

DAY 5
Turkey Lasagna   34

**DESSERT OF
THE MONTH**
Banana Chocolate
    Chip Bread   35

GROCERY LIST

Fresh Produce
Asparagus—1 1/2 pounds
Bananas, very ripe—4
Garlic—1 head
Lettuce, shredded—1 cup
Onions, yellow or white—2
Oregano—1 small bunch
Parsley—1 bunch
Tomato, large—1

Meat, Poultry, & Fish
Beef, ground, 95% lean—
    3/4 pound
Ham, reduced-sodium—
    1/2 cup
Tuna steaks, 4 ounces each—4
Turkey, ground, 93% lean—
    3/4 pound

Grains, Bread, & Pasta
Lasagna noodles, whole-
    wheat, no-boil—12
Oats, old-fashioned—small
    container
Shells, medium, whole-
    wheat—5 ounces
Tortillas, whole-wheat,
    low-carb (10 grams carb
    and more than 4 grams
    fiber)—8

Dairy & Cheese
Buttermilk, low-fat—1/4 cup
Cheese, cheddar, 75%
    reduced-fat—1 small bag
Cheese, mozzarella, part-
    skim, shredded—small bag
Cheese, Parmesan—1 wedge
Cheese, ricotta, fat-free—
    15 ounces
Eggs

Canned Goods & Sauces
Beans, Great Northern,
    16-ounce cans—2
Broth, chicken, fat-free, low-
    sodium, 14.5-ounce cans—2
Corn, creamed, 8-ounce
    can—1
Hot pepper sauce
Pasta sauce, marinara,
    reduced-sodium,
    24.5-ounce jars—2
Tomatoes, diced, no-salt-
    added, 14.5-ounce can—1

Frozen Foods
Spinach, chopped,
    9 ounces—1 bag

Staples, Seasonings, & Baking Needs
Baking powder
Baking soda
Bay leaves
Black pepper, ground
Cayenne pepper
Chili powder
Cumin
Flour, all-purpose
Nonstick cooking spray
Oil, canola
Oil, olive
Onion salt
Salt
Splenda Sugar Blend
Sugar substitute

Miscellaneous
Chocolate chips, semisweet,
    mini—1/3 cup
Corn muffin mix, 8.5-ounce
    box—1
Olives, Kalamata—1/2 cup

Ham and White Bean Soup

Makes: 6 servings   *Serving Size: 1 cup*   *Prep Time: 12 minutes*

nonstick cooking spray
1 medium onion, finely diced
1/2 cup chopped, cooked, reduced-sodium ham
2 14.5-ounce cans fat-free, low-sodium chicken broth
2 16-ounce cans Great Northern beans, rinsed and drained
1/2 tsp ground black pepper
1 bay leaf

1 Spray a large soup pot with cooking spray. Add onion and sauté with chopped ham 2 minutes over medium-high heat. Add all remaining ingredients and bring to a boil.

2 Reduce heat and simmer 15 minutes. Remove bay leaf before serving.

Exchanges/Choices
1 1/2 Starch   1 Lean Meat

Calories 145
　Calories from Fat 5
Total Fat . . . . 0.5 g
　Saturated Fat . . . . 0.2 g
　Trans Fat . . . . 0.0 g
Cholesterol . . . . 5 mg
Sodium . . . . 600 mg
Potassium . . . . 550 mg
Total Carbohydrate . . . . . . 24 g
　Dietary Fiber . . . . 7 g
　Sugars . . . . 4 g
Protein . . . . 12 g
Phosphorus . . . . 210 mg

Dietitian's Tip

Rinsing canned beans helps remove some of the sodium.

Quick Creamy Cornbread

Makes: 8 servings   *Serving Size: 1 slice*   *Prep Time: 5 minutes*

1   8.5-ounce box corn muffin mix
1   egg
1   8-ounce can creamed corn
    nonstick cooking spray

1 Preheat oven to 400°F. In a medium mixing bowl, combine corn muffin mix, egg, and creamed corn.

2 Pour batter into an 8 × 8-inch baking pan coated with cooking spray. Bake 20–25 minutes.

3 Cool. Cut into 8 slices.

Exchanges/Choices
1 1/2 Starch

Calories 110
   Calories from Fat 20
Total Fat . . . . .2.5 g
   Saturated Fat . . . . .1.3 g
   Trans Fat . . . . .0.0 g
Cholesterol. . . . . 20 mg
Sodium . . . . 330 mg
Potassium. . . . . 80 mg
Total Carbohydrate . . . . . . 26 g
   Dietary Fiber . . . . 1 g
   Sugars . . . . 7 g
Protein . . . . 3 g
Phosphorus . . . . 175 mg

Chef's Tip

Cornbread can't get much easier than this. The creamed corn adds a unique texture to this bread.

Quick Tacos

Makes: 8 servings   *Serving Size: 1 taco*   *Prep Time: 5 minutes*

3/4	pound 95% lean ground beef
2/3	cup water
1	tsp cumin
1	Tbsp chili powder
1/4	tsp cayenne pepper
1	tsp onion salt
8	whole-wheat, low-carb tortillas (10 grams carb and more than 4 grams fiber)
1/2	cup shredded, 75% reduced-fat cheddar cheese
1	cup shredded lettuce
1	large tomato, diced
	hot pepper sauce (optional)

1 Brown beef in a large nonstick skillet over medium-high heat until thoroughly cooked and no longer pink. Drain fat.

2 Add water, cumin, chili powder, cayenne pepper, and onion salt. Simmer 2–4 minutes.

3 Warm tortillas. Fill each tortilla with 1/4 cup taco meat, 1 Tbsp cheese, lettuce, tomato, and hot pepper sauce.

Exchanges/Choices
1/2 Starch   2 Lean Meat

Calories 130
  Calories from Fat 45
Total Fat . . . . .5.0 g
  Saturated Fat . . . . .1.4 g
  Trans Fat . . . . .0.1 g
Cholesterol. . . . . 30 mg
Sodium . . . . 455 mg
Potassium. . . . . 250 mg
Total Carbohydrate . . . . . . 12 g
  Dietary Fiber . . . . 8 g
  Sugars . . . . 1 g
Protein . . . . 16 g
Phosphorus . . . . 160 mg

Dietitian's Tip

If you need to watch your sodium intake, use onion powder instead of onion salt.

Spinach Pasta Shells

Makes: 5 servings   *Serving Size: 1 cup*   *Prep Time: 20 minutes*

5   ounces uncooked whole-wheat medium shell pasta (about 2 cups)
9   ounces frozen, chopped spinach
2   Tbsp olive oil, divided
4   garlic cloves, minced
1/4 cup freshly grated Parmesan cheese

1 Cook pasta according to package directions, omitting salt. While pasta is cooking, defrost spinach in microwave. Squeeze all liquid from spinach.

2 In a medium nonstick skillet, sauté spinach in 1 Tbsp olive oil over medium-high heat for about 5 minutes. Add garlic and Parmesan cheese; sauté 1 minute.

3 Drain pasta. Add spinach mixture and 1 Tbsp olive oil to pasta and toss.

Exchanges/Choices
1 1/2 Starch   1 Fat

Calories 170
  Calories from Fat 65
Total Fat . . . . .7.0 g
  Saturated Fat . . . . .1.2 g
  Trans Fat . . . . .0.0 g
Cholesterol. . . . . 0 mg
Sodium . . . . 75 mg
Potassium. . . . . 165 mg
Total Carbohydrate . . . . . . 23 g
  Dietary Fiber . . . . 4 g
  Sugars . . . . 1 g
Protein . . . . 7 g
Phosphorus . . . . 105 mg

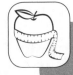

Dietitian's Tip

Olive oil is a great source of monounsaturated fat and is good for you (in the right portion sizes!).

Tuna with Tomatoes and Olives GF LC

Makes: 4 servings *Serving Size: 1 tuna steak* *Prep Time: 10 minutes*

nonstick cooking spray
4 4-ounce tuna steaks
1 tsp olive oil
1 large onion, thinly sliced (about 1 1/2 cups)
1 14.5-ounce can no-salt-added diced tomatoes with juice
1/2 cup Kalamata olives, pitted and chopped
2 Tbsp chopped fresh oregano (or 1 Tbsp dried oregano)
1 packet sugar substitute
1/4 tsp ground black pepper

1 Coat a large sauté pan with cooking spray. Over medium-high heat, sear tuna on each side about 2 minutes. Remove from pan.

2 Add olive oil to pan. Add onion and cook for about 5 minutes or until beginning to brown. Reduce heat to low. Add tomatoes, olives, and oregano and simmer for another 3 minutes. Mix in sugar substitute and black pepper.

3 Add tuna back to mixture, cover, and cook 3 more minutes.

Exchanges/Choices
2 Vegetable   3 Lean Meat
1 Fat

Calories 275
  Calories from Fat 115
Total Fat . . . . 13.0 g
  Saturated Fat . . . . 2.1 g
  Trans Fat . . . . 0.0 g
Cholesterol. . . . . 40 mg
Sodium . . . . 355 mg
Potassium. . . . . 560 mg
Total Carbohydrate . . . . . . 11 g
  Dietary Fiber . . . . 3 g
  Sugars . . . . 5 g
Protein . . . . 27 g
Phosphorus . . . . 315 mg

Dietitian's Tip

Tuna is a great source of omega-3 fatty acids, which have been found to help protect against heart disease.

Roasted Asparagus GF LC

Makes: 6 servings   *Serving Size: 1/6 recipe*   *Prep Time: 5 minutes*

1 1/2   pounds fresh asparagus
      nonstick cooking spray
  1   Tbsp olive oil
 1/4   cup freshly grated Parmesan
      cheese

1 Preheat oven to 450°F. Wash asparagus and cut off ends. Coat a baking dish with cooking spray.

2 Place asparagus in baking dish, drizzle with olive oil, and sprinkle with Parmesan cheese.

3 Bake 15 minutes.

Exchanges/Choices
1 Vegetable   1/2 Fat

Calories 45
  Calories from Fat 25
Total Fat . . . . .3.0 g
  Saturated Fat . . . . .0.8 g
  Trans Fat . . . . .0.0 g
Cholesterol. . . . . 0 mg
Sodium . . . . 55 mg
Potassium. . . . . 130 mg
Total Carbohydrate . . . . 2 g
  Dietary Fiber . . . . 1 g
  Sugars . . . . 1 g
Protein . . . . 2 g
Phosphorus . . . . 50 mg

Dietitian's Tip

Parmesan cheese can add a lot of flavor to many foods without adding too much fat.

Turkey Lasagna

Makes: 10 servings   *Serving Size: 1/10 recipe*   *Prep Time: 15 minutes*

nonstick cooking spray
3/4	pound 93% lean ground turkey
2	24.5-ounce jars reduced-sodium marinara pasta sauce
2/3	cup shredded part-skim mozzarella cheese, divided
15	ounces fat-free ricotta cheese
3	Tbsp freshly grated Parmesan cheese
1	egg, slightly beaten
1/4	cup chopped fresh parsley
12	no-boil whole-wheat lasagna noodles

1 Preheat oven to 350°F. Coat a 13 × 9 × 2-inch glass baking dish with cooking spray.

2 In a large saucepan, cook turkey over medium-high heat until browned. Drain fat. Lower heat to medium and add pasta sauce. Cook for 5 minutes.

3 In a medium bowl, mix together 1/2 cup mozzarella, ricotta, Parmesan, egg, and parsley.

4 Spread 1 cup pasta sauce on bottom of baking dish. Arrange noodles side by side on top of sauce, overlapping slightly. Spread 1/4 cup cheese mixture on top of noodles.

5 Repeat layering with pasta sauce, noodles, and cheese mixture 2 more times.

6 Top with remaining 3 noodles and 1 cup sauce. Cover lasagna with foil and bake 25 minutes. Uncover; top with remaining mozzarella cheese and bake additional 25 minutes or until cheese is light golden brown.

Exchanges/Choices

2 Starch   2 Lean Meat
1 Fat

Calories	290
Calories from Fat	100
Total Fat	11.0 g
Saturated Fat	2.5 g
Trans Fat	0.0 g
Cholesterol	65 mg
Sodium	480 mg
Potassium	640 mg
Total Carbohydrate	29 g
Dietary Fiber	4 g
Sugars	8 g
Protein	20 g
Phosphorus	295 mg

Chef's Tip

If you haven't used ground turkey before, you will be amazed how great it tastes in this recipe.

Banana Chocolate Chip Bread

Makes: 16 servings   *Serving Size: 1 slice*   *Prep Time: 15 minutes*

nonstick cooking spray
1 1/2 cups very ripe bananas, mashed (about 4 bananas)
2 Tbsp canola oil
1/4 cup low-fat buttermilk
4 egg whites
1 1/2 cups all-purpose flour
1/2 cup old-fashioned oats
1/4 cup Splenda Sugar Blend
2 tsp baking powder
1 tsp baking soda
1/2 tsp salt
1/3 cup mini semi-sweet chocolate chips (reserve 1 Tbsp)

1 Preheat oven to 350°F. Lightly spray an 8 × 4-inch loaf pan with cooking spray.

2 In a medium bowl, combine bananas, oil, buttermilk, and egg whites; mix well. Set aside.

3 In a large bowl, combine flour, oats, Splenda, baking powder, baking soda, and salt.

4 Make a well in the center of the dry ingredients. Add banana mixture to dry ingredients all at once and mix well.

5 Stir in all but 1 Tbsp of the chocolate chips to batter. Pour batter into loaf pan. Sprinkle reserved 1 Tbsp chocolate chips on top of batter.

6 Bake 50–60 minutes or until toothpick inserted in center comes out clean.

Exchanges/Choices
1 1/2 Carbohydrate   1/2 Fat

Calories 120
Calories from Fat 25
Total Fat . . . . .3.0 g
Saturated Fat . . . . .0.9 g
Trans Fat . . . . .0.0 g
Cholesterol. . . . . 0 mg
Sodium . . . . 215 mg
Potassium. . . . . 130 mg
Total Carbohydrate . . . . . . 21 g
Dietary Fiber . . . . 1 g
Sugars . . . . 8 g
Protein . . . . 3 g
Phosphorus . . . . 95 mg

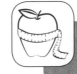

Dietitian's Tip

You'll love this low-fat chocolate version of banana bread.

FEBRUARY

American Heart Month

Did you know that diabetes and heart disease are linked? There is a lot you can do to reduce your risk, starting with how you eat. Try more chicken and fish, whole grains, fresh fruits, and crunchy vegetables—and get some exercise, too! This month will include tasty and healthy fish recipes along with other high-fiber, low-fat ideas. And you can even treat your Valentine to a romantic, yet healthy, meal. Don't forget to check out this month's delicious dessert recipe, Chocolate Mousse Pie.

Jalapeño Corn Muffins (page 54)

These light and scrumptious muffins are terrific with chili or hearty stews. Or make them for Sunday brunch and serve them in a pretty basket.

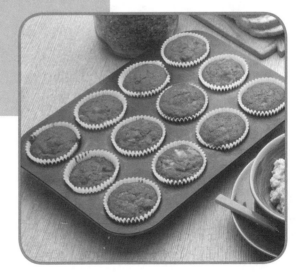

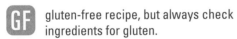 gluten-free recipe, but always check ingredients for gluten.

these recipes contain 15 grams of carbohydrate or less per serving.

NEW new recipe for the second edition.

FEBRUARY RECIPES

FEBRUARY

WEEK 1

DAY 1
Beef Tenderloin   40
Scalloped Potatoes   41

DAY 2
Turkey and Avocado
    Wraps   42
Confetti Pasta
    Salad   43

DAY 3
Penne with Chicken
    and Vegetables   44

DAY 4
Cantonese Chicken   45

DAY 5
Tuna Steaks with
    Balsamic Glaze   46

GROCERY LIST

Fresh Produce
Avocado—1
Bell pepper, green—1
Bell peppers, red—2
Broccoli—1–2 heads
Carrot—1
Celery—1–3 stalks
Cucumber—1
Lettuce—1 head
Onion, yellow, medium—1
Potatoes, russet, medium—6
Scallions—2
Squash, yellow, medium—2
Tomatoes—3

Meat, Poultry, & Fish
Beef, tenderloin steaks,
    4 ounces each—4
Chicken breasts, boneless,
    skinless—2 pounds
Tuna steaks, 5 ounces
    each—4
Turkey, deli, thinly sliced,
    no-added-salt—12 ounces

Grains, Bread, & Pasta
Penne pasta, whole-wheat—
    5 ounces
Rotini pasta, whole-wheat—
    9 ounces
Tortillas, low-carb, large
    (18 grams carb and
    12 grams fiber each)—4

Dairy & Cheese
Cheese, Parmesan—1 small
    block (1/4 cup grated)
Cheese, sharp cheddar,
    reduced-fat, shredded—
    1 bag
Half-and-half, fat-free—1 cup
Yogurt, plain, fat-free—
    1 container

Canned Goods & Sauces
Bean sprouts, 14.5-ounce
    can—1
Broth, chicken, fat-free,
    reduced-sodium,
    14.5-ounce can—1
Soy sauce, lite
Tomatoes, diced,
    no-salt-added,
    14-ounce can—1
Water chestnuts—1 cup

Frozen Foods
Peas—1 bag

Staples, Seasonings, & Baking Needs
Basil
Black pepper, ground
Chili powder
Cornstarch
Honey—1 jar
Nonstick cooking spray
Oil, olive
Oregano
Salt
Vinegar, balsamic
Vinegar, red wine

Miscellaneous
Wine, white

Beef Tenderloin GF LC

Makes: 4 servings   *Serving Size: 1 steak*   *Prep Time: 5 minutes*

4   4-ounce beef tenderloin steaks
1/2 tsp salt (optional)
1   tsp ground black pepper
     nonstick cooking spray

1 Preheat oven to 400°F. Trim visible fat from sides of meat. Season both sides of meat with salt and pepper.

2 Coat a large sauté pan with cooking spray. Over high heat, sear meat on both sides about 1 minute. Place steaks in baking pan.

3 Bake in oven for 15 minutes. Turn once halfway through baking.

National Women's Heart Health Day is February 1. Do the right thing for your heart by eating right and getting plenty of exercise.

Exchanges/Choices
3 Lean Meat

Calories	140
Calories from Fat	55
Total Fat	6.0 g
Saturated Fat	2.2 g
Trans Fat	0.0 g
Cholesterol	60 mg
Sodium	45 mg
Potassium	270 mg
Total Carbohydrate	0 g
Dietary Fiber	0 g
Sugars	0 g
Protein	21 g
Phosphorus	165 mg

Chef's Tip

After you remove the steaks from the oven, let them sit for 5 minutes before you cut them. This will allow the juices to redistribute themselves, providing maximum flavor!

Scalloped Potatoes

Makes: 6 servings   *Serving Size: 2/3 cup*   *Prep Time: 15 minutes*

6	medium russet potatoes
1	medium yellow onion, cut into thin strips
	nonstick cooking spray
1/4	tsp salt (optional)
1/4	tsp ground black pepper
1	cup fat-free half-and-half
1/2	cup shredded, reduced-fat sharp cheddar cheese, divided

1 Preheat oven to 400°F. Peel potatoes and slice into thin rounds.

2 Coat a large nonstick skillet with cooking spray and sauté onions and potatoes over medium-high heat until the onions turn clear.

3 Spray a pie pan or 8-inch round cake pan with cooking spray.

4 Place a thick layer (about half) of the potatoes and onions in the bottom of pan.

5 Add salt and pepper to half-and-half. Pour 1/2 cup of the half-and half over the potatoes. Sprinkle 1/4 cup of the cheese on top.

6 Add the remaining potatoes and pour 1/2 cup half-and-half over the potatoes and top with remaining cheese.

7 Bake for 40 minutes or until potatoes are soft.

Exchanges/Choices
2 Starch

Calories 160
  Calories from Fat 20
Total Fat . . . . .2.5 g
  Saturated Fat . . . . .1.5 g
  Trans Fat . . . . .0.0 g
Cholesterol. . . . . 5 mg
Sodium . . . . 120 mg
Potassium. . . . . 550 mg
Total Carbohydrate. . . . . . 29 g
  Dietary Fiber . . . . 2 g
  Sugars . . . . 5 g
Protein . . . . 6 g
Phosphorus . . . . 175 mg

Dietitian's Tip

Try fat-free half-and-half in any recipe where you want creaminess without added fat.

Turkey and Avocado Wraps

Makes: 4 servings   *Serving Size: 1 wrap*   *Prep Time: 25 minutes*

1/2	avocado
3	Tbsp fat-free plain yogurt
1/4	tsp chili powder
2	cups chopped lettuce
2	small tomatoes, seeded and finely diced
4	large low-carb tortillas (18 grams carb and 12 grams fiber each)
12	ounces thinly sliced no-added-salt deli turkey
1	cucumber, thinly sliced

1 In a small bowl, mash the avocado with a fork. Add yogurt and chili powder to avocado and mix well.

2 In a medium bowl, toss lettuce and tomato together.

3 Spread 1 1/2 Tbsp of avocado on tortillas. Add 3 ounces turkey, 1/4 lettuce and tomato mixture, and 5 slices cucumber to tortillas.

4 Fold in the left and right side of the tortillas until the edges are about 1 inch apart and then roll from the top down. Repeat this process for remaining 3 wraps.

Exchanges/Choices
1 Starch   1 Vegetable
3 Lean Meat

Calories 245
  Calories from Fat 65
Total Fat . . . . .7.0 g
  Saturated Fat . . . . .0.9 g
  Trans Fat . . . . .0.0 g
Cholesterol. . . . . 45 mg
Sodium . . . . 395 mg
Potassium. . . . . 660 mg
Total Carbohydrate . . . . . . 29 g
  Dietary Fiber . . . . 15 g
  Sugars . . . . 8 g
Protein . . . . 31 g
Phosphorus . . . . 380 mg

Dietitian's Tip

Avocados are a good source of potassium, a mineral that helps the body's fluids stay in balance.

Confetti Pasta Salad

Makes: 6 servings   *Serving Size: 1 cup*   *Prep Time: 20 minutes*

Dressing
- 1/4 cup red wine vinegar
- 2   tsp olive oil
- 1/4 tsp dried basil
- 1/4 tsp salt (optional)
- 1/4 tsp ground black pepper

Salad
- 5   ounces uncooked whole-wheat rotini pasta (about 2 cups)
- 1   cup fresh or frozen peas
- 1   cup finely diced carrot
- 1   green bell pepper, finely diced
- 1   tomato, seeded and finely diced

1 In a small bowl, whisk together all the dressing ingredients; set aside.

2 Cook pasta according to package directions, omitting salt. Drain pasta in colander and run under cold water for a few minutes to cool.

3 In a medium bowl, toss together pasta, peas, carrots, peppers, and tomatoes.

4 Drizzle dressing over the salad and toss again to coat.

Exchanges/Choices
1 1/2 Starch   1 Vegetable

Calories	140
Calories from Fat	20
Total Fat	2.0 g
Saturated Fat	0.3 g
Trans Fat	0.0 g
Cholesterol	0 mg
Sodium	45 mg
Potassium	225 mg
Total Carbohydrate	24 g
Dietary Fiber	5 g
Sugars	4 g
Protein	6 g
Phosphorus	90 mg

Dietitian's Tip

Feel free to add cooked chicken or shrimp to this dish for protein. Most green, deep yellow, and orange vegetables are great sources of vitamin A, which is important for healthy skin and eyes.

Penne with Chicken and Vegetables

Makes: 6 servings   *Serving Size: about 2 cups*   *Prep Time: 15 minutes*

9   ounces uncooked whole-wheat penne pasta
    nonstick cooking spray
1   pound boneless, skinless chicken breasts, cut into 1-inch strips
1   Tbsp olive oil
2   cups broccoli florets
2   medium red bell peppers, sliced into thin strips
2   medium yellow squash, sliced
1   14-ounce can no-salt-added diced tomatoes, juice drained
1/4 cup white wine
1/2 tsp dried basil
1/2 tsp dried oregano
1/4 tsp salt (optional)
1/4 tsp ground black pepper
1/4 cup freshly grated Parmesan cheese

1 Cook pasta according to package directions, omitting salt.

2 Coat a large nonstick skillet with cooking spray. Over medium-high heat, cook chicken strips for about 3–5 minutes or until done. Remove from pan and set aside.

3 Add olive oil to pan. Sauté broccoli, red peppers, and squash for 3–4 minutes. Add tomatoes, wine, herbs, salt, and pepper. Cook for 5–7 more minutes.

4 Toss chicken and vegetable mixture with drained, cooked penne pasta. Sprinkle with Parmesan cheese.

Exchanges/Choices

2 Starch   2 Vegetable
2 Lean Meat

Calories	315
Calories from Fat	55
Total Fat	6.0 g
Saturated Fat	1.5 g
Trans Fat	0.0 g
Cholesterol	45 mg
Sodium	120 mg
Potassium	605 mg
Total Carbohydrate	42 g
Dietary Fiber	7 g
Sugars	6 g
Protein	25 g
Phosphorus	275 mg

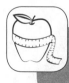

Dietitian's Tip

This tasty meal provides protein, carbohydrate, and veggies in one dish.

Cantonese Chicken LC

Makes: 4 servings   *Serving Size: 1/4 recipe*   *Prep Time: 15 minutes*

nonstick cooking spray
1   pound boneless, skinless chicken breasts, cut into 1-inch cubes
1   cup chopped celery
1   cup sliced, drained water chestnuts
1   14.5-ounce can bean sprouts, rinsed and drained
1   14.5-ounce can fat-free, low-sodium chicken broth
5   tsp lite soy sauce
1 1/2   Tbsp cornstarch
1/2   tsp salt (optional)
1/4   tsp ground black pepper

1 Coat a large nonstick skillet with cooking spray. Over medium-high heat, cook chicken for 6 minutes or until chicken is cooked through. Remove chicken from pan.

2 Add celery, water chestnuts, and bean sprouts; stir-fry for about 3 minutes.

3 In a medium bowl, whisk broth, soy sauce, and cornstarch together. Add broth mixture to pan. Bring to a boil; reduce heat and simmer for 5 minutes. Add salt and pepper. Add chicken back to pan and heat through.

4 Serve over brown rice if desired.

Exchanges/Choices
2 Vegetable   3 Lean Meat

Calories 185
　Calories from Fat 25
Total Fat . . . . .3.0 g
　Saturated Fat . . . . .0.8 g
　Trans Fat . . . . .0.0 g
Cholesterol. . . . . 65 mg
Sodium . . . . 585 mg
Potassium. . . . . 435 mg
Total Carbohydrate . . . . . . 11 g
　Dietary Fiber . . . . 2 g
　Sugars . . . . 3 g
Protein . . . . 27 g
Phosphorus . . . . 235 mg

Chef's Tip

Using a wok for this recipe helps the veggies cook evenly without getting mushy. If you don't have a wok, use a large skillet.

Tuna Steaks with Balsamic Glaze GF LC

Makes: 4 servings   *Serving Size: 1 tuna steak*   *Prep Time: 5 minutes*

nonstick cooking spray
4   5-ounce tuna steaks
1/2   tsp salt (optional)
1/4   tsp ground black pepper
3/4   cup balsamic vinegar
1   Tbsp honey
2   scallions, sliced diagonally

1 Coat a large nonstick skillet with cooking spray. Season each side of tuna steaks with salt and pepper. Place tuna steaks in pan and cook over medium-high heat for about 3–4 minutes on each side. Remove from heat.

2 In a small saucepan, combine balsamic vinegar and honey over medium heat. Bring to a low boil and cook until liquid is reduced by half (about 10 minutes). Stir frequently.

3 Spoon balsamic mixture over tuna steaks and top with scallions.

Exchanges/Choices
1 Carbohydrate   4 Lean Meat

Calories 255
  Calories from Fat 65
Total Fat . . . . 7.0 g
  Saturated Fat . . . . 1.7 g
  Trans Fat . . . . 0.0 g
Cholesterol . . . . 50 mg
Sodium . . . . 65 mg
Potassium . . . . 420 mg
Total Carbohydrate . . . . . . 13 g
  Dietary Fiber . . . . 0 g
  Sugars . . . . 11 g
Protein . . . . 32 g
Phosphorus . . . . 360 mg

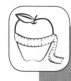

Dietitian's Tip

This recipe proves fish is easy to cook! You don't want to miss out on the benefits of all those heart-healthy omega-3 fatty acids.

FEBRUARY

WEEK 2

DAY 1
Veggie Pizza   48

DAY 2
Beef Fajitas   49

DAY 3
Oysters Rockefeller   50

DAY 4
Honey-Mustard Pork
     Chops   51
Pasta Cabbage
     Stir-Fry   52

DAY 5
Tuna Salad with
     Chickpeas   53
Jalapeño Corn
     Muffins   54

GROCERY LIST

Fresh Produce
Bell peppers, green—3
Bell peppers, red—3
Broccoli—1 head
Cabbage—1 small head
Celery—2 stalks
Cucumber—1
Garlic—2 cloves
Lemon—1
Mushrooms—1 pint
Onions, yellow or white—3
Pepper, jalapeño—1
Salad greens—4 cups
Squash, yellow—1
Tomato—1

Meat, Poultry, & Fish
Flank steak—2/3 pound
Oysters, fresh, shucked—
     1 pound
Pork chops, bone-in, center-
     cut, 5 ounces each—4
Tuna, chunk, flavor-fresh
     in 6.4-ounce pouches,
     packed in water—2

Grains, Bread, & Pasta
Bread crumbs, whole-
     wheat—1/4 cup
Linguine, whole-wheat—
     8 ounces
Pizza crust, whole-wheat,
     12-inch prepackaged—1
Tortillas, low-carb (10 grams
     carb and more than
     4 grams fiber)—8

Dairy & Cheese
Buttermilk, low-fat—1 cup
Cheese, cheddar, reduced-fat,
     shredded—1/2 cup
Cheese, mozzarella, part-
     skim, shredded—1/2 cup
Cheese, Parmesan, freshly
     grated—1 Tbsp
Eggs
Half-and-half, fat-free—1 cup
Margarine, trans-fat-free
Yogurt, fat-free, plain—
     3 Tbsp

Canned Goods & Sauces
Chickpeas (garbanzo
     beans)—1 cup
Mayonnaise, light—1 jar

Frozen Foods
Spinach, chopped—1 bag

Staples, Seasonings, & Baking Needs
Baking powder
Black pepper, ground
Cayenne pepper
Chili powder
Cornmeal
Cumin
Flour, all-purpose
Honey
Mustard, Dijon
Nonstick cooking spray
Oil, canola
Oil, olive
Red pepper flakes
Salt

Miscellaneous
Wine, white

Veggie Pizza

Makes: 4 servings   *Serving Size: 2 slices*   *Prep Time: 20 minutes*

1 tsp olive oil
1 cup broccoli florets
1 yellow squash, sliced (about 1 cup)
1 cup sliced mushrooms
1 red bell pepper, sliced into thin strips
2 garlic cloves, minced
1 12-inch prepackaged whole-wheat pizza crust
1/2 cup shredded part-skim mozzarella cheese
1/4 tsp ground black pepper
1/4 tsp crushed red pepper flakes

Salad

4 cups salad greens
1 medium tomato, sliced
1/2 medium cucumber, sliced

1 Preheat oven to 450°F. Add olive oil to a large nonstick skillet over medium heat. Add broccoli, squash, mushrooms, and red bell pepper; sauté for 3 minutes. Add garlic and sauté 30 more seconds.

2 Place pizza crust on a baking sheet. Spread the veggie mixture evenly over the pizza. Sprinkle with cheese, black pepper, and red pepper flakes.

3 Bake pizza in oven for 20 minutes or until the cheese begins to lightly brown.

4 Prepare a salad and serve it on the side.

Exchanges/Choices

2 Starch   2 Vegetable
1 Med-Fat Meat

Calories	270
Calories from Fat	70
Total Fat	8.0 g
Saturated Fat	3.2 g
Trans Fat	0.0 g
Cholesterol	10 mg
Sodium	455 mg
Potassium	715 mg
Total Carbohydrate	43 g
Dietary Fiber	9 g
Sugars	8 g
Protein	14 g
Phosphorus	305 mg

Dietitian's Tip

Eating pizza can be a great way to sneak even more vegetables into your meal plan.

Beef Fajitas

Makes: 4 servings   *Serving Size: 2 fajitas*   *Prep Time: 15 minutes*

nonstick cooking spray

2/3 pound flank steak, cut against the grain into 2-inch strips

1 tsp canola oil

2 green bell peppers, sliced into thin strips

1 medium onion, sliced into thin strips

1/4 cup water

1/2 Tbsp chili powder

1/4 tsp cayenne pepper

1/4 tsp cumin

1/2 tsp salt (optional)

1/2 tsp ground black pepper

8 low-carb tortillas (10 grams carb and more than 4 grams fiber)

1 Coat a large nonstick skillet with cooking spray. Cook beef over medium-high heat for about 3 minutes. Remove from pan and set aside.

2 Add oil to the pan and heat. Add green pepper and onion; cook for about 7 minutes or until beginning to brown. Add meat and any juices back to pan and cook another 2 minutes.

3 Add water and spices, including salt and pepper. Bring to a boil; reduce heat, and simmer until water evaporates. Serve with tortillas.

Exchanges/Choices

1 Starch   1 Vegetable
3 Lean Meat

Calories	245
Calories from Fat	80
Total Fat	9.0 g
Saturated Fat	1.8 g
Trans Fat	0.0 g
Cholesterol	25 mg
Sodium	465 mg
Potassium	440 mg
Total Carbohydrate	28 g
Dietary Fiber	16 g
Sugars	3 g
Protein	26 g
Phosphorus	225 mg

Chef's Tip

To cut "against the grain" means to slice the meat in the opposite direction of the lines—the grain—in the meat.

Oysters Rockefeller

Makes: 2 servings   *Serving Size: about 6 oysters*   *Prep Time: 15 minutes*

nonstick cooking spray
2 tsp light trans-fat-free margarine
2 Tbsp all-purpose flour
1 cup fat-free half-and-half
1/4 tsp salt (optional)
1/4 tsp ground black pepper
1/4 cup chopped, frozen spinach, thawed and drained
1/4 cup whole-wheat bread crumbs
1 Tbsp freshly grated Parmesan cheese
1 pound fresh oysters, shucked and with juice
2 Tbsp white wine

1 Preheat oven to 350°F. Coat an 8-inch pie or cake pan with cooking spray; set aside.

2 In a small nonstick skillet, melt margarine over medium heat. Add flour to margarine, stirring constantly. Cook for 2–3 minutes to make a roux.

3 In a small saucepan, bring half-and-half to a low boil over medium-high heat. Add roux, salt, and pepper to half-and-half while whisking. Boil for 2 minutes; stir in spinach and cook 2 more minutes.

4 In a small bowl, combine bread crumbs and Parmesan cheese; set aside.

5 Line the bottom of the pie or cake pan with the oysters and their juice. Sprinkle wine over the oysters. Pour spinach and sauce mixture over the oysters and sprinkle bread crumb mixture over the top.

6 Bake for 20 minutes or until oysters are done.

Exchanges/Choices
2 Carbohydrate   1 Lean Meat
1/2 Fat

Calories	220
Calories from Fat	55
Total Fat	6.0 g
Saturated Fat	2.3 g
Trans Fat	0.0 g
Cholesterol	30 mg
Sodium	305 mg
Potassium	435 mg
Total Carbohydrate	30 g
Dietary Fiber	2 g
Sugars	11 g
Protein	11 g
Phosphorus	295 mg

Chef's Tip

You can buy oysters already shucked in the fresh seafood department. You can also find frozen shucked oysters in the frozen food section.

Honey-Mustard Pork Chops GF LC

Makes: 4 servings   *Serving Size: 1 pork chop*   *Prep Time: 10 minutes*

1/4   cup Dijon mustard
1   Tbsp honey
1/4   tsp ground black pepper
4   5-ounce bone-in, center-cut
     pork chops
     nonstick cooking spray

1 Preheat oven to 400°F. In a small bowl, combine Dijon mustard, honey, and pepper.

2 Place pork chops in a baking dish coated with cooking spray. Pour mustard mixture over pork chops and spread to coat.

3 Bake pork chops in oven 30 minutes or until done.

Keep your heart healthy this month with low-fat, high-fiber foods and plenty of vegetables!

Exchanges/Choices
1/2 Carbohydrate
3 Lean Meat

Calories 170
  Calories from Fat 55
Total Fat . . . . .6.0 g
  Saturated Fat . . . . .2.2 g
  Trans Fat . . . . .0.0 g
Cholesterol. . . . . 60 mg
Sodium . . . . 405 mg
Potassium. . . . . 280 mg
Total Carbohydrate . . . . 7 g
  Dietary Fiber . . . . 1 g
  Sugars . . . . 5 g
Protein . . . . 21 g
Phosphorus . . . . 140 mg

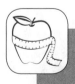

Dietitian's Tip

Mustard, a free food in the exchange system, adds great flavor without adding extra fat or calories.

Pasta Cabbage Stir-Fry

Makes: 10 servings   *Serving Size: 1/2 cup*   *Prep Time: 25 minutes*

8	ounces uncooked whole-wheat linguine
1/2	Tbsp olive oil
1	small onion, thinly sliced
4	cups shredded cabbage
1/4	tsp salt (optional)
1/4	tsp ground black pepper

1 Cook pasta according to package directions, omitting salt; drain.

2 Add oil to a large nonstick skillet over medium-high heat. Add onion to pan and cook for 3–5 minutes or until translucent.

3 Add cabbage to pan and stir-fry for 10 minutes or until cabbage is softened and beginning to brown. Add salt and pepper.

4 Add cooked pasta to pan and toss with cabbage mixture; sauté 3 more minutes.

Exchanges/Choices
1 Starch   1 Vegetable

Calories 100
  Calories from Fat 10
Total Fat . . . . .1.0 g
  Saturated Fat . . . . .0.2 g
  Trans Fat . . . . .0.0 g
Cholesterol . . . . 0 mg
Sodium . . . . 5 mg
Potassium . . . . 85 mg
Total Carbohydrate . . . . :. 19 g
  Dietary Fiber . . . . 3 g
  Sugars . . . . 2 g
Protein . . . . 4 g
Phosphorus . . . . 55 mg

Chef's Tip

If you don't cook cabbage very often, you might want to reconsider. Stir-frying cabbage with pasta and onions makes a great accompaniment to grilled or broiled meat.

Tuna Salad with Chickpeas GF LC NEW

Makes: 7 servings   *Serving Size: 1/2 cup*   *Prep Time: 10 minutes*

3	Tbsp fat-free plain yogurt
1/4	cup light mayonnaise
1/2	lemon, juiced
1/2	large red bell pepper, diced
2	medium celery stalks, diced
1/4	cup onion, finely diced
1	cup canned chickpeas (garbanzo beans), rinsed and drained
2	6.4-ounce flavor-fresh chunk tuna pouches, in water
1/4	tsp ground black pepper

1 In a small bowl, whisk together yogurt, mayonnaise, and lemon juice.

2 In a medium bowl, combine remaining ingredients. Pour mayonnaise mixture over tuna and mix well.

3 Serve tuna salad on your choice of lettuce or whole-wheat bread or crackers.

Exchanges/Choices
1/2 Starch   2 Lean Meat

Calories 125
   Calories from Fat 25
Total Fat . . . . .3.0 g
   Saturated Fat . . . . .0.5 g
   Trans Fat . . . . .0.0 g
Cholesterol. . . . . 25 mg
Sodium . . . . 335 mg
Potassium. . . . . 320 mg
Total Carbohydrate . . . . . . 10 g
   Dietary Fiber . . . . 3 g
   Sugars . . . . 3 g
Protein . . . . 15 g
Phosphorus . . . . 145 mg

Dietitian's Tip

This salad is full of flavor and crunch. It is made lighter by mixing fat-free plain yogurt and light mayonnaise—you'll be surprised when you can't taste the difference.

Jalapeño Corn Muffins

Makes: 12 muffins   *Serving Size: 1 muffin*   *Prep Time: 13 minutes*

1 1/4 cups all-purpose flour
3/4 cup cornmeal
2 tsp baking powder
1/2 tsp salt
2 eggs
1 cup low-fat buttermilk
1 Tbsp canola oil
1 jalapeño pepper, minced
1 red bell pepper, minced
1 green bell pepper, minced
1/2 cup reduced-fat shredded cheddar cheese

1 Preheat oven to 400°F. In a large mixing bowl, sift together flour, cornmeal, baking powder, and salt. Set aside.

2 In a medium mixing bowl, whisk eggs. Add buttermilk and oil; mix well.

3 Add jalapeño pepper, red pepper, green pepper, and cheese to dry ingredients and toss well to coat. Make a well in the center of the dry ingredients.

4 Pour wet ingredients into the well and gently combine just until dry ingredients are moistened. Batter will be thick and lumpy.

5 Spray a muffin pan or line with paper muffin cups. Fill muffin cups 2/3 full. Bake for 25 minutes or until golden brown.

Exchanges/Choices
1 1/2 Starch   1/2 Fat

Calories 130
  Calories from Fat 30
Total Fat . . . . .3.5 g
  Saturated Fat . . . . .1.1 g
  Trans Fat . . . . .0.0 g
Cholesterol . . . . 35 mg
Sodium . . . . 230 mg
Potassium . . . . 135 mg
Total Carbohydrate . . . . . . 20 g
  Dietary Fiber . . . . 1 g
  Sugars . . . . 2 g
Protein . . . . 5 g
Phosphorus . . . . 170 mg

Chef's Tip

These muffins are perfect for the holiday season because the bits of red and green pepper make them look very festive.

FEBRUARY

WEEK 3

DAY 1
Lemon Herb Tilapia
with Zucchini   56

DAY 2
Broiled BBQ
Chicken   57
Sugar Snap Peas   58

DAY 3
Salsa Turkey
Meatloaf   59

DAY 4
Marinated Flank
Steak   60
Garlic and Herb-Mashed
Parsnips   61

DAY 5
Spanish Chicken with
Quinoa   62

GROCERY LIST

Fresh Produce
Bell pepper, yellow or
orange—1
Cilantro—1 bunch
Garlic—1 large head
Limes—4
Onions, yellow or white—3
Parsley—1 small bunch
Parsnips, medium—8
Sugar snap peas, whole—
3 cups
Tarragon—1 small bunch
Zucchini—2 small

Meat, Poultry, & Fish
Chicken breast halves, bone
in, skin removed—
1 3/4 pounds
Chicken breasts, boneless,
skinless—1 pound
Flank steak—1 pound
Tilapia fillets, 4 ounces
each—4
Turkey, ground, 93% lean—
3/4 pound

Grains, Bread, & Pasta
Oats, old-fashioned—1/2 cup
Quinoa—1/2 cup

Dairy & Cheese
Egg
Margarine, trans-fat-free
Milk, fat-free

Canned Goods & Sauces
Barbecue sauce,
low-sodium—1 small
bottle (3/4 cup)
Broth, chicken, fat-free,
low-sodium, 14.5-ounce
can—1
Salsa—3/4 cup
Soy sauce, lite

Staples, Seasonings, & Baking Needs
Basil
Black pepper, ground
Cornstarch
Nonstick cooking spray
Oil, olive
Oregano
Paprika
Salt
Sesame seeds
Tarragon
Thyme

Miscellaneous
Lemon juice—1 small bottle

Lemon Herb Tilapia with Zucchini GF LC

Makes: 4 servings   Serving Size: 1 tilapia fillet and 1/2 cup zucchini   Prep Time: 25 minutes

1/2 cup lemon juice
3   garlic cloves, minced
1   tsp dried basil
1   tsp dried tarragon
1   tsp dried oregano
1   tsp dried thyme
4   4-ounce tilapia fillets
     nonstick cooking spray
2   small zucchini, thinly sliced
     lengthwise
1   Tbsp trans-fat-free margarine
1/4 tsp salt (optional)
1/4 tsp ground black pepper

1 Preheat oven to 400°F. Combine lemon juice, garlic, and herbs in a medium bowl. Add fish, cover, and marinate in the refrigerator for 15 minutes.

2 Remove fish from marinade (reserve the marinade). Spray a 12 × 12-inch sheet of aluminum foil with cooking spray.

3 Place 2 fillets of fish on the sheet of aluminum foil. Top with half of zucchini. Repeat layering with another layer of fish, then remaining zucchini.

4 Sprinkle chunks of margarine over the top of fish and drizzle 1/4 cup of the marinade over the top. Sprinkle with salt and pepper.

5 Bring foil sides up on both sides and seal. Place on baking sheet and bake in oven for 20 minutes.

Exchanges/Choices
1 Vegetable   3 Lean Meat

Calories 150
  Calories from Fat 45
Total Fat . . . . .5.0 g
  Saturated Fat . . . . .1.5 g
  Trans Fat . . . . .0.0 g
Cholesterol. . . . . 50 mg
Sodium . . . . 85 mg
Potassium. . . . . 535 mg
Total Carbohydrate . . . . 5 g
  Dietary Fiber . . . . 1 g
  Sugars . . . . 2 g
Protein . . . . 23 g
Phosphorus . . . . 205 mg

Chef's Tip

Cooking with aluminum foil (packet cooking) is a quick, easy, and low-fat method.

Broiled BBQ Chicken

Makes: 4 servings   *Serving Size: 1 chicken breast half*   *Prep Time: 5 minutes*

1 3/4   pounds chicken breast halves, bone in, skin removed
  1/2   tsp ground black pepper
  3/4   cup bottled low-sodium barbecue sauce (reserve 1/4 cup)

1 Preheat oven broiler. Season all sides of each chicken breast with black pepper. Place chicken breast side down in broiler for 10 minutes. Turn chicken over and coat well with 1/2 cup of sauce. Broil for 5 more minutes.

2 Remove chicken from broiler and coat with remaining 1/4 cup of sauce.

Exchanges/Choices
1 1/2 Carbohydrate
4 Lean Meat

Calories 265
  Calories from Fat 35
Total Fat . . . . 4.0 g
  Saturated Fat . . . . 1.1 g
  Trans Fat . . . . 0.0 g
Cholesterol . . . . 90 mg
Sodium . . . . 440 mg
Potassium . . . . 385 mg
Total Carbohydrate . . . . . . 23 g
  Dietary Fiber . . . . 0 g
  Sugars . . . . 18 g
Protein . . . . 33 g
Phosphorus . . . . 250 mg

Chef's Tip

This barbecued chicken couldn't be easier—try it outside on the grill in the summer, too!

Sugar Snap Peas LC

Makes: 6 servings　　　　　*Serving Size: 1/2 cup*　　　　　*Prep Time: 1 minute*

1/2 tsp olive oil

3 cups whole sugar snap peas, washed and dried

1 tsp sesame seeds

1 tsp lite soy sauce

1 Add oil to a medium nonstick skillet over medium-high heat. Add peas and stir-fry for 2 minutes. Sprinkle with sesame seeds and stir-fry for 2 more minutes.

2 Drizzle peas with soy sauce and stir-fry for 1 more minute.

Exchanges/Choices
1 Vegetable

Calories	25
Calories from Fat	5
Total Fat	0.5 g
Saturated Fat	0.1 g
Trans Fat	0.0 g
Cholesterol	0 mg
Sodium	35 mg
Potassium	60 mg
Total Carbohydrate	4 g
Dietary Fiber	1 g
Sugars	2 g
Protein	1 g
Phosphorus	25 mg

Chef's Tip

Sesame seeds provide a lot of flavor—and toasting them enhances that flavor even more.

Salsa Turkey Meatloaf LC

Makes: 6 servings   *Serving Size: 1/6 recipe*   *Prep Time: 10 minutes*

	nonstick cooking spray
3/4	pound 93% lean ground turkey
1	egg
1/2	cup old-fashioned oats
1	finely diced onion
1	garlic clove, minced
3/4	cup salsa, divided

1 Preheat oven to 400°F. Coat a 5 × 9-inch loaf pan with cooking spray. In a large mixing bowl, combine turkey, egg, oats, onion, garlic, and 1/2 cup salsa. Mix thoroughly.

2 Place turkey mixture in loaf pan and spread evenly. Top with remaining 1/4 cup salsa. Bake for 50–60 minutes.

Exchanges/Choices
1/2 Carbohydrate
2 Lean Meat

Calories	145
Calories from Fat	55
Total Fat	6.0 g
Saturated Fat	1.5 g
Trans Fat	0.1 g
Cholesterol	70 mg
Sodium	240 mg
Potassium	295 mg
Total Carbohydrate	9 g
Dietary Fiber	2 g
Sugars	2 g
Protein	14 g
Phosphorus	165 mg

Chef's Tip

Who said meatloaf has to be boring? Serve this zesty dish with Smashed Potatoes (page 167).

Marinated Flank Steak GF LC

Makes: 4 servings   *Serving Size: 1 steak*   *Prep Time: 20 minutes*

4 limes, juiced (about 1/2 cup lime juice)
1/2 cup whole cilantro leaves
2 garlic cloves, sliced
1 pound flank steak, cut into 4 4-ounce steaks
1/2 tsp salt (optional)
1/2 tsp ground black pepper

1 Prepare an indoor or outdoor grill.

2 Combine lime juice, cilantro, and garlic in a large bowl. Add steaks and marinate for 15 minutes in the refrigerator.

3 Remove steaks from marinade. Season meat on both sides with salt and pepper. Grill over medium-high heat for 5–7 minutes on each side.

4 Slice thinly against the grain to serve.

Exchanges/Choices
3 Lean Meat

Calories 155
  Calories from Fat 55
Total Fat . . . . .6.0 g
  Saturated Fat . . . . .2.5 g
  Trans Fat . . . . .0.0 g
Cholesterol. . . . . 40 mg
Sodium . . . . 50 mg
Potassium. . . . . 305 mg
Total Carbohydrate . . . . 2 g
  Dietary Fiber . . . . 0 g
  Sugars . . . . 0 g
Protein . . . . 22 g
Phosphorus . . . . 180 mg

Dietitian's Tip

The bold flavors of cilantro, lime juice, and garlic make a great-tasting dish without added fat.

Garlic and Herb-Mashed Parsnips GF

Makes: 4 servings   *Serving Size: 1/2 cup*   *Prep Time: 15 minutes*

8   medium parsnips, peeled and cubed
4   whole garlic cloves, peeled
3   Tbsp fat-free milk
1   tsp chopped fresh parsley
1   tsp chopped fresh tarragon
1/2   tsp salt
1/4   tsp ground black pepper

1 Fill a large saucepan 2/3 full with water and bring to a boil. Add parsnips and garlic cloves. Boil for 10–15 minutes or until parsnips are soft. Drain.

2 In a medium bowl, add all ingredients and, with an electric mixer or a whisk, beat until puréed.

February is Black History Month. Learn more about a famous African American today!

Exchanges/Choices
2 Starch

Calories	150
Calories from Fat	5
Total Fat	0.5 g
Saturated Fat	0.1 g
Trans Fat	0.0 g
Cholesterol	0 mg
Sodium	315 mg
Potassium	755 mg
Total Carbohydrate	35 g
Dietary Fiber	7 g
Sugars	10 g
Protein	3 g
Phosphorus	150 mg

Chef's Tip

If you don't like the flavor of tarragon, try basil in this recipe instead.

Spanish Chicken with Quinoa

Makes: 4   *Serving Size: 4 ounces chicken and 1/2 cup quinoa*   *Prep Time: 15 min*

1/2	cup quinoa
1	14.5-ounce can fat-free, low-sodium chicken broth, divided nonstick cooking spray
2	medium onions, thinly sliced
1	large yellow or orange bell pepper, thinly sliced
1	pound boneless, skinless chicken breasts
1	Tbsp cornstarch
1	Tbsp minced garlic
2	Tbsp smoked paprika
1	tsp dried thyme
1	tsp salt (optional)
1/2	tsp ground black pepper

1 Preheat oven to 375°F.

2 Rinse quinoa in a colander under cold water. Combine rinsed quinoa and 1 cup chicken broth in a medium saucepan. Bring to a boil, and then reduce to a simmer and cover. Cook for 15 minutes or until quinoa is tender.

3 Coat a 9 × 13 baking dish with cooking spray. Layer the onions and the bell pepper strips in the bottom of the pan. Place the chicken breasts on top of the vegetables.

4 In a small bowl, whisk together remaining cold chicken broth, cornstarch, garlic, paprika, thyme, salt (optional), and pepper. Pour this mixture over the chicken and bake for 15 minutes.

5 Baste the chicken with sauce and return to the oven for an additional 15–20 minutes or until the chicken's internal temperature is 165°F.

6 Serve one chicken breast over 1/2 cup quinoa and top with sauce and vegetables.

Exchanges/Choices

1 Starch   3 Vegetable
3 Lean Meat

Calories	275
Calories from Fat	40
Total Fat	4.5 g
Saturated Fat	1.0 g
Trans Fat	0.0 g
Cholesterol	65 mg
Sodium	320 mg
Potassium	685 mg
Total Carbohydrate	29 g
Dietary Fiber	4 g
Sugars	6 g
Protein	30 g
Phosphorus	335 mg

Chef's Tip

Contrary to popular belief, Spanish food typically isn't spicy hot. If you'd like to add a little heat to this dish, whisk 1/2 tsp cayenne pepper into the sauce before pouring it over the chicken. If you can't find smoked paprika, regular Spanish paprika will work just as well in this recipe.

FEBRUARY
WEEK 4

DAY 1
Sausage and Potato
  Soup   64

DAY 2
Ratatouille with Rotini
  65

DAY 3
Salmon Patties with
  Lemon Sauce   66

DAY 4
Hearty Turkey Burgers
  67
Cajun French Fries
  68

DAY 5
Chicken Vesuvio   69
Pear Salad with
  Almonds   70

**DESSERT OF
THE MONTH**
Chocolate Mousse
  Pie   71

GROCERY LIST

Fresh Produce
Bell pepper, green—1
Carrot—1 small
Celery—1 stalk
Garlic—1 head
Lemons—2
Lettuce, romaine—1 head
Mushrooms, sliced—1 pint
Onion, red—1 small
Onions, yellow or white—2
Parsley—1 small bunch
Pears, medium—2
Potatoes, russet, medium—10
Tomato—1 large
Zucchini, medium—2

Meat, Poultry, & Fish
Chicken breast halves,
  bone-in, with skin—3
Turkey, ground, lean—
  1 pound
Turkey sausage, lean,
  smoked—2 links

Grains, Bread, & Pasta
Hamburger buns,
  whole-wheat—6
Oats, old-fashioned—1 cup
Rotini pasta, whole-wheat—
  8 ounces

Dairy & Cheese
Cheese, goat, crumbled—
  1 1/2 ounces
Cheese, Parmesan—3 Tbsp
Eggs
Margarine, trans-fat-free
Milk, fat-free—2 2/3 cups

Canned Goods & Sauces
Broth, chicken, fat-free, low-
  sodium, 14.5-ounce cans—4
Salad dressing, Italian,
  fat-free—1 bottle

Salmon, 14.75-ounce can—1
Tomato sauce, 15-ounce
  can—1
Tomatoes, diced, no-salt-
  added, 14.5-ounce can—1

Frozen Foods
Peas—1/2 cup
Whipped topping, fat-free,
  8-ounce container—1

**Staples, Seasonings,
& Baking Needs**
Basil
Bay leaves
Black pepper, ground
Cayenne pepper
Chili powder
Cumin
Flour, all-purpose
Garlic salt
Mustard, Dijon
Nonstick cooking spray
Oil, canola
Oil, olive
Onion, dried minced
Oregano
Parsley
Rosemary
Sage
Salt

Miscellaneous
Almonds—2 ounces
Chocolate chips, semisweet,
  mini—1 1/2 Tbsp
Orange juice—1/2 cup
Pie crust, 9-inch
  prepackaged—1
Pudding mix, chocolate,
  sugar-free, fat-free,
  1.4-ounce package—2
Wine, white

Sausage and Potato Soup

Makes: 8 servings   *Serving Size: about 1 cup*   *Prep Time: 20 minutes*

nonstick cooking spray
2 cups lean smoked turkey sausage, sliced
1 1/2 cups diced onion
1/2 cup diced celery
1/2 cup diced carrot
2 Tbsp all-purpose flour
5 1/2 cups fat-free, low-sodium chicken broth
4 medium russet potatoes, peeled and diced
1/2 tsp dried sage
1/2 tsp ground black pepper
1 bay leaf
1 cup fat-free milk

1 Coat a large soup pot with cooking spray. Cook sausage for 2 minutes. Add onion, celery, and carrots and cook another 5–7 minutes or until beginning to brown.

2 Add flour, stirring well. Cook for 2 minutes. Add broth, potatoes, sage, black pepper, and bay leaf. Bring to a boil, scraping brown bits at the bottom of the pan. Reduce heat and simmer until potatoes are done (about 20 minutes).

3 Add milk and simmer 2 more minutes; do not boil. Remove bay leaf before serving.

Exchanges/Choices
1 Starch   1 Vegetable
1 Lean Meat

Calories	155
Calories from Fat	20
Total Fat	2.0 g
Saturated Fat	1.1 g
Trans Fat	0.0 g
Cholesterol	30 mg
Sodium	420 mg
Potassium	510 mg
Total Carbohydrate	20 g
Dietary Fiber	2 g
Sugars	5 g
Protein	10 g
Phosphorus	150 mg

Chef's Tip

There's nothing better than homemade soup on a cold winter night!

Ratatouille with Rotini

Makes: 6 servings   *Serving Size: 1 1/2 cups*   *Prep Time: 15 minutes*

8	ounces uncooked whole-wheat rotini pasta
1	Tbsp olive oil
1	medium onion, finely chopped
1 1/2	cups green bell pepper, cut into thin strips
2	medium zucchini, thinly sliced
1 1/2	cups sliced mushrooms
4	garlic cloves, minced
1	15-ounce can tomato sauce
1	14.5-ounce can no-salt-added diced tomatoes
1	tsp dried basil
1/2	tsp ground black pepper
3	Tbsp freshly grated Parmesan cheese

1 Cook pasta according to package directions, omitting salt; drain.

2 Heat oil in a large nonstick skillet or wok. Over medium-high heat, sauté onion and green pepper until onion is clear. Add zucchini and mushrooms and sauté about 5 more minutes.

3 Add garlic, tomato sauce, and diced tomatoes. Stir in basil and black pepper.

4 Reduce heat and bring to a low boil for 25 minutes. Combine ratatouille with cooked rotini pasta. Sprinkle with Parmesan cheese.

Exchanges/Choices

2 Starch   2 Vegetable
1/2 Fat

Calories 230
  Calories from Fat 35
Total Fat . . . . .4.0 g
  Saturated Fat . . . . .0.9 g
  Trans Fat . . . . .0.0 g
Cholesterol. . . . . 0 mg
Sodium . . . . 445 mg
Potassium. . . . . 725 mg
Total Carbohydrate . . . . . . 41 g
  Dietary Fiber . . . . 8 g
  Sugars . . . . 8 g
Protein . . . . 10 g
Phosphorus . . . . 185 mg

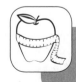

Dietitian's Tip

If you'd like a little protein with this meal, add some turkey or chicken Italian sausage.

Salmon Patties with Lemon Sauce LC

Makes: 4 patties   *Serving Size: 1 patty*   *Prep time: 15 minutes*

Salmon Patties

1	14.75-ounce can salmon
2	egg whites
1/2	tsp ground black pepper
1/4	cup old-fashioned oats
2	tsp Dijon mustard
1	Tbsp dried parsley

Lemon Sauce

1	lemon, juiced
2	Tbsp trans-fat-free margarine
1	tsp chopped fresh parsley

1 In a medium bowl, combine all patty ingredients. Divide into 4 equal servings. Shape into 1/4-inch-thick patties.

2 Coat a large nonstick skillet with cooking spray. Cook patties over medium heat for about 5 minutes on each side or until golden brown.

3 To prepare sauce, combine lemon juice, margarine, and parsley in a saucepan and simmer 5 minutes.

4 Serve 2 tsp sauce over each salmon patty.

Exchanges/Choices

1/2 Carbohydrate   3 Lean Meat
1/2 Fat

Calories	190
Calories from Fat	80
Total Fat	9.0 g
Saturated Fat	2.2 g
Trans Fat	0.0 g
Cholesterol	40 mg
Sodium	595 mg
Potassium	405 mg
Total Carbohydrate	5 g
Dietary Fiber	1 g
Sugars	1 g
Protein	20 g
Phosphorus	305 mg

Dietitian's Tip

Salmon is another great source of heart-healthy omega-3 fatty acids—and it's easy to make!

Hearty Turkey Burgers

Makes: 6 servings   *Serving Size: 1 burger*   *Prep Time: 10 minutes*

1	pound lean ground turkey
1	egg
3/4	cup old-fashioned oats
1/2	cup minced fresh mushrooms
2	Tbsp dried minced onion
1/2	tsp garlic salt
1/2	tsp ground black pepper
6	whole-wheat hamburger buns
6	lettuce leaves
6	medium tomato slices
6	medium red onion slices

1 Prepare an indoor or outdoor grill. Combine first 7 ingredients in a bowl. Divide turkey into 6 equal portions, shaping each into a patty 1/2 inch thick.

2 Place patties on grill rack; grill 7 minutes on each side or until done. (Or coat a large nonstick skillet with cooking spray and cook patties over medium heat for 3–4 minutes per side, or until juices run clear).

3 Serve burgers on whole-wheat hamburger buns, layered with lettuce, tomato, and onion.

Exchanges/Choices

2 Starch   2 Lean Meat
1 Fat

Calories	300
Calories from Fat	90
Total Fat	10.0 g
Saturated Fat	2.4 g
Trans Fat	0.1 g
Cholesterol	90 mg
Sodium	380 mg
Potassium	475 mg
Total Carbohydrate	33 g
Dietary Fiber	5 g
Sugars	6 g
Protein	22 g
Phosphorus	320 mg

Dietitian's Tip

You can substitute a whole-wheat sandwich thin for the hamburger bun and lower the carbs to 20 grams per serving.

Cajun French Fries GF

Makes: 6 servings   *Serving Size: 1/6 recipe*   *Prep Time: 10 minutes*

6 medium russet potatoes (6 ounces each), peeled and sliced into eighths
1 Tbsp canola oil
1/4 tsp cayenne pepper
1 tsp chili powder
1/2 tsp cumin
1/2 tsp salt (optional)
1/4 tsp ground black pepper
nonstick cooking spray

1 Preheat oven to 350°F.

2 Combine potatoes and oil in a large bowl and toss well to coat. In a small bowl, combine cayenne pepper, chili powder, cumin, salt, and black pepper. Sprinkle over potatoes and toss well until all potatoes are coated with seasoning.

3 Coat a large baking sheet with cooking spray. Spread potatoes evenly on baking sheet. Bake for 30 minutes or until golden brown and crispy.

Exchanges/Choices
1 1/2 Starch

Calories 125
  Calories from Fat 20
Total Fat . . . . .2.5 g
  Saturated Fat . . . . .0.2 g
  Trans Fat . . . . .0.0 g
Cholesterol. . . . . 0 mg
Sodium . . . . 10 mg
Potassium. . . . . 435 mg
Total Carbohydrate . . . . . . 24 g
  Dietary Fiber . . . . 2 g
  Sugars . . . . 2 g
Protein . . . . 2 g
Phosphorus . . . . 55 mg

Dietitian's Tip

Feel free to try sweet potatoes in this recipe.

Chicken Vesuvio LC

Makes: 3 servings   *Serving Size: 1 chicken breast*   *Prep Time: 25 minutes*

3 chicken breast halves, bone-in, skin on
1/4 cup all-purpose flour
1 Tbsp olive oil
3 garlic cloves, minced
1 14.5-ounce can fat-free, low-sodium chicken broth
2 tsp lemon juice
1/4 cup white wine
1 tsp dried oregano
1 tsp dried rosemary
1/2 cup frozen peas
1/2 tsp salt (optional)
1/4 tsp ground black pepper

1 Preheat oven to 400°F. Remove all excess fat from chicken, leaving the skin on. Dredge the skin side of the chicken in flour and set aside.

2 Add oil to a large nonstick skillet over high heat. Place chicken flour side down in skillet to brown (about 5–6 minutes). Remove chicken from pan and set aside.

3 In the same skillet, reduce heat to medium and add the garlic for 30 seconds. Add chicken broth, lemon juice, and wine and cook until liquid is reduced by half. Add the herbs and cook for 1 more minute.

4 Place the chicken skin side up in a medium metal baking pan. Add the chicken broth mixture to the pan, making sure to avoid pouring broth over the top of the chicken. (The liquid should not cover the browned skin). Bake in oven for 30 minutes.

5 Take out of oven. Sprinkle with salt and pepper. Pour liquid into the skillet and bring to a boil and reduce by half.

6 Add the frozen peas to the liquid and immediately remove from heat.

7 Serve each breast with 1/2 cup of the broth and peas.

Exchanges/Choices

1 Starch   3 Med-Fat Meat

Calories 310
  Calories from Fat 110
Total Fat . . . . .12.0 g
  Saturated Fat . . . . .2.8 g
  Trans Fat . . . . .0.0 g
Cholesterol . . . . 80 mg
Sodium . . . . 425 mg
Potassium . . . . 410 mg
Total Carbohydrate . . . . . . 13 g
  Dietary Fiber . . . . 2 g
  Sugars . . . . 2 g
Protein . . . . 33 g
Phosphorus . . . . 265 mg

Chef's Tip

You can easily double this recipe when company's coming.

Pear Salad with Almonds GF

Makes: 6 servings   *Serving Size: 1 serving*   *Prep Time: 15 minutes*

1/2	cup fat-free Italian dressing
1/2	cup orange juice
12	ounces chopped romaine lettuce
2	ounces sliced almonds, toasted
1 1/2	ounces goat cheese, crumbled
2	medium pears, peeled and diced

1 In a small bowl, whisk together dressing and orange juice; set aside.

2 In a large salad bowl, toss together remaining ingredients.

3 Drizzle dressing over salad and toss again to coat.

Exchanges/Choices
1 Fruit   1 1/2 Fat

Calories	140
Calories from Fat	65
Total Fat	7.0 g
Saturated Fat	1.5 g
Trans Fat	0.0 g
Cholesterol	5 mg
Sodium	265 mg
Potassium	340 mg
Total Carbohydrate	17 g
Dietary Fiber	4 g
Sugars	11 g
Protein	5 g
Phosphorus	110 mg

Chef's Tip

To toast almonds, place them in a small nonstick skillet over low heat and toast for about 4 minutes or until they begin to brown.

Chocolate Mousse Pie

Makes: 8 servings　　　*Serving Size: 1 piece*　　　*Prep Time: 5 minutes*

1	9-inch prepackaged pie crust
2	1.4-ounce packages sugar-free fat-free chocolate pudding mix
1 2/3	cups fat-free milk
1	8-ounce container fat-free whipped topping, divided
1 1/2	Tbsp mini semi-sweet chocolate chips

1 Preheat oven to 400°F. Bake pie crust according to package directions. Remove from oven and cool thoroughly.

2 In a medium bowl, whisk together pudding mix and milk. Fold half (4 ounces) of whipped topping into pudding mixture and fold until fully blended.

3 Spread pudding mixture into pie crust and top with remaining whipped topping. Sprinkle top with chocolate chips.

Exchanges/Choices
2 Carbohydrate　　　1 Fat

Calories 190
　Calories from Fat 55
Total Fat . . . . .6.0 g
　Saturated Fat . . . . .2.0 g
　Trans Fat . . . . .0.0 g
Cholesterol . . . . 0 mg
Sodium . . . . 455 mg
Potassium . . . . 155 mg
Total Carbohydrate . . . . . . 29 g
　Dietary Fiber . . . . 1 g
　Sugars . . . . 13 g
Protein . . . . 3 g
Phosphorus . . . . 170 mg

Chef's Tip

Your Valentine will never guess how easy it was to make this dessert!

MARCH

National Nutrition Month®

Eating a variety of foods is a key component of good nutrition. This month's recipes prove that good nutrition does not mean boring. In addition to March being National Nutrition Month, it is also the time to celebrate Registered Dietitian Day! If you haven't already seen a registered dietitian (or RD), now is a good time to make an appointment and see what an RD can do to help individualize healthy eating guidelines for your specific needs. If you have diabetes, be sure to find an RD who is also a certified diabetes educator (CDE).

Bleu Cheese-Crusted Steak (page 139)
Basil Mashed Potatoes (page 122)
Honey Tarragon Carrots (page 169)

This meal is fabulous for serving to dinner guests. It's hearty, with just the right balance of flavors!

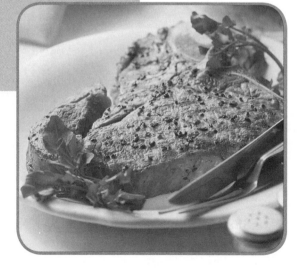

GF gluten-free recipe, but always check ingredients for gluten.

LC these recipes contain 15 grams of carbohydrate or less per serving.

NEW new recipe for the second edition.

MARCH RECIPES

MARCH
WEEK 1

DAY 1
Chopped BBQ Chicken
Salad 76

DAY 2
Spice-Rubbed Pork
Chops 77
Roasted Parmesan
Zucchini 78

DAY 3
Chicken, Mango, and
Black Bean Lettuce
Wraps 79

DAY 4
Alfredo Orange Roughy
and Rice 80

DAY 5
Cream of Broccoli
Soup 81
Cheesy Breadsticks 82

GROCERY LIST

Fresh Produce
Bell pepper, green, large—1
Bell pepper, red, large—1
Broccoli—2–3 heads
Garlic—2 cloves
Lettuce, butter (Bibb)—
1 head
Lettuce, romaine—1 head
Mango—1
Onion, red, medium—1
Onion, red, small—1
Pepper, jalapeño, medium—1
Tomatoes—2
Zucchini, large—2

Meat, Poultry, & Fish
Chicken breasts, boneless,
skinless—2 pounds
Orange roughy fillets,
4 ounces each—4
Pork chops, bone-in,
5 ounces each—4
Turkey bacon—5 slices

Grains, Bread, & Pasta
Breadsticks, refrigerated,
ready-made in a can
(12 breadsticks)—1 can
Rice, brown—1 small bag

Dairy & Cheese
Cheese, cheddar, reduced-fat,
shredded—1/2 cup
Cheese, Parmesan—small
block
Half-and-half, fat-free—
1 pint + 1 cup

Canned Goods & Sauces
Barbecue sauce—1/4 cup
Beans, black, 15-ounce
can—1
Broth, chicken, fat-free,
low-sodium, 14.5-ounce
cans—3
Salad dressing, Ranch,
fat-free—1/2 cup

Staples, Seasonings, & Baking Needs
Black pepper, ground
Cayenne pepper
Chili powder
Cornstarch
Garlic salt
Nonstick cooking spray
Paprika
Oil, olive
Oregano
Salt
Splenda Sugar Blend
Vinegar, red wine

Miscellaneous
Wine, white, dry

Chopped BBQ Chicken Salad NEW

Makes: 5 servings   *Serving Size: 2 cups*   *Prep Time: 20 min*

nonstick cooking spray
1   pound boneless, skinless chicken breasts
1/4   cup barbeque sauce
5   slices turkey bacon, cooked crisp, chopped
4   cups chopped red cabbage
4   cups chopped romaine lettuce
1/2   medium red onion (or 1 small), small dice
1   large green bell pepper, small dice
2   tomatoes, seeded and small dice
1/2   tsp salt (optional)
1/2   tsp ground black pepper
1/2   cup fat-free Ranch salad dressing

1 Preheat oven to 375°F.

2 Coat a baking sheet with cooking spray. Line the sheet with chicken breast and brush each generously with barbeque sauce. Bake for 30 minutes or until internal temperature of chicken is 165°F. Set aside to cool.

3 In a large salad bowl, toss together bacon, cabbage, lettuce, onion, bell pepper, tomatoes, salt, and pepper.

4 Once chicken is cool, chop into small pieces and toss with the salad ingredients.

5 Pour dressing over salad and toss gently to coat.

Exchanges/Choices
1 Carbohydrate   2 Vegetable
2 Lean Meat

Calories	215
Calories from Fat	45
Total Fat	5.0 g
Saturated Fat	1.3 g
Trans Fat	0.0 g
Cholesterol	50 mg
Sodium	595 mg
Potassium	685 mg
Total Carbohydrate	24 g
Dietary Fiber	4 g
Sugars	11 g
Protein	20 g
Phosphorus	235 mg

Chef's Tip

If you want to eat this salad over a couple of days, leave the dressing off and keep in an airtight container. Dress the salad as needed. This recipe works great with leftover chicken from the grill!

Spice-Rubbed Pork Chops GF LC

Makes: 4 servings　　　*Serving Size: 1 pork chop*　　　*Prep Time: 5 minutes*

1　Tbsp dried oregano
2　Tbsp paprika
1　tsp cayenne pepper
1　tsp chili powder
1/2　tsp salt (optional)
1/2　tsp ground black pepper
4　5-ounce bone-in pork chops
　　nonstick cooking spray

1 In a small bowl, combine the first six ingredients and stir well.

2 Rub one side of each pork chop well with spice mixture.

3 Coat a large nonstick skillet with cooking spray. Over medium-high heat, place each chop spice side down and cook for four minutes on each side or until done.

Exchanges/Choices
3 Lean Meat

Calories 155
　Calories from Fat 55
Total Fat . . . . .6.0 g
　Saturated Fat . . . . .2.3 g
　Trans Fat . . . . .0.0 g
Cholesterol . . . . 60 mg
Sodium . . . . 50 mg
Potassium . . . . 365 mg
Total Carbohydrate . . . . . . 3 g
　Dietary Fiber . . . . 2 g
　Sugars . . . . 0 g
Protein . . . . 21 g
Phosphorus . . . . 140 mg

Chef's Tip

To make these pork chops even spicier, add 1/2 tsp crushed red pepper flakes to the rub.

Roasted Parmesan Zucchini GF LC

Makes: 5 servings   *Serving Size: 1/2 cup*   *Prep Time: 5 minutes*

nonstick cooking spray
2 large zucchini, sliced into 2-inch wedges
2 tsp olive oil
1/2 tsp garlic salt (optional)
3 Tbsp freshly grated Parmesan cheese

1 Preheat oven to 450°F. Coat a roasting pan with cooking spray.

2 Place zucchini in pan. Drizzle olive oil over zucchini and sprinkle evenly with garlic salt and Parmesan cheese.

3 Roast for about 20 minutes.

Exchanges/Choices
1 Vegetable   1/2 Fat

Calories 45
  Calories from Fat 20
Total Fat . . . . 2.5 g
  Saturated Fat . . . . 0.7 g
  Trans Fat . . . . 0.0 g
Cholesterol . . . . 0 mg
Sodium . . . . 55 mg
Potassium . . . . 340 mg
Total Carbohydrate . . . . 4 g
  Dietary Fiber . . . . 1 g
  Sugars . . . . 2 g
Protein . . . . 3 g
Phosphorus . . . . 70 mg

Chef's Tip

Roasting vegetables enhances their flavor quickly, making the flavor more concentrated and sweet.

Chicken, Mango, and Black Bean Lettuce Wraps GF NEW

Makes: 5 servings   *Serving Size: 2/3 cup or two lettuce wraps*   *Prep Time: 10 minutes*

1 pound boneless, skinless chicken breasts, cooked and chopped

1 15.5-ounce can black beans, rinsed and drained

1 mango, peeled, diced, and pitted, juice reserved (1 Tbsp of juice)

1/2 small red onion, diced

1 medium jalapeño pepper, seeded and minced

1 large red bell pepper, seeded and diced

2 Tbsp red wine vinegar

1 Tbsp olive oil

1 tsp Splenda Sugar Blend

10 butter (Bibb) lettuce leaves, washed and dried

1 Combine all ingredients in a medium bowl except lettuce. Refrigerate for at least 1 hour, or up to a day to marinate.

2 Fill each lettuce leaf with 1/3 cup of salad mixture and fold over to make a wrap. Repeat for remaining lettuce leaves.

Exchanges/Choices

1/2 Starch	1/2 Fruit
1 Vegetable	3 Lean Meat

Calories 240
 Calories from Fat 45
Total Fat . . . . .5.0 g
 Saturated Fat . . . . .1.1 g
 Trans Fat . . . . .0.0 g
Cholesterol. . . . . 50 mg
Sodium . . . . 110 mg
Potassium. . . . . 560 mg
Total Carbohydrate . . . . . . 23 g
 Dietary Fiber . . . . 6 g
 Sugars . . . . 10 g
Protein . . . . 24 g
Phosphorus . . . . 235 mg

Chef's Tip

Be careful when cutting the jalapeño peppers. The seeds and veins inside the peppers are where the heat resides. Consider wearing gloves during this step and be careful not to touch your face or eyes when handling hot peppers. If jalapeños are too hot for you, substitute with a green bell pepper.

Alfredo Orange Roughy and Rice

Makes: 4 servings   *Serving Size: 1 fillet and 1/2 cup rice*   *Prep Time: 5 minutes*

nonstick cooking spray
4   4-ounce orange roughy fillets
2   garlic cloves, minced
1/2   cup dry white wine
1   pint fat-free half-and-half
1/2   cup freshly grated Parmesan cheese
1/2   tsp salt (optional)
1/8   tsp ground black pepper
2   cups cooked brown rice

1 Coat a large sauté pan with cooking spray. Over medium-high heat, sear fish on both sides about 2 minutes.

2 Remove fish from pan and set aside. Spray pan again with cooking spray; add garlic. Cook for about 30 seconds; do not let it brown.

3 Add wine; cook until liquid evaporates by half. Add half-and-half and Parmesan cheese; simmer for about 4 minutes.

4 Add fish back to pan and add salt and pepper. Simmer for 2 more minutes.

5 Serve over brown rice.

Exchanges/Choices
1 1/2 Starch   1 Fat-Free Milk
2 Lean Meat

Calories	315
Calories from Fat	55
Total Fat	6.0 g
Saturated Fat	2.7 g
Trans Fat	0.0 g
Cholesterol	85 mg
Sodium	325 mg
Potassium	465 mg
Total Carbohydrate	34 g
Dietary Fiber	2 g
Sugars	6 g
Protein	29 g
Phosphorus	415 mg

Chef's Tip

Steamed asparagus would be a great addition to this meal.

Cream of Broccoli Soup LC

Makes: 8 servings   *Serving Size: 1 cup*   *Prep Time: 10 minutes*

4	cups broccoli florets
1	Tbsp olive oil
1	cup finely diced onion
3	14.5-ounce cans fat-free, low-sodium chicken broth
2	Tbsp cornstarch
1	cup fat-free half-and-half
3/4	tsp salt (optional)
1/2	tsp ground black pepper

1 Coarsely chop broccoli florets in food processor or chopper.

2 Heat oil in a large soup pot over medium-high heat. Add broccoli and onions and cook for 3 minutes.

3 Add broth and bring to a boil. Reduce heat and simmer for 15 minutes or until broccoli and onions are soft.

4 In a small bowl, combine the cornstarch and half-and-half and whisk. Add this mixture (called a slurry) to the soup and bring back to a boil.

5 Reduce to a simmer for 5 more minutes; add salt and pepper.

Exchanges/Choices
1/2 Carbohydrate   1/2 Fat

Calories 70
  Calories from Fat 20
Total Fat . . . . 2.0 g
  Saturated Fat . . . . 0.5 g
  Trans Fat . . . . 0.0 g
Cholesterol . . . . 0 mg
Sodium . . . . 420 mg
Potassium . . . . 330 mg
Total Carbohydrate . . . . 9 g
  Dietary Fiber . . . . 1 g
  Sugars . . . . 4 g
Protein . . . . 4 g
Phosphorus . . . . 100 mg

Dietitian's Tip

Cream soups are typically higher in fat than broth-based soups, but using fat-free half-and-half in this recipe adds creaminess without adding fat.

Cheesy Breadsticks LC

Makes: 12 servings   *Serving Size: 1 breadstick*   *Prep Time: 5 minutes*

nonstick cooking spray
1   can ready-made refrigerated breadsticks (12 breadsticks)
1/2   cup reduced-fat shredded cheddar cheese

1 Preheat oven to 375°F. Coat a large baking sheet with cooking spray. Place breadsticks on baking sheet and spray lightly with cooking spray.

2 Sprinkle cheese over each breadstick and bake for 15 minutes.

Exchanges/Choices
1 Starch

Calories 80
  Calories from Fat 20
Total Fat . . . . .2.0 g
  Saturated Fat . . . . .0.8 g
  Trans Fat . . . . .0.0 g
Cholesterol. . . . . 5 mg
Sodium . . . . 230 mg
Potassium. . . . . 20 mg
Total Carbohydrate . . . . . . 13 g
  Dietary Fiber . . . . 0 g
  Sugars . . . . 2 g
Protein . . . . 3 g
Phosphorus . . . . 45 mg

Chef's Tip

Reduced-fat versions of cheeses, rather than fat-free versions, work better in recipes like this because they melt better.

MARCH

WEEK 2

DAY 1
Shrimp Egg Fu
   Yung   84
Edamame Salad   85

DAY 2
Chicken Gyros   86
Fruit Salad   87

DAY 3
Spinach Lasagna   88

DAY 4
Beef Stroganoff   89

DAY 5
White Chicken
   Chili   90

GROCERY LIST

Fresh Produce
Bell pepper, orange—1
Bell pepper, red—1
Bell pepper, yellow—1
Blueberries—1 cup
Cantaloupe—1 cup
Carrots, medium—2
Cucumber—1
Garlic—1 small head
Grapes, green—1 cup
Mushrooms, sliced—1 pint
Onions, red, small—1
Onions, yellow or white—2
Strawberries—1 cup
Tomato—1

Meat, Poultry, & Fish
Beef tenderloin tips,
   boneless—1 pound
Chicken breasts, boneless,
   skinless—2 pounds
Shrimp—1 cup

Grains, Bread, & Pasta
Lasagna, whole-wheat,
   no-boil noodles—1 box
   (12 noodles)
Pocket pita halves, whole-
   wheat—5
Ronzoni Healthy Harvest
   Whole Grain egg
   noodles—5 ounces

Dairy & Cheese
Cheese, mozzarella, part-skim,
   shredded—1 1/3 cups
Cheese, Parmesan—1 small
   block
Cheese, ricotta, fat-free,
   15-ounce container—1
Egg
Egg substitute—4 ounces
Sour cream, fat-free—1/2 cup
Yogurt, plain, fat-free—1 cup

Canned Goods & Sauces
Bean sprouts—1 cup
Beans, black, 15-ounce cans—2
Beans, Great Northern,
   16-ounce cans—2
Broth, beef, reduced-fat, low-
   sodium, 14.5-ounce can—1
Broth, chicken, reduced-fat,
   low-sodium, 14.5-ounce
   cans—1 1/2
Chickpeas (garbanzo beans),
   15-ounce can—1
Chilies, green, mild, 4-ounce
   can—1
Pasta sauce, marinara, low-
   sodium—5 cups (40 ounces)
Soy sauce, lite

Frozen Foods
Edamame, shelled, 16-ounce
   bag—1
Spinach, chopped, 10-ounce
   package—1

Staples, Seasonings, & Baking Needs
Black pepper, ground
Cornstarch
Flour, all-purpose
Lemon juice
Mustard, Dijon
Nonstick cooking spray
Oil, olive
Oregano
Paprika
Salt
Splenda Sugar Blend
Sugar substitute
Vinegar, apple cider

Miscellaneous
Wine, white

Shrimp Egg Fu Yung LC

Makes: 4 servings   *Serving Size: 1 patty*   *Prep Time: 10 minutes*

nonstick cooking spray
1/4 cup minced onion
1 cup canned bean sprouts, drained and rinsed
4 ounces egg substitute
1 egg
3 Tbsp all-purpose flour
1 cup cooked shrimp, diced
1/2 tsp salt (optional)
1 Tbsp cornstarch
1 packet sugar substitute
2 tsp lite soy sauce
1 1/2 cups fat-free, low-sodium chicken broth (12 ounces)

1 Coat a large nonstick skillet with cooking spray over medium heat. Add onion and bean sprouts. Sauté until onion turns clear. Set aside to cool.

2 In a medium bowl, whisk the egg substitute and egg together. Add flour, onion, bean sprouts, shrimp, and salt to eggs and stir well.

3 Over medium-high heat, pour batter by 1/2 cups into same pan to form patties and cook well on both sides until golden brown, about 4 minutes each side. Remove patties from pan and set aside.

4 In a small bowl, combine cornstarch, sugar substitute, soy sauce, and chicken broth. Mix well. Add this mixture to the hot pan and bring to a boil; reduce heat and simmer 5 minutes to make a gravy.

5 Pour the gravy over patties and serve.

Exchanges/Choices
1/2 Carbohydrate
2 Lean Meat

Calories 125
 Calories from Fat 20
Total Fat . . . . .2.0 g
 Saturated Fat . . . . .0.7 g
 Trans Fat . . . . .0.0 g
Cholesterol . . . . 125 mg
Sodium . . . . 550 mg
Potassium . . . . 230 mg
Total Carbohydrate . . . . . . 10 g
 Dietary Fiber . . . . 1 g
 Sugars . . . . 2 g
Protein . . . . 15 g
Phosphorus . . . . 175 mg

Chef's Tip

Your dinner guests will never know this dish didn't come from a Chinese restaurant!

Edamame Salad GF NEW

Makes: 10 servings   *Serving Size: 1/10 recipe*   *Prep Time: 20 minutes*

1 16-ounce bag frozen, shelled edamame, thawed

Dressing

3/4 cup apple cider vinegar
1/4 cup fat-free, low-sodium chicken or vegetable broth
3 Tbsp olive oil
2 Tbsp Splenda Sugar Blend
1/2 tsp paprika
1/2 tsp salt (optional)
1/2 tsp ground black pepper

Salad

1 yellow bell pepper, small dice
1 orange bell pepper, small dice
1 red bell pepper, small dice
1 small red onion, small dice
2 15-ounce cans black beans, drained and rinsed
1 15-ounce can chickpeas (garbanzo beans), drained and rinsed

1 Cook edamame according to package directions. Drain and rinse in cold water to stop cooking process. Set aside.

2 In a large salad bowl, whisk together dressing ingredients.

3 Add cooked and cooled edamame and remaining salad ingredients to dressing and toss gently to coat.

4 Refrigerate for at least 1 hour before serving.

Chef's Tip

This salad is best when made the day before and allowed to marinate overnight.

Exchanges/Choices

1 Starch	1 Vegetable
1 Lean Meat	1 Fat

Calories 210
  Calories from Fat 65
Total Fat . . . . .7.0 g
  Saturated Fat . . . . .1.0 g
  Trans Fat . . . . .0.0 g
Cholesterol . . . . 0 mg
Sodium . . . . 120 mg
Potassium . . . . 590 mg
Total Carbohydrate . . . . . . 26 g
  Dietary Fiber . . . . 9 g
  Sugars . . . . 6 g
Protein . . . . 12 g
Phosphorus . . . . 200 mg

MyFoodAdvisor

This is an original recipe from the American Diabetes Association's online nutrition resource, **Recipes for Healthy Living**—your one-stop shop for diabetes-friendly recipes, meal plans, and other nutrition tips. Sign up today for the FREE *Recipes for Healthy Living* newsletter and to get access to the website by visiting **www.diabetes.org/recipes**.

Chicken Gyros

Makes: 5 servings   *Serving Size: 1 gyro*   *Prep Time: 15 minutes*

1/4 cup lemon juice
1 tsp dried oregano
1 pound boneless, skinless chicken breasts, thinly sliced into strips
   nonstick cooking spray
1/4 tsp salt (optional)
1/4 tsp ground black pepper
5 whole-wheat pocket pita halves
1 cup diced tomato

Sauce

1 cup fat-free plain yogurt
1 cup peeled, seeded, and grated cucumber
1 garlic clove, minced

1 In a medium bowl, combine lemon juice and oregano. Add chicken and marinate in the refrigerator for 15 minutes.

2 Remove the chicken from the marinade (reserve 1 Tbsp of the marinade).

3 Coat a large nonstick skillet with cooking spray and heat over medium-high heat. Add chicken strips and reserved marinade to pan and sauté for 4–5 minutes or until the chicken is done. Add salt and pepper.

4 In a medium bowl, combine all sauce ingredients.

5 Fill each pita with even amounts of chicken, tomatoes, and sauce.

Exchanges/Choices
1 Starch   1/2 Carbohydrate
3 Lean Meat

Calories	215
Calories from Fat	25
Total Fat	3.0 g
Saturated Fat	0.8 g
Trans Fat	0.0 g
Cholesterol	55 mg
Sodium	230 mg
Potassium	465 mg
Total Carbohydrate	22 g
Dietary Fiber	3 g
Sugars	5 g
Protein	25 g
Phosphorus	285 mg

Chef's Tip

You can grate the peeled cucumber using the large hole on your cheese grater, or pulse the cucumber in a blender or food processor for 30 seconds.

Fruit Salad GF

Makes: 4 servings   *Serving Size: 1 cup*   *Prep Time: 15 minutes*

1 cup cubed cantaloupe
1 cup sliced strawberries
1 cup green grapes
1 cup blueberries

Combine all ingredients and toss gently.

Exchanges/Choices
1 Fruit

Calories 75
  Calories from Fat 0
Total Fat . . . . .0.0 g
  Saturated Fat . . . . .0.1 g
  Trans Fat . . . . .0.0 g
Cholesterol. . . . . 0 mg
Sodium . . . . 10 mg
Potassium. . . . . 270 mg
Total Carbohydrate . . . . . . 19 g
  Dietary Fiber . . . . 2 g
  Sugars . . . . 15 g
Protein . . . . 1 g
Phosphorus . . . . 30 mg

Dietitian's Tip

Fruit is a sweet end to a great meal.

Spinach Lasagna

Makes: 10 servings   *Serving Size: 1 slice*   *Prep Time: 12 minutes*

nonstick cooking spray
1 egg
1 1/3 cups shredded part-skim mozzarella cheese, divided
1 15-ounce container fat-free ricotta cheese
1/4 cup freshly grated Parmesan cheese
1 10-ounce package frozen chopped spinach, thawed and drained
5 cups jarred low-sodium marinara pasta sauce
12 whole-wheat no-boil lasagna noodles

1 Preheat oven to 350°F. Coat a 13 × 9 × 2-inch glass baking dish with cooking spray.

2 In a medium bowl, mix together egg, 1 cup mozzarella, ricotta, and Parmesan cheese. Add spinach and mix well.

3 Spread 1 cup pasta sauce on bottom of baking dish. Arrange noodles side by side on top of sauce, overlapping slightly. Spread 1 cup spinach and cheese mixture on top of noodles.

4 Repeat layering with pasta sauce, noodles, and spinach and cheese mixture 3 more times.

5 Top with remaining 3 noodles and 1 cup sauce. Cover lasagna with foil and bake 25 minutes. Uncover; top with remaining 1/3 cup mozzarella cheese, and bake an additional 25–35 minutes or until cheese is light golden brown.

Exchanges/Choices

2 Starch   1 Lean Meat
1 Fat

Calories	245
Calories from Fat	70
Total Fat	8.0 g
Saturated Fat	2.5 g
Trans Fat	0.0 g
Cholesterol	45 mg
Sodium	475 mg
Potassium	555 mg
Total Carbohydrate	29 g
Dietary Fiber	5 g
Sugars	7 g
Protein	15 g
Phosphorus	275 mg

Chef's Tip

Using no-boil noodles really saves time in this recipe.

Beef Stroganoff

Makes: 5 servings   *Serving Size: 1/5 recipe*   *Prep Time: 15 minutes*

5	ounces uncooked Ronzoni Healthy Harvest Whole Grain egg noodles
2	tsp olive oil
1	pound boneless beef tenderloin tips, sliced into 2-inch strips
1 1/2	cups sliced mushrooms
1/2	cup minced onion
1	Tbsp all-purpose flour
1/2	cup dry white wine
1	tsp Dijon mustard
1	14.5-ounce can fat-free, low-sodium beef broth
1/2	cup fat-free sour cream
1/4	tsp salt (optional)
1/4	tsp ground black pepper

1 Cook noodles according to package directions, omitting salt.

2 Add oil to a large sauté pan over high heat. Add meat and sauté for about 3 minutes. Remove meat from pan. Add mushrooms and onion and sauté for 5 minutes or until beginning to brown.

3 Add flour and cook for 1 minute. Add wine to deglaze pan; cook for 2 minutes. Add Dijon mustard and beef broth; bring to a boil. Reduce heat and simmer for 5 minutes.

4 Add beef and any juices back to broth and simmer for 3 more minutes. Add sour cream, salt (optional), and pepper; simmer for 30 seconds.

5 Serve over whole-grain egg noodles.

Exchanges/Choices
2 Starch   2 Lean Meat
1/2 Fat

Calories	275
Calories from Fat	65
Total Fat	7.0 g
Saturated Fat	2.3 g
Trans Fat	0.0 g
Cholesterol	50 mg
Sodium	250 mg
Potassium	465 mg
Total Carbohydrate	29 g
Dietary Fiber	4 g
Sugars	3 g
Protein	23 g
Phosphorus	265 mg

Chef's Tip

Save prep time by buying presliced mushrooms.

White Chicken Chili

Makes: 7 servings   *Serving Size: 1 cup*   *Prep Time: 10 minutes*

nonstick cooking spray
1   pound boneless, skinless chicken breasts, cut into 1-inch cubes
1   medium onion, finely diced
2   medium carrots, finely diced
3   garlic cloves, minced
2   16-ounce cans Great Northern beans
1   cup fat-free, low-sodium chicken broth
1   4-ounce can mild green chilies, diced
1/2   tsp ground black pepper

1 Coat a large soup pot with cooking spray. Add chicken and cook over medium-high heat until lightly brown. Remove chicken from pan and set aside.

2 Spray pan again with cooking spray. Sauté onion and carrots about 4 minutes until onion turns clear.

3 Add all remaining ingredients and chicken and stir. Bring to a boil, reduce heat, and simmer 15 minutes.

Exchanges/Choices
1 Starch   1 Vegetable
2 Lean Meat

Calories	205
Calories from Fat	20
Total Fat	2.5 g
Saturated Fat	0.6 g
Trans Fat	0.0 g
Cholesterol	40 mg
Sodium	560 mg
Potassium	700 mg
Total Carbohydrate	21 g
Dietary Fiber	6 g
Sugars	4 g
Protein	21 g
Phosphorus	295 mg

Chef's Tip

Canned green chilies are an easy way to add great flavor to recipes.

MARCH
WEEK 3

DAY 1
Linguine with Red
    Clam Sauce   92

DAY 2
Tuna Melt   93

DAY 3
Turkey Divan with
    Broccoli   94
Irish Vegetables   95

DAY 4
Portobello Mushroom
    Pizza   96

DAY 5
Spinach and Pine Nut
    Stuffed Chicken   97
Rice Pilaf   98

GROCERY LIST

Fresh Produce
Basil—1 small bunch
Broccoli—2 heads
Cabbage—1 medium head
Carrots, large—4
Carrots, medium—1
Celery—2 stalks
Garlic—1 head
Lettuce—1 head
Mushrooms, portobello,
    large—4
Onions, yellow or white,
    medium—2

Meat, Poultry, & Fish
Chicken breasts, boneless,
    skinless, 4 ounces each—4
Turkey, ground, 93% lean—
    1/2 pound
Turkey breast, boneless,
    skinless—1 pound

Grains, Bread, & Pasta
English muffins, whole-wheat,
    halves—5
Linguine, whole-wheat—
    1 box (16 ounces)
Rice, brown—1 bag

Dairy & Cheese
Cheese, cheddar,
    75% reduced-fat,
    shredded—1 bag
Cheese, mozzarella, part-
    skim, shredded—3/4 cup
Cheese, Parmesan—1 small
    block
Milk, fat-free—2 cups

Canned Goods & Sauces
Broth, chicken, fat-free,
    low-sodium, 14.5-ounce
    cans—2
Clams, minced, with juice,
    6.5-ounce cans—3
Pasta sauce, low-sodium—
    1 1/2 cups
Tomato sauce—1 cup
Tomatoes, crushed, 28-ounce
    can—1
Tuna, packed in water,
    6-ounce cans—2

Frozen Foods
Spinach—1/2 cup

Staples, Seasonings, & Baking Needs
Bay leaf
Black pepper, ground
Flour, all-purpose
Mustard, Dijon
Nonstick cooking spray
Oil, olive
Onion powder
Paprika
Red pepper flakes
Salt
Thyme

Miscellaneous
Italian seasoning herb mix
Mayonnaise, light
Pine nuts—1/4 cup
Wine, white

Linguine with Red Clam Sauce

Makes: 8 servings   *Serving Size: 1 cup*   *Prep Time: 10 minutes*

16	ounces uncooked whole-wheat linguine
2	tsp olive oil
2	garlic cloves, minced
3	6.5-ounce cans minced clams with juice (drain one can only)
1/2	cup white wine
1	28-ounce can crushed tomatoes
1/4	tsp salt (optional)
1/4	tsp ground black pepper
1/4	tsp crushed red pepper flakes
1	cup tomato sauce
1	Tbsp chopped fresh basil

1 Cook pasta according to package directions, omitting salt. Drain.

2 Add oil to a large nonstick skillet over medium-high heat. Add garlic and sauté 30 seconds.

3 Add clams (with juice) and wine. Turn heat to high and cook for about 10 minutes or until liquid is reduced by half.

4 Add all remaining ingredients except basil and simmer 10 minutes. Remove from heat and add basil.

5 Serve sauce over linguine noodles.

Exchanges/Choices

2 1/2 Starch   2 Vegetable
1 Lean Meat

Calories	310
Calories from Fat	25
Total Fat	3.0 g
Saturated Fat	0.4 g
Trans Fat	0.0 g
Cholesterol	20 mg
Sodium	385 mg
Potassium	690 mg
Total Carbohydrate	52 g
Dietary Fiber	8 g
Sugars	7 g
Protein	19 g
Phosphorus	285 mg

Chef's Tip

A green leaf or spinach salad would be a great addition to this meal.

Tuna Melt

Makes: 5 servings   *Serving Size: 1 tuna melt*   *Prep Time: 5 minutes*

2   6-ounce cans tuna packed in water, drained
1/4   cup light mayonnaise
1/4   tsp ground black pepper
1/4   tsp onion powder
2   tsp Dijon mustard
5   whole-wheat English muffin halves
2/3   cup shredded 75% reduced-fat cheddar cheese

1 Preheat oven to 400°F. In a medium mixing bowl, combine tuna, mayonnaise, pepper, onion powder, and Dijon mustard.

2 Spread 1/4 cup tuna mixture on top of each muffin half and top with about 2 Tbsp cheese.

3 Place muffins on baking sheet and bake 10 minutes.

Exchanges/Choices
1 Starch   2 Lean Meat

Calories 185
    Calories from Fat 55
Total Fat . . . . 6.0 g
    Saturated Fat . . . . 1.4 g
    Trans Fat . . . . 0.0 g
Cholesterol . . . . 35 mg
Sodium . . . . 600 mg
Potassium . . . . 235 mg
Total Carbohydrate . . . . . . 16 g
    Dietary Fiber . . . . 2 g
    Sugars . . . . 4 g
Protein . . . . 20 g
Phosphorus . . . . 265 mg

Dietitian's Tip

A fruit salad would be a great side dish for this meal.

Turkey Divan with Broccoli

Makes: 6 servings   *Serving Size: 1/6 recipe*   *Prep Time: 15 minutes*

nonstick cooking spray
4   cups broccoli florets
1   pound boneless, skinless turkey breast, cubed
2   cups cooked brown rice
2   cups fat-free milk
1 1/2   Tbsp all-purpose flour
3/4   cup shredded reduced-fat cheddar cheese
1/2   tsp salt (optional)
1/4   tsp ground black pepper

1 Preheat oven to 350°F. Coat a 9 × 9-inch glass baking dish with cooking spray.

2 Steam broccoli florets until tender-crisp. In a large bowl, combine steamed broccoli, turkey breast, and rice. Spread into the prepared baking dish.

3 Whisk together milk and flour in a small bowl. In a medium saucepan, bring milk and flour mixture to a boil. Reduce heat and add cheese, salt, and pepper. Simmer for 1 minute or until all cheese is melted.

4 Pour cheese sauce over turkey, broccoli, and rice mixture and stir. Bake for 30 minutes or until turkey is done and sauce is bubbly.

Exchanges/Choices
1 Starch   1 Vegetable
3 Lean Meat

Calories 245
   Calories from Fat 40
Total Fat . . . . 4.5 g
   Saturated Fat . . . . 2.1 g
   Trans Fat . . . . 0.0 g
Cholesterol . . . . 55 mg
Sodium . . . . 205 mg
Potassium . . . . 545 mg
Total Carbohydrate . . . . . . 23 g
   Dietary Fiber . . . . 2 g
   Sugars . . . . 5 g
Protein . . . . 28 g
Phosphorus . . . . 410 mg

Chef's Tip

This is a great dish to serve if you have turkey left over from Thanksgiving.

Irish Vegetables

Makes: 4 servings　　　　*Serving Size: 1/4 recipe*　　　　*Prep Time: 10 minutes*

1	medium head cabbage, cut into 4 wedges
4	large carrots, peeled and cut into large chunks
1	medium onion, peeled and cut into eighths
1	14.5-ounce can fat-free, low-sodium chicken broth
3	cups water
3	garlic cloves, sliced in half
1/2	tsp salt (optional)
1/2	tsp ground black pepper

1 In a large soup pot, add all ingredients. Bring to a boil; reduce heat and simmer 35 minutes or until cabbage is tender.

2 Serve vegetables in a bowl with 1/4 cup of liquid served over them.

Exchanges/Choices
4 Vegetable

Calories	115
Calories from Fat	0
Total Fat	0.0 g
Saturated Fat	0.1 g
Trans Fat	0.0 g
Cholesterol	0 mg
Sodium	135 mg
Potassium	765 mg
Total Carbohydrate	25 g
Dietary Fiber	8 g
Sugars	13 g
Protein	5 g
Phosphorus	115 mg

Dietitian's Tip

These low-carb vegetables can be a great filler when cutting back on calories for weight loss.

Portobello Mushroom Pizza LC NEW

Makes: 4 servings　　　*Serving Size: 1 mushroom*　　　*Prep Time: 15 minutes*

4	large portobello mushrooms
1	Tbsp olive oil
	nonstick cooking spray
1/2	pound 93% lean ground turkey
1	Tbsp Italian seasoning herb mix (mixture of basil, oregano, parsley)
1	tsp crushed red pepper flakes
2	garlic cloves, minced
1/2	tsp ground black pepper
1 1/2	cups low-sodium jarred pasta sauce
3/4	cup shredded part-skim mozzarella cheese
12	lettuce leaves

1 Preheat oven to 375°F.

2 Prepare the mushrooms by cutting off the stem and scraping off the gills on the underside of the mushroom with a small spoon, keeping the mushroom intact. Place the prepared mushrooms scraped side up on a baking sheet and set aside.

3 Add olive oil and a generous amount of cooking spray to a large sauté pan over medium-high heat. Add turkey, Italian seasoning, crushed red pepper flakes, garlic, and black pepper and sauté until turkey is cooked through, about 7–9 minutes.

4 Add pasta sauce to the turkey mixture and sauté until heated through, about 2 minutes. Divide the turkey mixture evenly among the four mushrooms, top each with 3 Tbsp mozzarella cheese, and bake for 10–12 minutes.

5 On four plates, serve each filled mushroom on top of 3 lettuce leaves.

Exchanges/Choices

1/2 Starch	1 Vegetable
2 Med-Fat Meat	1/2 Fat

Calories	230
Calories from Fat	110
Total Fat	12.0 g
Saturated Fat	3.5 g
Trans Fat	0.1 g
Cholesterol	55 mg
Sodium	210 mg
Potassium	860 mg
Total Carbohydrate	13 g
Dietary Fiber	3 g
Sugars	8 g
Protein	21 g
Phosphorus	345 mg

Chef's Tip

If you don't have Italian seasoning herb mix, make your own with 1 tsp dried basil, 1 tsp dried oregano, and 1 tsp dried parsley.

▲.American Diabetes Association.
MyFoodAdvisor

This is an original recipe from the American Diabetes Association's online nutrition resource, **Recipes for Healthy Living**—your one-stop shop for diabetes-friendly recipes, meal plans, and other nutrition tips. Sign up today for the FREE *Recipes for Healthy Living* newsletter and to get access to the website by visiting **www.diabetes.org/recipes**.

Spinach and Pine Nut Stuffed Chicken GF LC

Makes: 4 servings   *Serving Size: 1 chicken breast*   *Prep Time: 15 minutes*

1/4   cup pine nuts
4   4-ounce boneless, skinless chicken breasts
1 1/2 Tbsp freshly grated Parmesan cheese
1/2   cup frozen spinach, thawed and drained
2   garlic cloves, minced
1/2   tsp salt (optional)
1/2   tsp ground black pepper
1   tsp paprika
       nonstick cooking spray

1 Preheat oven to 350°F.

2 In a small nonstick sauté pan, sauté pine nuts over medium-high heat for 2–3 minutes to toast. Set aside.

3 Place one chicken breast on a cutting board and cover with plastic wrap. Pound meat with a meat tenderizer or rolling pin until it is about 1/4 inch thick. Repeat this process for the other breasts. Set aside.

4 In a medium bowl, combine toasted pine nuts, Parmesan cheese, spinach, and garlic. Spread 3 Tbsp of this mixture on one side of the pounded chicken breast. Roll breast and secure the seam with a toothpick. Repeat procedure for remaining chicken breasts.

5 Sprinkle all sides of rolled chicken breasts with salt, pepper, and paprika.

6 Coat a glass or metal baking dish with cooking spray and place chicken in dish seam side down. Bake for 30 minutes or until chicken is done.

7 To serve, remove toothpicks and slice each piece into 5 rounds. Serve over Rice Pilaf (see recipe, page 98).

Exchanges/Choices
4 Lean Meat

Calories 200
    Calories from Fat 80
Total Fat . . . . .9.0 g
    Saturated Fat . . . . .1.5 g
    Trans Fat . . . . .0.0 g
Cholesterol. . . . . 65 mg
Sodium . . . . 100 mg
Potassium. . . . . 340 mg
Total Carbohydrate . . . . 3 g
    Dietary Fiber . . . . 1 g
    Sugars . . . . 1 g
Protein . . . . 27 g
Phosphorus . . . . 250 mg

Chef's Tip

For added flavor, bring 1 cup of balsamic vinegar to a boil and cook until it's reduced by half. Drizzle a little of the vinegar over each chicken breast after it has been sliced.

Rice Pilaf

Makes: 5 servings   *Serving Size: 2/3 cup*   *Prep Time: 10 minutes*

1	tsp olive oil
1	medium carrot, finely diced
2	medium celery stalks, finely diced
1	medium onion, finely diced
1	cup uncooked brown rice
3	cups fat-free, low-sodium chicken broth
1/2	tsp dried thyme
1	bay leaf
1/2	tsp salt (optional)
1/4	tsp ground black pepper

1 Add oil to a medium saucepan. Sauté carrots, celery, and onion over medium-high heat for about 3 minutes or until onions begin to turn clear.

2 Add rice to the mixture and stir constantly over heat for 2 minutes. Add remaining ingredients except salt and pepper and bring to a boil.

3 Reduce heat to low and simmer, covered. Cook for 10 minutes. Add salt and pepper and remove bay leaf. Fluff rice with a fork.

Exchanges/Choices

2 Starch   1 Vegetable

Calories	175
Calories from Fat	20
Total Fat	2.0 g
Saturated Fat	0.4 g
Trans Fat	0.0 g
Cholesterol	0 mg
Sodium	335 mg
Potassium	320 mg
Total Carbohydrate	34 g
Dietary Fiber	3 g
Sugars	3 g
Protein	5 g
Phosphorus	160 mg

Dietitian's Tip

If you are feeling adventurous, substitute quinoa for rice in this recipe. Quinoa is a healthy grain with protein.

MARCH

WEEK 4

GROCERY LIST

Fresh Produce
Carrot—1
Celery—1 head
Garlic—1 head
Lemon—2
Lettuce, iceberg—1 head
Lettuce, romaine—1 large head
Mushrooms—2 pints
Onions, yellow or white—2
Parsley—1 bunch
Potatoes, red, diced—3 cups
Rosemary—1 sprig
Tomatoes, large—2

Meat, Poultry, & Fish
Beef tenderloin steaks,
    4 ounces each—4
Chicken, whole, fryer,
    3 pounds—2
Chicken breast strips,
    precooked, flavored (lemon
    pepper or garlic herb),
    10-ounce package—1
Fish, white (such as cod)—
    1/2 pound
Mussels, live—1/2 pound
Shrimp, peeled and
    deveined—1 pound
Turkey bacon—4 slices

Grains, Bread, & Pasta
Baguette, whole-wheat—
    16 ounce
Farfalle pasta, whole-wheat—
    1 box
Tortillas, corn—10–12

Dairy & Cheese
Cheese, Asiago—1 wedge
Cheese, cheddar or Colby,
    75% reduced-fat, shredded—
    1 1/4 cups
Cheese, Parmesan—1 block
Egg
Egg substitute—1 cup
Half-and-half, fat-free—2 cups
Margarine, trans-fat-free
Milk, fat-free—1/2 cup
Sour cream, fat-free—1/2 cup

Canned Goods & Sauces
Broth, chicken, fat-free,
    low-sodium, 14.5-ounce
    cans—2
Green chilies, chopped,
    4-ounce cans—2
Mushroom stems and pieces,
    12- to 14-ounce can—1
Pasta sauce, marinara,
    reduced-sodium, 16-ounce
    jar—1
Salad dressing, bleu cheese,
    lite—1 bottle
Salad dressing, Italian, lite—
    1 bottle
Soup, cream of chicken,
    condensed, low-fat,
    10.75-ounce cans—2
Tomatoes, diced, no-salt-
    added, 15-ounce can—1

Staples, Seasonings, & Baking Needs
Baking powder
Basil
Black pepper, ground
Black peppercorns, whole
Cayenne pepper
Chili powder
Cumin
Flour, all-purpose
Nonstick cooking spray
Oil, olive
Paprika
Poppy seeds
Sage
Salt
Splenda Sugar Blend
Sugar, powdered
Thyme
Vanilla extract

Miscellaneous
Wine, white

Blackened Beef Tenderloin GF LC

Makes: 4 servings *Serving Size: 1 steak* *Prep Time: 5 minutes*

2	Tbsp paprika
1	tsp cayenne pepper
1	Tbsp chili powder
1	tsp cumin
1/2	tsp salt (optional)
1/2	tsp ground black pepper
4	4-ounce beef tenderloin steaks nonstick cooking spray

1 In a small bowl, combine first six ingredients and stir well.

2 Rub one side of each steak well with spice mixture.

3 Coat a large nonstick skillet with cooking spray. Over medium-high heat, place each steak spice side down and cook for 6 minutes on each side.

Exchanges/Choices
3 Lean Meat

Calories	160
Calories from Fat	65
Total Fat	7.0 g
Saturated Fat	2.3 g
Trans Fat	0.0 g
Cholesterol	60 mg
Sodium	65 mg
Potassium	395 mg
Total Carbohydrate	3 g
Dietary Fiber	2 g
Sugars	1 g
Protein	22 g
Phosphorus	185 mg

Chef's Tip

If you like your steaks less spicy, reduce the cayenne pepper to 1/2 tsp.

Savory Mushroom Bread Pudding

Makes: 9 servings *Serving Size: 1/3 cup* *Prep Time: 25 minutes*

nonstick cooking spray
2 tsp olive oil
4 cups chopped fresh mushrooms
2 garlic cloves, minced
1 tsp dried sage
1 tsp dried basil
1/2 tsp salt (optional)
1/4 tsp ground black pepper
1 cup egg substitute
1 egg
1/2 cup fat-free milk
2 cups fat-free half-and-half
1/3 cup grated Asiago cheese
1 16-ounce whole-wheat baguette or hearty whole-grain bread, cubed
2 Tbsp freshly grated Asiago cheese

1 Preheat oven to 350°F. Generously coat an 8 × 8-inch baking dish with cooking spray. Set aside.

2 In a large nonstick sauté pan, heat oil over medium-high heat. Add mushrooms and garlic. Sauté until all liquid evaporates and mushrooms begin to brown. Remove from heat.

3 Add dried herbs, salt, and pepper and mix well; set aside to cool.

4 In a medium bowl, whisk egg substitute and egg together. Add milk, half-and-half, and 1/3 cup grated cheese and whisk well. Add bread to egg mixture and stir to coat well. Let sit for 5 minutes.

5 Fold mushroom mixture into bread mixture. Pour into prepared pan. Sprinkle with 2 Tbsp grated cheese. Bake for 45 minutes or until pudding is brown and puffed.

Exchanges/Choices
1 1/2 Starch   1/2 Fat-Free Milk
1 Med-Fat Meat

Calories	230
Calories from Fat	55
Total Fat	6.0 g
Saturated Fat	2.4 g
Trans Fat	0.0 g
Cholesterol	30 mg
Sodium	385 mg
Potassium	400 mg
Total Carbohydrate	29 g
Dietary Fiber	4 g
Sugars	7 g
Protein	14 g
Phosphorus	290 mg

Chef's Tip

Just a touch of Asiago cheese adds great flavor to this bread pudding.

Chicken Cacciatore LC

Makes: 6 servings   *Serving Size: 1/6 recipe*   *Prep Time: 15 minutes*

1   3-pound fryer chicken, cut into 8 pieces
      nonstick cooking spray
1   16-ounce jar reduced-sodium marinara pasta sauce
1   cup sliced mushrooms
2   garlic cloves, minced
1/4 cup freshly grated Parmesan cheese

1 Preheat oven to 350°F.

2 Remove skin from chicken and trim any excess fat.

3 Coat a 9-inch glass baking dish with cooking spray and place chicken in bottom of dish.

4 In a medium bowl, combine pasta sauce, mushrooms, and garlic. Pour sauce over chicken. Sprinkle chicken with Parmesan cheese.

5 Bake for 35 minutes.

Go to www.diabetes.org to find out more about the American Diabetes Association Alert Day, a one-day call to action held on the fourth Tuesday of March for people to find out if they are at risk for diabetes. Go ahead—take the Risk Test!

Exchanges/Choices
1/2 Starch   3 Lean Meat
1/2 Fat

Calories	210
Calories from Fat	80
Total Fat	9.0 g
Saturated Fat	2.0 g
Trans Fat	0.0 g
Cholesterol	70 mg
Sodium	260 mg
Potassium	475 mg
Total Carbohydrate	7 g
Dietary Fiber	1 g
Sugars	3 g
Protein	25 g
Phosphorus	195 mg

Chef's Tip
If you can't find a cut-up fryer in the meat department racks, the butcher will cut one up for you.

Enchilada Casserole

Makes: 12 servings   *Serving Size: 1 slice*   *Prep Time: 35 minutes*

Broth

- **1/2** cup chopped onion
- **1/2** cup chopped celery
- **6** whole black peppercorns
- **1** rosemary sprig
- **1** 3-pound whole chicken

Casserole

- nonstick cooking spray
- **1** large onion, chopped
- **2** 10.75-ounce cans low-fat condensed cream of chicken soup
- **2** 4-ounce cans chopped green chilies
- **1** 15-ounce can no-salt-added diced tomatoes, drained
- **1** 12- to 14-ounce can mushroom stems and pieces, undrained
- **10–12** corn tortillas, cut into eighths
- **1 1/4** cups shredded 75% reduced-fat cheddar or Colby cheese

1 Preheat oven to 350°F. Fill a large soup pot 2/3 full with water. Add onion, celery, peppercorns, and rosemary. Remove neck and giblet bag from cavity of chicken. Rinse chicken and place in the soup pot and cook over high heat until boiling. Reduce heat and simmer 30 minutes or until chicken is done.

2 Remove chicken and strain broth through colander. Remove fat from broth. Reserve 1 3/4 cups for use in this recipe. Save remaining broth for another use. Remove skin from chicken and pull meat from bones into chunks.

3 Coat a medium nonstick skillet with cooking spray over medium-high heat. Sauté remaining onion until slightly brown.

4 In large bowl, combine chicken, reserved broth, soup, sautéed onion, green chilies, tomatoes, and mushrooms. Mix well.

5 Coat an extra-large casserole dish (at least 10 × 15) with cooking spray. Cover bottom of casserole with half of the tortillas. Spoon half of chicken mixture over the tortillas and top with half of the cheese. Repeat process, ending with cheese. Bake for 45 minutes.

Exchanges/Choices

1 Starch	1 Vegetable
2 Lean Meat	1 Fat

Calories 235
  Calories from Fat 70
Total Fat . . . . .8.0 g
  Saturated Fat . . . . .2.6 g
  Trans Fat . . . . .0.0 g
Cholesterol. . . . . 45 mg
Sodium . . . . 595 mg
Potassium. . . . . 380 mg
Total Carbohydrate . . . . . . 20 g
  Dietary Fiber . . . . 3 g
  Sugars . . . . 3 g
Protein . . . . 21 g
Phosphorus . . . . 265 mg

Chef's Tip

Serve this satisfying dish with salsa, fat-free sour cream, and black olives as garnishes.

Tossed Salad with Chicken and Pasta

Makes: 4 servings   *Serving Size: 1/4 recipe*   *Prep Time: 10 minutes*

2 1/2   cups cooked whole-wheat
        farfalle pasta
    6   cups shredded romaine lettuce
    1   large tomato, seeded and diced
    1   10-ounce package precooked,
        flavored chicken breast strips
        (try lemon pepper or garlic
        herb)
  1/4   cup light Italian dressing

In a large salad bowl, toss together all ingredients.

Exchanges/Choices

1 1/2 Starch   1 Vegetable
1 Lean Meat

Calories 195
  Calories from Fat 35
Total Fat . . . . .4.0 g
  Saturated Fat . . . . .0.8 g
  Trans Fat . . . . .0.0 g
Cholesterol. . . . . 35 mg
Sodium . . . . 415 mg
Potassium. . . . . 455 mg
Total Carbohydrate . . . . . . 26 g
  Dietary Fiber . . . . 4 g
  Sugars . . . . 3 g
Protein . . . . 17 g
Phosphorus . . . . 220 mg

Chef's Tip

Precooked chicken breast strips are near the packaged lunchmeats at most grocery stores. This product is higher in sodium than plain chicken breasts, though.

Seafood Stew

Makes: 6 servings   *Serving Size: 1 1/2 cups*   *Prep Time: 25 minutes*

1   Tbsp olive oil
1   cup diced carrot
1   cup diced celery
1   cup diced onion
2   garlic cloves, minced
3   cups unpeeled diced red potatoes
1/2 cup white wine
2   14.5-ounce cans fat-free, low-sodium chicken broth

1   tsp dried thyme
2   Tbsp chopped fresh parsley
1/2 tsp salt (optional)
1/2 tsp ground black pepper
1/2 pound live mussels, cleaned (see Chef's Tip)
1/2 pound peeled and deveined shrimp
1/2 pound white fish (such as cod), cubed

1   Add oil to a large soup pot over medium-high heat. Add carrots, celery, onion, and garlic and sauté until onion turns clear.

2   Add potatoes and sauté for 2 more minutes. Add wine and cook until liquid is reduced by half.

3   Add chicken broth, thyme, parsley, salt, and pepper; bring to a boil.

4   Reduce heat to a simmer for 20 minutes or until potatoes are soft. Add mussels, shrimp, and fish; simmer for 5 minutes or until shrimp is done and mussels have opened.

Exchanges/Choices

1 1/2 Starch   1 Vegetable
2 Lean Meat

Calories	235
Calories from Fat	35
Total Fat	4.0 g
Saturated Fat	0.8 g
Trans Fat	0.0 g
Cholesterol	80 mg
Sodium	410 mg
Potassium	800 mg
Total Carbohydrate	27 g
Dietary Fiber	3 g
Sugars	5 g
Protein	21 g
Phosphorus	290 mg

Chef's Tip

Live mussels in the shell should be closed when you purchase them at the store. Wash them under cold water and remove the beard (the stringy substance) attached to the shell. Discard any open mussels. The mussels will open when they are cooked.

Wedge Salad LC NEW

Makes: 4 servings   *Serving Size: 1/4 recipe*   *Prep Time: 5 minutes*

1 head iceberg lettuce, quartered
1 large tomato, quartered
4 slices turkey bacon, cooked crisp and chopped
1/4 cup light bleu cheese dressing

1 Place 1/4 of iceberg lettuce, 1/4 tomato, and 1/4 chopped turkey bacon on a salad plate.

2 Drizzle 1 Tbsp of bleu cheese dressing over the top.

3 Repeat for remaining quarters.

National Doctor's Day is March 30 every year— thank your doctor for helping you feel better!

Exchanges/Choices

1 Vegetable	1 Fat

Calories	95
Calories from Fat	55
Total Fat	6.0 g
Saturated Fat	1.2 g
Trans Fat	0.0 g
Cholesterol	10 mg
Sodium	345 mg
Potassium	365 mg
Total Carbohydrate	8 g
Dietary Fiber	2 g
Sugars	4 g
Protein	4 g
Phosphorus	130 mg

Dietitian's Tip

Remember, half your plate should be filled with low-carb veggies, such as lettuce, tomatoes, broccoli, spinach, and cauliflower. These foods can help fill you up without raising your blood glucose too much.

Lemon Poppy Seed Bundt Cake

Makes: 16 servings   *Serving Size: 1 slice*   *Prep Time: 25 minutes*

Cake

	nonstick cooking spray
2	cups all-purpose flour
1 1/2	tsp baking powder
1/4	tsp salt (optional)
1/2	cups + 8 tsp Splenda Sugar Blend
1/2	cup trans-fat-free margarine, softened
2	eggs
1	egg white
1 1/2	tsp vanilla extract
1	Tbsp lemon rind
1	Tbsp lemon juice
1/2	cup fat-free sour cream
1/4	cup poppy seeds

Glaze

1/2	cup powdered sugar
1	Tbsp lemon juice
1	tsp water

1 Preheat oven to 325°F. Coat a Bundt pan with cooking spray. In a medium bowl, sift together flour, baking powder, and salt. Set aside.

2 In a large bowl, beat sugar and margarine with an electric mixer at medium speed until well blended. Add eggs and egg white, one at a time. Beat well. Add vanilla, lemon rind, and lemon juice; beat 30 seconds.

3 Add part of flour mixture to sugar mixture and beat. Add part of sour cream to sugar mixture and beat. Continue alternating between adding flour and sour cream to sugar mixture. Beat at low speed until well blended.

4 Stir in poppy seeds. Spoon batter into Bundt pan and bake for 35 minutes or until a toothpick inserted in center comes out clean. Let cool.

5 In a small bowl, whisk together powdered sugar, lemon juice, and water until glaze consistency is formed. Drizzle glaze over cooled cake.

Exchanges/Choices

2 Carbohydrate	1 Fat

Calories	175
Calories from Fat	55
Total Fat	6.0 g
Saturated Fat	1.6 g
Trans Fat	0.0 g
Cholesterol	25 mg
Sodium	100 mg
Potassium	60 mg
Total Carbohydrate	26 g
Dietary Fiber	1 g
Sugars	12 g
Protein	3 g
Phosphorus	100 mg

Chef's Tip

Make sure this cake is completely cool before you drizzle the glaze over it; otherwise, the glaze will melt into the cake.

APRIL

Spring into Health

Get some physical activity and enjoy the spring weather with a great bike ride. Tour de Cure® is the American Diabetes Association's signature cycling fundraising event, taking place in more than 44 states nationwide. Ride a tour route that is breezy and easy or challenging and tough. If it's 10 miles or 100—you decide! Call 1-800-DIABETES for more info.

Chicken Fajita Pizza (page 150)

You could also make this delicious pizza with beef or pork strips. The bell pepper adds a festive touch.

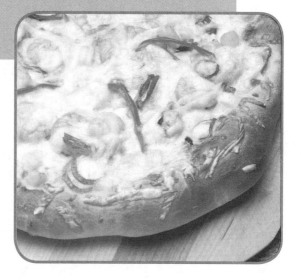

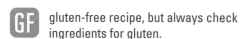 **GF** gluten-free recipe, but always check ingredients for gluten.

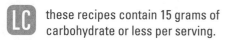 **LC** these recipes contain 15 grams of carbohydrate or less per serving.

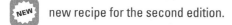 **NEW** new recipe for the second edition.

APRIL RECIPES

APRIL
WEEK 1

GROCERY LIST

Fresh Produce
Asparagus—2 bunches
Bell pepper, green—1
Bell peppers, red—2
Broccoli—3 heads
Carrots, large—2
Eggplant, medium—1
Garlic—1 head
Mushrooms, button—1 quart
Onion, yellow or white—1
Orange—1 large
Rosemary—1 bunch
Scallions—1 bunch
Shallot, small—1
Squash, yellow, small—1
Zucchini, small—3

Meat, Poultry, & Fish
Chicken breasts, boneless,
   skinless, 4 ounces each—4
Tuna steaks, 4 ounces each—4
Veal rib chops, bone in, 6
   ounces each—4

Grains, Bread, & Pasta
Rice, brown—1 box or small
   bag
Tortellini, cheese, whole-
   wheat, 9-ounce
   package—1

Canned Goods & Sauces
Broth, chicken, fat-free,
   low-sodium, 14.5-ounce
   cans—3
Soy sauce, lite

Staples, Seasonings, & Baking Needs
Black pepper, ground
Cornstarch
Flour, all-purpose
Garlic salt
Honey
Nonstick cooking spray
Oil, olive
Oil, sesame
Red pepper flakes
Salt
Sesame seeds
Splenda Brown Sugar Blend
Vinegar, apple cider
Vinegar, red wine

Miscellaneous
Juice, orange—1 1/2 cups
Tofu, extra-firm, 12-ounce
   packages—2

Broccoli Tofu Stir-Fry

Makes: 4 servings   *Serving Size: 2 cups*   *Prep Time: 10 minutes*

- **2** 12-ounce packages extra-firm tofu, drained and cut into 1-inch squares
- **2** tsp olive oil, divided
- **2** tsp sesame oil, divided
- **2** Tbsp lite soy sauce
- **4** cups broccoli florets
- **2** tsp cornstarch
- **3** cups fat-free, low-sodium chicken broth
- **3** tsp sesame seeds, toasted
- **1/4** tsp crushed red pepper flakes
- **1/2** tsp ground black pepper
- **2 2/3** cups cooked brown rice

1 Sauté tofu in 1 tsp olive oil and 1 tsp sesame oil in a wok or large sauté pan until golden brown on all sides. Add soy sauce and sauté for 1 more minute.

2 Remove tofu from pan and add remaining olive and sesame oil; sauté broccoli until tender-crisp.

3 In a small bowl, whisk together cornstarch and chicken broth.

4 Return tofu to the pan and add broth and the remaining ingredients except rice.

5 Simmer for 5–10 minutes or until sauce begins to thicken. Serve over white or brown rice.

April is National Soy Foods Month.

Exchanges/Choices
2 Starch   1 Vegetable
2 Med-Fat Meat

Calories 335
  Calories from Fat 90
Total Fat . . . . .10.0 g
  Saturated Fat . . . . .1.7 g
  Trans Fat . . . . .0.0 g
Cholesterol . . . . 5 mg
Sodium . . . . 470 mg
Potassium . . . . 710 mg
Total Carbohydrate . . . . . . 40 g
  Dietary Fiber . . . . 5 g
  Sugars . . . . 4 g
Protein . . . . 21 g
Phosphorus . . . . 365 mg

Chef's Tip

If you've never tried tofu, this is a great first recipe. The keys are to make sure the tofu isn't too thick and to cook it until golden brown, so the texture is just right.

Orange Chicken

Makes: 4 servings   *Serving Size: 1 chicken breast*   *Prep Time: 10 minutes*

nonstick cooking spray

4   4-ounce boneless, skinless chicken breasts

1   Tbsp Splenda Brown Sugar Blend

1/4   cup water

2   Tbsp apple cider vinegar

1 1/2   cups fresh orange juice

2   Tbsp grated orange peel

2   Tbsp shallots, minced (1 small shallot)

1 1/2   cups fat-free, low-sodium chicken broth

1 Preheat oven to 350°F.

2 Coat a shallow baking dish with cooking spray. Arrange chicken breasts in the bottom of the pan and bake for 30 minutes.

3 In a medium saucepan, mix Splenda Brown Sugar Blend and water over medium heat until sugar dissolves. Bring to a boil and boil until syrup begins to reduce, about 6 minutes. Whisk in vinegar, orange juice, orange peel, and shallots. Boil until reduced by half, about 15 minutes.

4 Add broth and boil another 20–25 minutes until reduced to about 1 cup liquid. Pour 1/4 cup sauce over each breast.

Exchanges/Choices

1 Fruit   3 Lean Meat

Calories 195
  Calories from Fat 25
Total Fat . . . . 3.0 g
  Saturated Fat . . . . 0.9 g
  Trans Fat . . . . 0.0 g
Cholesterol . . . . 65 mg
Sodium . . . . 95 mg
Potassium . . . . 490 mg
Total Carbohydrate . . . . . . 15 g
  Dietary Fiber . . . . 1 g
  Sugars . . . . 10 g
Protein . . . . 26 g
Phosphorus . . . . 210 mg

Chef's Tip

Be sure when you grate the orange peel not to include any of the white part (pith) of the peel, which is bitter.

Roasted Vegetables

Makes: 8 servings   *Serving Size: 1/8 of recipe*   *Prep Time: 25 minutes*

	nonstick cooking spray
1	medium eggplant, peeled and medium dice
2	zucchini, medium dice
2	large carrots, peeled and medium dice
1	onion, peeled and cut into eighths
1	red bell pepper, medium dice
1	bunch asparagus, trimmed and cut into 1-inch pieces
1	quart button mushrooms, stemmed and halved
1	Tbsp sesame oil
2	Tbsp minced garlic
2	Tbsp lite soy sauce
1/4	tsp ground black pepper

1 Preheat oven to 400°F. Coat two baking sheets with cooking spray.

2 Toss all ingredients in a large bowl, and arrange in a single layer on both pans.

3 Bake for 30 minutes or until vegetables are tender and golden brown.

Exchanges/Choices
3 Vegetable   1/2 Fat

Calories 90
 Calories from Fat 20
Total Fat . . . . .2.5 g
 Saturated Fat . . . . .0.4 g
 Trans Fat . . . . .0.0 g
Cholesterol. . . . . 0 mg
Sodium . . . . 160 mg
Potassium. . . . . 560 mg
Total Carbohydrate . . . . . . 16 g
 Dietary Fiber . . . . 5 g
 Sugars . . . . 7 g
Protein . . . . 4 g
Phosphorus . . . . 110 mg

Chef's Tip

If you want to change the flavor of this recipe, you can use olive oil instead of sesame oil and rosemary instead of soy sauce.

Tortellini Primavera

Makes: 7 servings   *Serving Size: 1 cup*   *Prep Time: 15 minutes*

1   9-ounce package whole-wheat cheese tortellini
      nonstick cooking spray

1 2/3 Tbsp olive oil, divided

2   cups broccoli florets

1   medium green bell pepper, thinly sliced

1   medium red bell pepper, thinly sliced

1   small zucchini, thinly sliced

1   small yellow squash, thinly sliced

1   tsp garlic salt (optional)

1 Cook tortellini according to package directions. Drain.

2 Coat a large nonstick skillet with cooking spray. Add 1 Tbsp olive oil and heat over medium-high heat. Add broccoli, green pepper, red pepper, zucchini, and squash and sauté for 5–7 minutes or until peppers begin to soften.

3 Add cooked tortellini to skillet and sauté another 2 minutes. Drizzle 2 tsp olive oil over entire mixture and sprinkle with garlic salt. Toss well to coat.

Exchanges/Choices

1 Starch   1 Vegetable
1 Fat

Calories 165	
Calories from Fat 65	
Total Fat . . . . 7.0 g	
Saturated Fat . . . . 1.5 g	
Trans Fat . . . . 0.0 g	
Cholesterol . . . . 20 mg	
Sodium . . . . 180 mg	
Potassium . . . . 270 mg	
Total Carbohydrate . . . . . . 20 g	
Dietary Fiber . . . . 4 g	
Sugars . . . . 3 g	
Protein . . . . 7 g	
Phosphorus . . . . 115 mg	

Dietitian's Tip

You can really lower your carb intake by adding a lot of veggies to pasta dishes.

Marinated Veal Chops GF LC

Makes: 4 servings   *Serving Size: 1 veal chop*   *Prep Time: 25 minutes*

2	Tbsp olive oil
2	Tbsp red wine vinegar
1 1/2	Tbsp chopped fresh rosemary (or 2 tsp dried rosemary)
2	large garlic cloves, minced
1/2	tsp salt (optional)
1/4	tsp ground black pepper
4	6-ounce bone-in veal rib chops

1 Prepare an indoor or outdoor grill.

2 In a medium bowl, whisk together all ingredients except chops. Place chops in shallow baking dish and pour marinade over chops.

3 Marinate for 20 minutes in the refrigerator.

4 Grill chops over medium-high heat, about 5–6 minutes per side.

Exchanges/Choices

3 Lean Meat   1 1/2 Fat

Calories	200
Calories from Fat	110
Total Fat	12.0 g
Saturated Fat	2.5 g
Trans Fat	0.0 g
Cholesterol	90 mg
Sodium	60 mg
Potassium	210 mg
Total Carbohydrate	1 g
Dietary Fiber	0 g
Sugars	0 g
Protein	21 g
Phosphorus	135 mg

Chef's Tip

Rosemary is the signature flavor in this dish, but you can use any other herb if you prefer.

Asparagus with Scallions GF LC

Makes: 4 servings   *Serving Size: 5–6 spears*   *Prep Time: 5 minutes*

1	bunch asparagus (about 22 spears), ends trimmed
2	tsp olive oil
	nonstick cooking spray
2	garlic cloves, minced
3	scallions, chopped
1/4	tsp salt (optional)

1 Steam asparagus until tender-crisp.

2 Add oil and a generous amount of cooking spray to a large nonstick skillet over medium-high heat. Add garlic and scallions and sauté for 30 seconds.

3 Add asparagus and sauté 3 more minutes. Season with salt and serve hot.

Exchanges/Choices

1 Vegetable	1/2 Fat

Calories	45
Calories from Fat	20
Total Fat	2.5 g
Saturated Fat	0.4 g
Trans Fat	0.0 g
Cholesterol	0 mg
Sodium	15 mg
Potassium	220 mg
Total Carbohydrate	5 g
Dietary Fiber	2 g
Sugars	1 g
Protein	2 g
Phosphorus	50 mg

Dietitian's Tip

Asparagus is a great source of folic acid.

Tuna Steaks GF LC

Makes: 4 servings *Serving Size: 1 tuna steak* *Prep Time: 10 minutes*

nonstick cooking spray
4 4-ounce tuna steaks
1/2 tsp salt (optional)
1/4 tsp ground black pepper
4 garlic cloves, minced
2 Tbsp honey
1 tsp olive oil

1 Preheat oven to 350°F.

2 Coat a shallow baking dish with cooking spray. Season tuna steaks on both sides with salt (optional) and pepper. Set aside.

3 In blender, purée garlic, honey, and olive oil until smooth. Place tuna steaks in baking dish and brush garlic purée on top of each steak, coating generously. Bake for 20 minutes.

Exchanges/Choices
1/2 Carbohydrate
4 Lean Meat

Calories	205
Calories from Fat	55
Total Fat	6.0 g
Saturated Fat	1.5 g
Trans Fat	0.0 g
Cholesterol	40 mg
Sodium	45 mg
Potassium	295 mg
Total Carbohydrate	10 g
Dietary Fiber	0 g
Sugars	9 g
Protein	26 g
Phosphorus	280 mg

Dietitian's Tip

Are you eating two servings of fish per week? If not, try this recipe for starters. The American Heart Association recommends two servings of fish per week, preferably a fatty fish such as tuna or salmon.

DAY 1
Chicken and Vegetables
with Cashews   120

DAY 2
Herb-Rubbed Pork
Tenderloin   121
Basil Mashed Potatoes
122

DAY 3
Pasta Spinach
Carbonara   123

DAY 4
Grilled Chimichurri
Salmon   124
Cauliflower Florets
with Lemon Mustard
Butter   125

DAY 5
Turkey Salad   126

GROCERY LIST

Fresh Produce
Basil—1 bunch
Broccoli—1 large head
Carrots, medium—2
Cauliflower—1 large head
Celery—1 head
Garlic—1 head
Lemon—1
Onion, yellow or white—1
Oregano—1 bunch
Parsley, Italian (flat leaf)—
    1 bunch
Pea pods—2 cups
Potatoes, Idaho, medium—4
Scallions—1 bunch

Meat, Poultry, & Fish
Chicken breasts, boneless,
    skinless—1 pound
Pork tenderloin—1 pound
Salmon fillets, skinless,
    4 ounces each—4
Turkey bacon—7 slices
Turkey breast—12 ounces

Grains, Bread, & Pasta
Farfalle pasta, whole-
    wheat—8 ounces
Sandwich thins, whole-wheat
    (100 calories, 5 grams
    fiber, 22 grams carb)—6

Dairy & Cheese
Cheese, Parmesan—1 small
    block
Margarine, trans-fat-free
Milk, fat-free—1 cup
Yogurt, plain, fat-free—
    1/2 cup

Canned Goods & Sauces
Broth, chicken, fat-free,
    low-sodium, 14.5-ounce
    can—1
Soy sauce, lite

Frozen Foods
Spinach, 10-ounce
    package—1

Staples, Seasonings, & Baking Needs
Black pepper, ground
Cornstarch
Mayonnaise, light
Mustard, Dijon
Nonstick cooking spray
Oil, olive
Oil, sesame
Red pepper flakes
Salt
Tarragon
Vinegar, red wine

Miscellaneous
Brandy
Cashews—1/4 cup
Tofu, firm, silken—6 ounces

Chicken and Vegetables with Cashews LC

Makes: 6 servings   *Serving Size: 1 cup*   *Prep Time: 10 minutes*

1	14.5-ounce can fat-free, low-sodium chicken broth
4	cups water
1	pound boneless, skinless chicken breasts
2	tsp sesame oil
	nonstick cooking spray
2	medium carrots, sliced into thin sticks
2	medium celery stalks, chopped
2	cups pea pods
3	cups broccoli florets
1/4	cup cashews
2	Tbsp cold water
1	Tbsp cornstarch
1	Tbsp lite soy sauce
1/4	tsp crushed red pepper flakes
1/2	tsp salt (optional)

1 In a large soup pot, bring broth and water to a boil. Reduce to a low simmer and add chicken breast. Simmer the chicken breast for 20 minutes. Remove from liquid and reserve 1 cup of the broth.

2 Using a fork, shred the chicken meat and set aside.

3 Add sesame oil and a generous amount of cooking spray to a large nonstick skillet or wok over medium-high heat. Add carrots, celery, pea pods, and broccoli, and stir-fry 3–4 minutes. Add cashews and chicken to skillet.

4 In a small bowl, whisk together cold water, cornstarch, soy sauce, crushed red pepper, and salt (optional). Whisk in reserved chicken broth. Pour liquid over vegetables and chicken. Bring to a boil and reduce heat to simmer for 2 minutes.

5 Serve over rice or by itself.

Exchanges/Choices
2 Vegetable   2 Lean Meat
1/2 Fat

Calories	175
Calories from Fat	55
Total Fat	6.0 g
Saturated Fat	1.3 g
Trans Fat	0.0 g
Cholesterol	45 mg
Sodium	380 mg
Potassium	495 mg
Total Carbohydrate	10 g
Dietary Fiber	3 g
Sugars	3 g
Protein	20 g
Phosphorus	205 mg

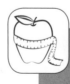

Dietitian's Tip

You should be eating 3–5 servings of vegetables each day. One serving is 1/2 cup cooked or 1 cup raw vegetables.

Herb-Rubbed Pork Tenderloin GF LC

Makes: 4 servings   *Serving Size: 3–4 ounces*   *Prep Time: 5 minutes*

2   Tbsp olive oil
2   Tbsp brandy or apple cider vinegar
1   Tbsp tarragon, dried
2   garlic cloves, minced
1   pound pork tenderloin
1/2 tsp salt (optional)
1/4 tsp ground black pepper

1 Preheat oven to 350°F.

2 In a small bowl, whisk together olive oil, brandy (or vinegar), tarragon, and garlic. Season pork tenderloin with salt (optional) and pepper on all sides.

3 Place tenderloin in a shallow baking dish. Pour sauce over tenderloin and turn several times to coat. Bake for 25–30 minutes or until done.

Exchanges/Choices
3 Lean Meat   1 Fat

Calories 190
  Calories from Fat 90
Total Fat . . . . .10.0 g
  Saturated Fat . . . . .1.9 g
  Trans Fat . . . . .0.0 g
Cholesterol. . . . . 60 mg
Sodium . . . . 40 mg
Potassium. . . . . 370 mg
Total Carbohydrate . . . . 1 g
  Dietary Fiber . . . . 0 g
  Sugars . . . . 0 g
Protein . . . . 22 g
Phosphorus . . . . 200 mg

Chef's Tip

Brandy or cider vinegars are classic flavors used with pork. Try them in marinades or sauces for instant hits!

Basil Mashed Potatoes GF

Makes: 6 servings   *Serving Size: 1/6 recipe*   *Prep Time: 10 minutes*

4 medium Idaho potatoes, peeled and cut into chunks
1 cup fat-free milk, heated
1/4 cup freshly grated Parmesan cheese
2 tsp olive oil
3 garlic cloves, peeled and sliced
1/2 tsp salt (optional)
1/4 tsp ground black pepper
1 cup basil leaves

1 Add potatoes to a large soup pot and cover with cold water. Bring to a boil and cook for 20 minutes or until potatoes are soft. Drain and return to the pot.

2 Pour fat-free milk over the potatoes and beat with an electric mixer on high until smooth (about 5 minutes).

3 Add remaining ingredients to a blender and purée until smooth. Fold basil mixture into potatoes.

Exchanges/Choices
1 1/2 Starch

Calories 120
 Calories from Fat 20
Total Fat . . . . 2.5 g
 Saturated Fat . . . . 0.8 g
 Trans Fat . . . . 0.0 g
Cholesterol . . . . 5 mg
Sodium . . . . 70 mg
Potassium . . . . 395 mg
Total Carbohydrate . . . . . . 20 g
 Dietary Fiber . . . . 2 g
 Sugars . . . . 3 g
Protein . . . . 4 g
Phosphorus . . . . 105 mg

Dietitian's Tip

If you want to decrease your carb intake further, try making this recipe with cauliflower instead of potatoes. You may be pleasantly surprised to find this low-carb substitute for potatoes.

Pasta Spinach Carbonara

Makes: 5 servings   *Serving Size: 1 cup*   *Prep Time: 15 minutes*

8	ounces uncooked whole-wheat farfalle pasta
6	ounces silken firm tofu
1/4	cup freshly grated Parmesan cheese
1/4	tsp ground black pepper
2	tsp olive oil
1	10-ounce package frozen spinach, thawed and drained
2	garlic cloves, minced
7	slices turkey bacon, cooked and chopped

1 Cook pasta according to package directions, omitting salt. Drain.

2 Combine tofu, Parmesan cheese, and pepper in a blender or food processor and process until smooth. Set aside.

3 Add oil to a large nonstick skillet over medium-high heat. Add spinach and cook 3 minutes. Add garlic and turkey bacon and cook 30 seconds.

4 Pour the tofu mixture in with the spinach and cook 1–2 minutes. Pour the tofu mixture over cooked pasta and toss to coat.

Exchanges/Choices

2 1/2 Starch
1 Med-Fat Meat

Calories	270
Calories from Fat	70
Total Fat	8.0 g
Saturated Fat	2.1 g
Trans Fat	0.0 g
Cholesterol	15 mg
Sodium	370 mg
Potassium	350 mg
Total Carbohydrate	38 g
Dietary Fiber	5 g
Sugars	2 g
Protein	15 g
Phosphorus	250 mg

Chef's Tip

Tofu can be used in many recipes to make a cream sauce or to provide a creamy texture—and it provides a little extra protein for those meatless dishes. Most people would be surprised to know this recipe contains tofu.

Grilled Chimichurri Salmon GF LC (NEW)

Makes: 4 servings   Serving Size: 1 salmon fillet and 2 Tbsp chimichurri   Prep Time: 15 minutes

Chimichurri

1	cup Italian (flat leaf) parsley
4	garlic cloves
2	Tbsp fresh oregano
1	Tbsp olive oil
1	Tbsp red wine vinegar
1/4	tsp ground black pepper
1/4	tsp crushed red pepper flakes

Salmon

4	4-ounce salmon fillets (skinless)
1	tsp salt (optional)
1/2	tsp ground black pepper nonstick cooking spray

1 Prepare an indoor or outdoor grill.

2 Add all chimichurri ingredients to blender or food processor and pulse until blended. Set aside.

3 Season both sides of the salmon fillets with salt (optional) and pepper. Spray both sides of the salmon with cooking spray and place on the indoor or outdoor grill. Grill for about 5–7 minutes on each side or until salmon is just cooked through.

4 Remove the salmon from the grill and evenly divide the chimichurri mixture over each salmon fillet.

Exchanges/Choices

4 Lean Meat   1 1/2 Fat

Calories	245
Calories from Fat	125
Total Fat	14.0 g
Saturated Fat	2.3 g
Trans Fat	0.0 g
Cholesterol	80 mg
Sodium	65 mg
Potassium	405 mg
Total Carbohydrate	2 g
Dietary Fiber	1 g
Sugars	0 g
Protein	26 g
Phosphorus	265 mg

Chef's Tip

The chimichurri sauce may separate while waiting for the salmon to grill. Be sure to stir it well before pouring over the salmon, to ensure even distribution of the ingredients.

Cauliflower Florets with Lemon Mustard Butter GF LC

Makes: 8 servings   *Serving Size: 1/2 cup*   *Prep Time: 10 minutes*

2   Tbsp trans-fat-free margarine, room temperature
1   Tbsp Dijon mustard
2   tsp grated lemon peel
1/4   cup scallions, chopped
1/4   tsp salt (optional)
4   cups cauliflower florets

1 In a small bowl, whisk together the first five ingredients.

2 Steam cauliflower florets until tender-crisp.

3 In a large saucepan, add cauliflower and margarine mixture over low heat. Toss gently until cauliflower is coated.

Exchanges/Choices
1 Vegetable   1/2 Fat

Calories 35
  Calories from Fat 20
Total Fat . . . . 2.5 g
  Saturated Fat . . . . 0.7 g
  Trans Fat . . . . 0.0 g
Cholesterol . . . . 0 mg
Sodium . . . . 80 mg
Potassium . . . . 140 mg
Total Carbohydrate . . . . . . 3 g
  Dietary Fiber . . . . 1 g
  Sugars . . . . 1 g
Protein . . . . 1 g
Phosphorus . . . . 20 mg

Chef's Tip

This great-tasting, low-fat sauce really perks up cauliflower.

Turkey Salad **NEW**

Makes: 6 servings   *Serving Size: 1 sandwich*   *Prep Time: 10 minutes*

12	ounces cooked turkey breast, cubed
2	Tbsp light mayonnaise
1/2	cup fat-free plain yogurt
3	celery stalks, finely diced
1/2	onion, finely diced
1	Tbsp Dijon mustard
6	whole-wheat sandwich thins (100 calories, 5 grams fiber, 22 grams carb)

1 In a medium bowl, combine all ingredients except sandwich thins.

2 Scoop 1/6 of salad onto 1 piece of sandwich thin and top with piece of sandwich thin. Repeat for remaining five sandwiches.

Exchanges/Choices
1 1/2 Starch   2 Lean Meat

Calories 210
  Calories from Fat 25
Total Fat . . . . 3.0 g
  Saturated Fat . . . . 0.3 g
  Trans Fat . . . . 0.0 g
Cholesterol . . . . 50 mg
Sodium . . . . 335 mg
Potassium . . . . 415 mg
Total Carbohydrate . . . . . . 25 g
  Dietary Fiber . . . . 6 g
  Sugars . . . . 5 g
Protein . . . . 23 g
Phosphorus . . . . 260 mg

Chef's Tip

This is a great way to use up leftover turkey!

APRIL

WEEK 3

GROCERY LIST

Fresh Produce
Avocado, small—1
Banana, medium—1
Bell pepper, green, large—1
Bell pepper, red, medium—1
Broccoli—1 head
Garlic—1 head
Mushrooms—1 pint
Mushrooms, portobello,
   large—2
Onions, yellow or white—2
Orange, medium—1
Salad greens, mixed—4 cups
Tomatoes, Roma (plum)—2

Meat, Poultry, & Fish
Chicken breasts, boneless,
   skinless, about 1 inch
   thick, 4 ounces each—4
Lamb stew meat, lean—
   1 1/2 pounds
Pork chops, bone-in, center-
   cut, 5 ounces each—4
Salami, reduced-fat—6 slices
Turkey, ground, 93% lean—
   1 pound

Grains, Bread, & Pasta
Hamburger buns, whole-
   wheat, 1 1/2 ounces
   each—6

Dairy & Cheese
Cheese, Parmesan—1 small
   block
Half-and-half, fat-free—1 pint
Soy milk—1 1/2 cups

Canned Goods & Sauces
Artichoke hearts, 15-ounce
   can—1
Broth, chicken, fat-free,
   low-sodium, 14.5-ounce
   cans—2
Tomatoes, crushed, 15-ounce
   can—1

Frozen Foods
Blueberries—1 small bag
Corn—1 small bag
Lima beans, 9-ounce bag—2
Peas—1 small bag
Strawberries—1 small bag

Staples, Seasonings, & Baking Needs
Black pepper, ground
Flour, all-purpose
Garlic salt
Honey
Lemon juice
Mustard, Dijon
Nonstick cooking spray
Oil, olive
Rosemary
Salt
Sugar substitute
Vinegar, red wine

Miscellaneous
Salsa
Tofu, firm, silken, 12.3-ounce
   box—1
Tofu, soft, silken, 12.3-ounce
   box—1

Citrus Honey Pork Chops GF LC

Makes: 4 servings　　　*Serving Size: 1 pork chop*　　　*Prep Time: 25 minutes*

4	5-ounce bone-in, center-cut pork chops (about 1 inch thick)
1/2	tsp salt (optional)
1/4	tsp ground black pepper
1	Tbsp olive oil
3	Tbsp honey
1/4	cup orange juice (juice of 1 medium orange)
1	Tbsp lemon juice
2	garlic cloves, minced
2	tsp dried rosemary

1 Prepare an indoor or outdoor grill. Season pork chops with salt (optional) and pepper.

2 In a small bowl, whisk together remaining ingredients. Place chops in marinade and refrigerate for 20 minutes.

3 Remove chops from marinade and grill 5 minutes on each side over medium-high heat or until done.

Exchanges/Choices
1 Carbohydrate　　　3 Lean Meat

Calories	200
Calories from Fat	70
Total Fat	8.0 g
Saturated Fat	2.5 g
Trans Fat	0.0 g
Cholesterol	60 mg
Sodium	45 mg
Potassium	295 mg
Total Carbohydrate	11 g
Dietary Fiber	0 g
Sugars	10 g
Protein	21 g
Phosphorus	130 mg

Chef's Tip
Fruit and citrus sauces go very well with pork, so don't be afraid to be creative.

Succotash GF

Makes: 8 servings *Serving Size: 1/2 cup* *Prep Time: 5 minutes*

2	9-ounce bags frozen lima beans
1	small onion, chopped
2	cups frozen corn
1/4	cup fat-free half-and-half
1/2	tsp salt (optional)
	dash of ground black pepper

1 Add lima beans and onion to a large saucepan and cover with cold water. Bring to a boil; reduce heat and simmer, covered, for 5 minutes.

2 Stir in corn and simmer, covered, for 4 more minutes. Drain and return to pan.

3 Add half-and-half, salt (optional), and pepper to pan and heat over medium heat, stirring occasionally until hot (about 2 minutes).

Exchanges/Choices
1 1/2 Starch

Calories	110
Calories from Fat	5
Total Fat	0.5 g
Saturated Fat	0.2 g
Trans Fat	0.0 g
Cholesterol	0 mg
Sodium	55 mg
Potassium	325 mg
Total Carbohydrate	22 g
Dietary Fiber	5 g
Sugars	3 g
Protein	5 g
Phosphorus	110 mg

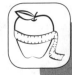

Dietitian's Tip

Lima beans are tasty! Although they are high in carb, they are loaded with fiber.

Chicken with Portobello Tofu Sauce LC

Makes: 4 servings   *Serving Size: 1 chicken breast and 1/2 cup sauce*   *Prep Time: 5 minutes*

1	Tbsp olive oil
2	large portobello mushrooms, diced
2	garlic cloves, minced
3/4	cup fat-free, low-sodium chicken broth, divided
1	12.3-ounce box silken soft tofu
2	Tbsp freshly grated Parmesan cheese nonstick cooking spray
4	4-ounce boneless, skinless chicken breasts
1/2	tsp salt (optional)
1/4	tsp ground black pepper

1 Preheat oven to 350°F.

2 In a large nonstick sauté pan, heat oil over medium heat. Add mushrooms and garlic and sauté for 2 minutes. Add 1/4 cup chicken broth and simmer for 5 minutes.

3 In a blender, purée the tofu and 1/2 cup chicken broth until smooth. Pour tofu mixture over mushrooms. Add Parmesan cheese and simmer 2 minutes, stirring consistently.

4 Coat a glass baking dish with cooking spray. Line chicken breasts along the pan. Pour the tofu and mushroom mixture over the top. Sprinkle with salt (optional) and pepper and bake for 20–25 minutes. Serve with brown rice.

Exchanges/Choices
1/2 Carbohydrate
4 Lean Meat

Calories	235
Calories from Fat	80
Total Fat	9.0 g
Saturated Fat	1.9 g
Trans Fat	0.0 g
Cholesterol	65 mg
Sodium	195 mg
Potassium	635 mg
Total Carbohydrate	6 g
Dietary Fiber	0 g
Sugars	2 g
Protein	31 g
Phosphorus	320 mg

Chef's Tip

There are two main types of tofu available. Water-packed (extra-firm or firm) is solid and dense and works well in stir-frys, soups, or grilled dishes. Silken tofu (extra-firm, firm, soft, or reduced-fat) is a creamy, custard-like product and works well in puréed or blended dishes and smoothies.

Southwest Turkey Burger

Makes: 6 servings   *Serving Size: 1 burger*   *Prep Time: 5 minutes*

1	pound 93% lean ground turkey
1/2	cup salsa, divided
1/2	cup frozen corn
1/2	tsp garlic salt
1/4	tsp ground black pepper
1/2	small avocado
6	whole-wheat hamburger buns (1 1/2 ounces each)

1 Prepare an indoor or outdoor grill.

2 In a large bowl, combine ground turkey, 6 Tbsp salsa, frozen corn, garlic salt, and pepper. Mix well. Divide into six equal portions and form into 1/2-inch-thick patties.

3 Place patties on grill rack; grill 7 minutes on each side or until done. (Or coat a large nonstick skillet with cooking spray and cook patties over medium heat for 3–4 minutes per side, or until juices run clear.)

4 In a small bowl, combine avocado and 2 Tbsp salsa and mash with a fork.

5 Place one patty and 1 Tbsp avocado mixture on a whole-wheat bun. Repeat for remaining five burgers.

Exchanges/Choices

2 Starch   2 Lean Meat
1 Fat

Calories	270
Calories from Fat	100
Total Fat	11.0 g
Saturated Fat	2.3 g
Trans Fat	0.1 g
Cholesterol	55 mg
Sodium	490 mg
Potassium	445 mg
Total Carbohydrate	27 g
Dietary Fiber	5 g
Sugars	5 g
Protein	20 g
Phosphorus	260 mg

Chef's Tip

You can also blend the avocado and salsa mixture in a blender or food processor for a smoother consistency.

Fruit Smoothies GF

Makes: 4 servings   *Serving Size: about 1 cup*   *Prep Time: 5 minutes*

1	12.3-ounce box silken firm tofu, drained
1 1/2	cups frozen strawberries (unsweetened)
1/2	cup frozen blueberries
1	medium banana
1 1/2	cups soy or fat-free milk
4–6	packets sugar substitute

Add all ingredients to a blender and purée on high until smooth.

April is Alcohol Awareness Month. If you enjoy a glass of beer or wine, that's fine . . . just avoid overindulging!

Exchanges/Choices
1 Fruit   1/2 Fat-Free Milk
1/2 Fat

Calories 150
  Calories from Fat 25
Total Fat . . . . .3.0 g
  Saturated Fat . . . . .0.4 g
  Trans Fat . . . . .0.0 g
Cholesterol. . . . . 0 mg
Sodium . . . . 65 mg
Potassium. . . . . 430 mg
Total Carbohydrate . . . . . . 23 g
  Dietary Fiber . . . . 3 g
  Sugars . . . . 14 g
Protein . . . . 8 g
Phosphorus . . . . 140 mg

Dietitian's Tip

This smoothie makes a quick, nutrient-packed breakfast.

Antipasto Salad LC

Makes: 6 servings   *Serving Size: 1 cup*   *Prep Time: 20 minutes*

Dressing

- **2** Tbsp olive oil
- **1/2** cup red wine vinegar
- **1** Tbsp Dijon mustard
- **1/2** cup water
- **1** Tbsp honey
- **1/2** tsp salt (optional)
- **1/4** tsp ground black pepper

Salad

- **2** cups mushrooms, stemmed and quartered
- **1** medium red bell pepper, sliced into thin strips
- **1** 15-ounce can artichoke hearts, drained and quartered
- **2** Roma (plum) tomatoes, diced
- **2** cups broccoli florets
- **6** slices reduced-fat salami, chopped
- **4** cups mixed salad greens

1 In a medium bowl, whisk together dressing ingredients. Set aside.

2 In a large salad bowl, toss together remaining ingredients except salad greens. Drizzle dressing over vegetables. Cover and refrigerate for 15 minutes.

3 Serve vegetables over salad greens.

Exchanges/Choices

2 Vegetable   1 1/2 Fat

Calories	125
Calories from Fat	55
Total Fat	6.0 g
Saturated Fat	1.2 g
Trans Fat	0.0 g
Cholesterol	5 mg
Sodium	400 mg
Potassium	495 mg
Total Carbohydrate	12 g
Dietary Fiber	4 g
Sugars	6 g
Protein	6 g
Phosphorus	115 mg

Dietitian's Tip

You can still enjoy the great taste of salami— just buy the reduced-fat version (2.5 grams of fat or less per serving).

Lamb Stew LC

Makes: 6 servings   *Serving Size: 1/6 recipe*   *Prep Time: 15 minutes*

1 1/2	pounds lean lamb stew meat, cut into 1-inch pieces
1	Tbsp all-purpose flour nonstick cooking spray
1	Tbsp olive oil
1	large green bell pepper, chopped
1	medium onion, chopped
2	garlic cloves, minced
1	15-ounce can crushed tomatoes
1	14.5-ounce can fat-free, low-sodium chicken broth
1	cup frozen peas
1/2	tsp salt (optional)
1/4	tsp ground black pepper

1 Place lamb in a large bowl. Sprinkle with flour and toss to coat. Coat a large soup pot with cooking spray and add oil. Add lamb and sauté over high heat until browned well.

2 Stir in pepper and onion and cook until onion turns clear. Add garlic, tomato, and broth and bring to a boil while scraping the brown bits at the bottom of the pan.

3 Reduce heat and simmer, covered, for 50 minutes. Stir in peas, salt (optional), and pepper and simmer 15 more minutes.

Exchanges/Choices
2 Vegetable   3 Lean Meat
1 Fat

Calories	240
Calories from Fat	80
Total Fat	9.0 g
Saturated Fat	2.5 g
Trans Fat	0.0 g
Cholesterol	75 mg
Sodium	340 mg
Potassium	655 mg
Total Carbohydrate	13 g
Dietary Fiber	3 g
Sugars	6 g
Protein	27 g
Phosphorus	250 mg

Chef's Tip

If you can't find lamb stew meat at your grocery store, ask your butcher to cube some lamb chops for you. Most butchers are happy to help!

APRIL
WEEK 4

DAY 1
Mediterranean Shrimp
Wrap   136

DAY 2
Corn Chowder   137

DAY 3
Chicken Fajitas   138

DAY 4
Bleu Cheese-Crusted
Steak   139
Garlic Butter
Mushrooms   140

DAY 5
Breaded Catfish   141
Buttery Peas   142

**DESSERT OF
THE MONTH**
Almond Joy Hot
Chocolate   143

GROCERY LIST

Fresh Produce
Bell pepper, green, large—1
Bell peppers, red, large—2
Carrots—2
Celery—2 stalks
Garlic—1 head
Lettuce, romaine—1 head
Mushrooms, button—1 pint
Onion, red, small—1
Onions, yellow or white—2
Pepper, jalapeño—1
Salad greens, mixed—4 cups
Tomatoes—2

Meat, Poultry, & Fish
Beef, tenderloin steaks,
4 ounces each—4
Catfish fillets, 4 ounces
each—4
Chicken breasts, boneless,
skinless—1 pound
Shrimp, cooked, peeled—
6 ounces

Grains, Bread, & Pasta
Bread crumbs, whole-
wheat—1/2 cup
Tortillas, whole-wheat,
low-carb, 10 inches—12

Dairy & Cheese
Almond milk—32 ounces
Cheese, bleu, reduced-fat—
small wedge
Cheese, feta—small package
Egg substitute—1/2 cup
Margarine, trans-fat-free

Canned Goods & Sauces
Broth, chicken, fat-free,
low-sodium, 14.5-ounce
cans—3

Frozen Foods
Corn—1 large bag
Peas—1-pound bag
Whipped topping, fat-free—
1 container

**Staples, Seasonings,
& Baking Needs**
Black pepper, ground
Chili powder
Flour, all-purpose
Garlic powder
Garlic salt
Lemon juice
Lime juice
Nonstick cooking spray
Oil, canola
Oil, olive
Salt
Splenda Sugar Blend
Thyme

Miscellaneous
Almonds, sliced
Cocoa powder
Coconut extract
Tofu, soft, silken, 12.3-ounce
box—1

Mediterranean Shrimp Wrap

Makes: 4 servings *Serving Size: 1 wrap* *Prep Time: 10 minutes*

Dressing
- 1 Tbsp olive oil
- 2 Tbsp lemon juice
- 1/4 tsp garlic powder
  Dash ground black pepper

Wraps
- 4 10-inch whole-wheat, low-carb tortillas
- 4 cups romaine lettuce, chopped
- 1 small onion, diced
- 1 cup diced tomato
- 4 ounces cooked, peeled shrimp, chilled
- 1 red bell pepper, sliced into strips
- 2 Tbsp crumbled feta cheese

1 In a small bowl, whisk together dressing ingredients.

2 Fill each tortilla with 1 cup romaine lettuce, 1/4 of the onions, 1/4 cup tomatoes, about 4 shrimp, 1/4 of the peppers, 1/2 Tbsp feta cheese, and 1/2 Tbsp dressing. Fold left and right sides of tortillas in until they touch and roll from the bottom to make the wrap.

Exchanges/Choices

1 Starch	1 Vegetable
1 Lean Meat	1 Fat

Calories	195
Calories from Fat	70
Total Fat	8.0 g
Saturated Fat	1.5 g
Trans Fat	0.1 g
Cholesterol	65 mg
Sodium	630 mg
Potassium	435 mg
Total Carbohydrate	27 g
Dietary Fiber	15 g
Sugars	6 g
Protein	17 g
Phosphorus	275 mg

Chef's Tip

Buy cooked, peeled shrimp—it really saves time!

Corn Chowder

Makes: 9 servings　　　　　　*Serving Size: 1 cup*　　　　　　*Prep Time: 10 minutes*

nonstick cooking spray
1　tsp olive oil
2　carrots, finely diced
2　celery stalks, finely diced
1　small onion, finely diced
1　jalapeño pepper, seeded and minced
3　14.5-ounce cans fat-free, low-sodium chicken broth
6　cups frozen corn
1/2　tsp chili powder
1　12.3-ounce box silken soft tofu
1/2　tsp salt (optional)
1/4　tsp ground black pepper

1 Coat a large soup pot with cooking spray. Add oil and heat over medium-high heat. Add carrots, celery, onion, and jalapeño pepper and sauté for 4 minutes or until onion begins to turn clear.

2 Add broth, corn, and chili powder and bring to a boil; reduce heat and simmer for 20 minutes.

3 In a blender (or with an immersion blender), blend 1 quart of soup and tofu. Add back to soup and simmer for 2 minutes. Season with salt (optional) and pepper.

Exchanges/Choices
1 1/2 Starch　　　1 Vegetable

Calories 140
　Calories from Fat 20
Total Fat . . . . 2.5 g
　Saturated Fat . . . . 0.3 g
　Trans Fat . . . . 0.0 g
Cholesterol . . . . 0 mg
Sodium . . . . 365 mg
Potassium . . . . 540 mg
Total Carbohydrate . . . . . . 26 g
　Dietary Fiber . . . . 4 g
　Sugars . . . . 6 g
Protein . . . . 7 g
Phosphorus . . . . 145 mg

Chef's Tip

For a balanced meal, serve this soup with a large green salad topped with walnuts.

Chicken Fajitas

Makes: 8 servings *Serving Size: 1 fajita* *Prep Time: 20 minutes*

1 pound boneless, skinless chicken breasts, sliced into 1-inch strips
1/4 cup fresh lime juice
2 garlic cloves, minced
1/2 tsp salt (optional)
1/4 tsp ground black pepper
  nonstick cooking spray
1 Tbsp canola oil
1 large onion, thickly sliced
1 large red bell pepper, thickly sliced
1 large green bell pepper, thickly sliced
8 whole-wheat, low-carb tortillas

1 Add chicken to a large bowl and drizzle with lime juice. Add garlic, salt (optional), and pepper and toss to coat. Marinate in the refrigerator for 15 minutes.

2 Coat a large nonstick skillet or wok with cooking spray and add oil. Heat over high heat and add chicken. Sauté 5–6 minutes until done or beginning to brown.

3 Remove chicken from pan and spray pan generously again with cooking spray. Add onion and peppers and sauté for 5 minutes. Add chicken back to pan and toss with vegetables. Serve in warm tortillas.

Exchanges/Choices

1/2 Starch 1 Vegetable
2 Lean Meat

Calories	155
Calories from Fat	45
Total Fat	5.0 g
Saturated Fat	0.6 g
Trans Fat	0.0 g
Cholesterol	35 mg
Sodium	240 mg
Potassium	260 mg
Total Carbohydrate	16 g
Dietary Fiber	8 g
Sugars	3 g
Protein	18 g
Phosphorus	150 mg

Chef's Tip

Garnish these fajitas with fat-free sour cream and salsa.

Bleu Cheese-Crusted Steak LC

Makes: 4 servings   *Serving Size: 1 steak*   *Prep Time: 2 minutes*

Steak

- **4** 4-ounce tenderloin steaks
- **1/2** tsp salt (optional)
- **1/4** tsp ground black pepper
  nonstick cooking spray
- **1 1/2** Tbsp reduced-fat bleu cheese

Salad

- **4** cups mixed salad greens
- **1** cup diced fresh tomatoes
- **1/4** cup chopped red onion

1 Preheat oven to 400°F. Season both sides of steak well with salt (optional) and pepper.

2 Coat a large oven-safe skillet with cooking spray. Sear steaks over high heat for 2 minutes on each side and transfer to oven. Bake for 10 minutes.

3 Remove from oven and sprinkle 1/2 Tbsp cheese on top of each steak. Return to oven and bake 2 more minutes.

4 Serve with a green salad on the side.

Exchanges/Choices

1 Vegetable   3 Lean Meat

Calories	170
Calories from Fat	55
Total Fat	6.0 g
Saturated Fat	2.5 g
Trans Fat	0.0 g
Cholesterol	60 mg
Sodium	90 mg
Potassium	490 mg
Total Carbohydrate	4 g
Dietary Fiber	2 g
Sugars	2 g
Protein	23 g
Phosphorus	200 mg

Dietitian's Tip

Although bleu cheese is high in fat, you only need to use a small amount because of its strong flavor.

Garlic Butter Mushrooms GF LC

Makes: 4 servings   *Serving Size: 1/3 cup*   *Prep Time: 5 minutes*

nonstick cooking spray
1   Tbsp trans-fat-free margarine
1   pint button mushrooms, stemmed and halved
3   garlic cloves, minced
3   Tbsp water
1/2   tsp salt (optional)

1 Coat a large nonstick skillet with cooking spray and add margarine; melt over medium-low heat.

2 Add mushrooms, stirring constantly. Cook for 2 minutes. Add garlic and water and sauté 10 more minutes or until almost all the liquid is evaporated and the mushrooms are cooked through. Add salt (optional), and serve.

National Volunteer Week is in April. Give of yourself this year. You'll get more in return!

Exchanges/Choices
1/2 Fat

Calories 30
　Calories from Fat 20
Total Fat . . . . .2.5 g
　Saturated Fat . . . . .0.6 g
　Trans Fat . . . . .0.0 g
Cholesterol. . . . . 0 mg
Sodium . . . . 25 mg
Potassium. . . . . 140 mg
Total Carbohydrate . . . . 2 g
　Dietary Fiber . . . . 0 g
　Sugars . . . . 1 g
Protein . . . . 1 g
Phosphorus . . . . 40 mg

Chef's Tip

This recipe also makes a great appetizer.

Breaded Catfish

Makes: 4 servings *Serving Size: 1 fillet* *Prep Time: 10 minutes*

1/3 cup all-purpose flour
1/2 cup egg substitute
1/2 tsp dried thyme
1/2 tsp salt (optional)
1/4 tsp ground black pepper
1/2 cup whole-wheat bread crumbs
4 4-ounce catfish fillets
nonstick cooking spray

1 Preheat oven to 350°F.

2 Place flour in a shallow dish. Place egg substitute in another shallow dish. Add thyme, salt (optional), and pepper to bread crumbs and place in a third shallow dish.

3 Dredge one fillet in flour, coating all sides. Dip into egg substitute and roll in bread crumb mixture, coating well. Repeat for remaining three fillets.

4 Coat a baking dish with cooking spray and line the bottom of pan with prepared fillets. Spray each fillet with more cooking spray. Bake for 25 minutes.

Exchanges/Choices
1 Starch   3 Lean Meat

Calories 240
  Calories from Fat 70
Total Fat . . . . .8.0 g
  Saturated Fat . . . . .1.7 g
  Trans Fat . . . . .0.1 g
Cholesterol . . . . 65 mg
Sodium . . . . 190 mg
Potassium . . . . 450 mg
Total Carbohydrate . . . . . . 17 g
  Dietary Fiber . . . . 2 g
  Sugars . . . . 1 g
Protein . . . . 24 g
Phosphorus . . . . 285 mg

Dietitian's Tip

This recipe is a great replacement for traditional fried catfish. The fat content is reduced dramatically because of the baking, but the great flavor still remains.

Buttery Peas GF LC

Makes: 7 servings   *Serving Size: 1/2 cup*   *Prep Time: 2 minutes*

nonstick cooking spray
1   Tbsp trans-fat-free margarine
1   pound frozen peas
1/2 tsp garlic salt (optional)

1 Coat a large nonstick skillet with cooking spray and melt margarine over medium-high heat.

2 Add frozen peas and sauté for 5 minutes. Add garlic salt (optional).

Exchanges/Choices
1/2 Starch   1/2 Fat

Calories 55
  Calories from Fat 15
Total Fat . . . . .1.5 g
  Saturated Fat . . . . .0.4 g
  Trans Fat . . . . .0.0 g
Cholesterol. . . . . 0 mg
Sodium . . . . 55 mg
Potassium. . . . . 65 mg
Total Carbohydrate. . . . . . 8 g
  Dietary Fiber . . . . 3 g
  Sugars . . . . 3 g
Protein . . . . 3 g
Phosphorus . . . . 45 mg

Chef's Tip

You can substitute fresh peas for frozen in this recipe.

Almond Joy Hot Chocolate GF LC (NEW)

Makes: 4 servings *Serving Size: 1 cup with 2 Tbsp whipped topping and 1 Tbsp sliced almonds* *Prep Time: 15 minutes*

1/4 cup sliced almonds
4 cups unsweetened almond milk
1/4 cup cocoa powder
1/4 cup Splenda Sugar Blend
1/2 tsp coconut extract
1/2 cup fat-free whipped topping

1 Add almonds to a dry sauté pan over medium-high heat and sauté until lightly toasted. Set aside to cool.

2 Add almond milk, cocoa powder, Splenda, and coconut extract to a blender and blend until incorporated and slightly foamy.

3 Add hot chocolate mixture to a saucepan over medium heat and bring to a simmer.

4 Add one cup of hot chocolate to a coffee mug, top with 2 Tbsp whipped topping and sprinkle with 1 Tbsp cooled, toasted almonds.

5 Repeat for three remaining coffee mugs.

Exchanges/Choices
1 Carbohydrate   1 Fat

Calories 105
  Calories from Fat 65
Total Fat . . . . 7.0 g
  Saturated Fat . . . . 0.9 g
  Trans Fat . . . . 0.0 g
Cholesterol. . . . . 0 mg
Sodium . . . . 190 mg
Potassium. . . . . 320 mg
Total Carbohydrate . . . . . . 11 g
  Dietary Fiber . . . . 3 g
  Sugars . . . . 5 g
Protein . . . . 3 g
Phosphorus . . . . 90 mg

Chef's Tip

If you have an immersion blender, add the almond milk, cocoa powder, Splenda, and coconut extract directly to the saucepan and blend with the immersion blender instead of using a regular blender.

MAY

Happy Cinco de Mayo

Celebrate Cinco de Mayo with a fiesta of Mexican-inspired dishes that have been transformed into healthy, delicious, lower-carb meals. In addition, this month has many tasty recipes that are good any time of year, such as the Crab Cakes, Asian Tuna Salad, and Beef Barley Soup, as well as the scrumptious dessert—Pretzel and Strawberry Delight.

Mango Salsa Chicken over Rice (page 190)
With its great blend of flavors, this dish is fun to make outdoors on the grill when the weather gets warm. Serve it with steamed fresh green beans and some fruit sorbet for dessert!

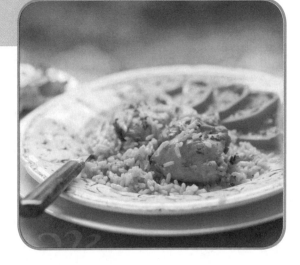

GF gluten-free recipe, but always check ingredients for gluten.

LC these recipes contain 15 grams of carbohydrate or less per serving.

NEW new recipe for the second edition.

MAY RECIPES

MAY
WEEK 1

DAY 1
Butterfly Steak 148
Berry Compote 149

DAY 2
Chicken Fajita
  Pizza 150

DAY 3
Tortilla Soup 151

DAY 4
Farfalle Pasta with
  Asiago Cheese
  Sauce 152

DAY 5
Crab Cakes 153
Wilted Lettuce
  Salad 154

GROCERY LIST

Fresh Produce
Bell peppers, green—2
Berries, mixed (strawberries,
  blueberries, and
  raspberries)—4 cups
Garlic—1 head
Lettuce, butter (Bibb)—
  1 large head
Mint—1 bunch
Onion, red—1
Onions, yellow or white—2
Salad greens, mixed—8 cups
Tomatoes, cherry—8

Meat, Poultry, & Fish
Beef tenderloin steaks,
  4 ounces each, about
  1 1/2–2 inches thick—4
Chicken breasts, boneless,
  skinless—1/2 pound
Turkey bacon—4 slices

Grains, Bread, & Pasta
Bread crumbs, whole-
  wheat—1/2 cup
Farfalle pasta, whole-
  wheat—8 ounces
Pizza crust, whole-wheat,
  12-inch prepackaged—1

Dairy & Cheese
Cheese, Asiago,
  shredded—1/2 cup
Cheese, mozzarella,
  part-skim, shredded—
  1 cup
Egg
Milk, fat-free—1 cup

Canned Goods & Sauces
Broth, chicken, fat-free,
  low-sodium, 14.5-ounce
  cans—7
Chilies, green, chopped,
  4-ounce cans—2
Crabmeat, lump, 6-ounce
  cans—2
Hot pepper sauce
Tomatoes, diced, no-salt-
  added, 15-ounce cans—2

Staples, Seasonings, & Baking Needs
Black pepper, ground
Flour, all-purpose
Lemon juice
Nonstick cooking spray
Oil, olive
Oregano
Red pepper flakes
Salt
Splenda Sugar Blend
Sugar
Vinegar, apple cider
Vinegar, balsamic

Miscellaneous
Chilies, red, dried
Salsa
Tortilla chips, baked—
  1 medium bag

Butterfly Steak GF LC

Makes: 4 servings   *Serving Size: 1 steak*   *Prep Time: 5 minutes*

4 4-ounce tenderloin steaks (about 1 1/2–2 inches thick)
1/2 tsp salt (optional)
1/4 tsp ground black pepper

1 Prepare an indoor or outdoor grill. Using a sharp knife, slice through steak lengthwise, leaving about 1/4 inch from the edge. Do not cut all the way through the steak. Fold steaks open at slit and season well with salt (optional) and pepper.

2 Grill over medium-high heat, about 5 minutes each side. Place steak on a plate cut side up. Serve with Berry Compote (page 149) on the side.

Exchanges/Choices
3 Lean Meat

Calories 140
  Calories from Fat 55
Total Fat . . . . 6.0 g
  Saturated Fat . . . . 2.2 g
  Trans Fat . . . . 0.0 g
Cholesterol . . . . 60 mg
Sodium . . . . 45 mg
Potassium . . . . 265 mg
Total Carbohydrate . . . . 0 g
  Dietary Fiber . . . . 0 g
  Sugars . . . . 0 g
Protein . . . . 21 g
Phosphorus . . . . 165 mg

Chef's Tip

Using a sharp knife is especially important in this recipe. A properly sharpened knife should slide right through your meat. And give the Berry Compote a try—it's really good with the steak!

Berry Compote GF

Makes: 4 servings   *Serving Size: 1/2 cup*   *Prep Time: 5 minutes*

1/2	cup water
2	Tbsp Splenda Sugar Blend
1	Tbsp lemon juice
1	Tbsp fresh mint leaves, chopped
1	tsp balsamic vinegar
4	cups mixed berries (strawberries, blueberries, and raspberries)

1 In a medium saucepan, bring water and Splenda to a boil; add lemon juice, mint, and balsamic vinegar and whisk.

2 Stir in berries and reduce to a simmer. Simmer for 10 minutes or until berries are broken down.

3 Serve with Butterfly Steak (page 148).

May is National Arthritis Awareness Month. Ask your doctor about taking nutritional supplements to help you feel better.

Exchanges/Choices
1 Fruit   1/2 Carbohydrate

Calories	95
Calories from Fat	5
Total Fat	0.5 g
Saturated Fat	0.0 g
Trans Fat	0.0 g
Cholesterol	0 mg
Sodium	0 mg
Potassium	190 mg
Total Carbohydrate	23 g
Dietary Fiber	5 g
Sugars	16 g
Protein	1 g
Phosphorus	30 mg

Dietitian's Tip

These berries are packed with vitamin C and are a great source of fiber, not to mention incredible flavor!

Chicken Fajita Pizza

Makes: 8 servings *Serving Size: 1 slice* *Prep Time: 15 minutes*

nonstick cooking spray
1/2 pound boneless, skinless chicken breasts, cut into chunks
1/4 tsp ground black pepper
1 green bell pepper, sliced into 1-inch strips
1/2 large onion, sliced
1 12-inch prepackaged whole-wheat pizza crust
1 1/2 cups salsa
1 cup shredded, part-skim mozzarella cheese

Salad
8 cups mixed salad greens
8 cherry tomatoes
1/4 cup chopped red onion

1 Preheat oven to 450°F. Coat a medium nonstick skillet with cooking spray and sauté chicken over medium-high heat for 5–6 minutes. Season with pepper.

2 When chicken is lightly browned, add green pepper and onion and sauté another 3 minutes.

3 Place pizza crust on baking sheet. Spread salsa over pizza crust.

4 Spoon chicken mixture over pizza crust and distribute evenly. Top with cheese. Bake 10 minutes or until pizza crust is crisp and cheese is melted.

5 Serve pizza with a side salad.

Exchanges/Choices

1 Starch	1 Vegetable
1 Lean Meat	1/2 Fat

Calories 190
 Calories from Fat 45
Total Fat . . . . 5.0 g
 Saturated Fat . . . . 2.4 g
 Trans Fat . . . . 0.0 g
Cholesterol. . . . . 25 mg
Sodium . . . . 575 mg
Potassium. . . . . 485 mg
Total Carbohydrate . . . . . . 24 g
 Dietary Fiber . . . . 5 g
 Sugars . . . . 5 g
Protein . . . . 15 g
Phosphorus . . . . 230 mg

Chef's Tip

For a great vegetarian version of this recipe, simply omit the chicken.

Tortilla Soup

Makes: 7 servings   *Serving Size: 1 cup*   *Prep Time: 10 minutes*

1	Tbsp olive oil
1	medium onion, chopped
1	15-ounce can no-salt-added diced tomatoes, with juice
4	garlic cloves, minced
1	4-ounce can chopped green chilies
2	dried red chilies
1/2	tsp dried oregano
3	14.5-ounce cans fat-free, low-sodium chicken broth
1/2	tsp salt (optional)
1/4	tsp ground black pepper
3 1/2	cups coarsely crushed baked tortilla chips

1 Add oil to a large soup pot over medium-high heat. Add onion and sauté for 4–5 minutes or until onion turns clear. Add tomatoes, garlic, and green chilies. Sauté for 2–3 minutes.

2 Add red chilies, oregano, chicken broth, salt (optional), and pepper. Bring to a boil. Reduce heat and simmer for 15 minutes. Remove red chilies from soup and discard. Serve each serving of soup with 1/2 cup crushed tortilla chips.

Have a great Cinco de Mayo, the Mexican Independence Day!

Exchanges/Choices
1 1/2 Starch   1 Vegetable

Calories	145
Calories from Fat	25
Total Fat	3.0 g
Saturated Fat	0.6 g
Trans Fat	0.0 g
Cholesterol	5 mg
Sodium	285 mg
Potassium	385 mg
Total Carbohydrate	26 g
Dietary Fiber	3 g
Sugars	3 g
Protein	5 g
Phosphorus	115 mg

Chef's Tip

Serve this soup with a Mexican side salad: shredded lettuce, black beans, reduced-fat shredded Mexican cheese, and a mixture of light Ranch dressing and salsa.

Farfalle Pasta with Asiago Cheese Sauce

Makes: 5 servings   *Serving Size: 1 cup*   *Prep Time: 5 minutes*

8	ounces uncooked whole-wheat farfalle pasta
1	Tbsp all-purpose flour
1	cup fat-free milk
	nonstick cooking spray
1	garlic clove, minced
1/4	tsp crushed red pepper flakes
1/4	tsp salt (optional)
1/8	tsp ground black pepper
1/2	cup shredded Asiago cheese

1 Cook pasta according to package directions, omitting salt; drain.

2 In a small bowl, whisk together flour and milk. Set aside.

3 Coat a medium saucepan generously with cooking spray. Add garlic and sauté for 30 seconds over low heat. Add crushed red pepper and stir for a few seconds.

4 Add flour and milk mixture and bring to a boil, whisking constantly; reduce to a simmer for 7–8 minutes, whisking occasionally. Stir in salt (optional) and pepper.

5 Toss cream sauce with cooked pasta. Sprinkle with Asiago cheese and toss.

Exchanges/Choices
2 1/2 Starch

Calories	205
Calories from Fat	20
Total Fat	2.5 g
Saturated Fat	1.4 g
Trans Fat	0.0 g
Cholesterol	5 mg
Sodium	80 mg
Potassium	185 mg
Total Carbohydrate	38 g
Dietary Fiber	4 g
Sugars	4 g
Protein	10 g
Phosphorus	210 mg

Chef's Tip

Feel free to add some cooked chicken breast to this recipe for added protein. The crushed red pepper flakes add just the right amount of zing for most people, but you can leave them out if you prefer.

Crab Cakes LC

Makes: 6 servings *Serving Size: 1 cake* *Prep Time: 10 minutes*

nonstick cooking spray
1/4 cup onion, minced
1/4 cup minced green bell pepper
2 6-ounce cans lump crabmeat, drained
1/2 cup whole-wheat bread crumbs
1 egg
1 egg white
1/2 tsp hot pepper sauce
1/2 tsp salt (optional)
1/4 tsp ground black pepper
1 Tbsp olive oil

1 Coat a small nonstick skillet with cooking spray over medium-high heat. Add onion and green pepper and sauté 2–3 minutes or until onion is clear. Set aside to cool.

2 In a medium bowl, combine crabmeat, bread crumbs, egg, egg white, hot pepper sauce, salt (optional), and pepper. Mix well. Stir in cooled onion and green pepper.

3 Form crab mixture into 1/2-inch-thick patties with your hands using a heaping 1/4 cup mixture for each patty.

4 Add oil and a generous amount of cooking spray to a large nonstick skillet over medium-high heat. Fry crab cakes about 4–5 minutes on each side or until golden brown.

5 If desired, serve each crab cake over a bed of Wilted Lettuce Salad (page 154).

National Running and Fitness Week is in May. Try walking first, then gradually increase your speed and distance until you are actually—yes—running!

Exchanges/Choices
1/2 Starch   1 Lean Meat
1/2 Fat

Calories	90
Calories from Fat	30
Total Fat	3.5 g
Saturated Fat	0.7 g
Trans Fat	0.0 g
Cholesterol	65 mg
Sodium	205 mg
Potassium	210 mg
Total Carbohydrate	7 g
Dietary Fiber	1 g
Sugars	1 g
Protein	8 g
Phosphorus	140 mg

Chef's Tip

You can mix a little hot sauce with low-fat or fat-free mayonnaise to make a nice sauce for crab cakes. Just serve a little dollop of the sauce on top of each cake.

Wilted Lettuce Salad LC

Makes: 6 servings　　　*Serving Size: 1/2 cup*　　　*Prep Time: 10 minutes*

7　cups butter (Bibb) lettuce, torn into pieces
4　slices turkey bacon
1　Tbsp olive oil
4　Tbsp apple cider vinegar
1　tsp sugar
1/4　cup fat-free, low-sodium chicken broth
1/4　tsp salt (optional)
　　Dash ground black pepper

1 Place lettuce in a large salad bowl.

2 In a small nonstick sauté pan, cook bacon over medium heat until crisp. Remove bacon from pan and chop into small pieces. Toss bacon with lettuce.

3 In a small bowl, whisk together remaining ingredients. In the bacon skillet, add dressing and bring to a boil. Reduce heat and simmer for 8–10 minutes or until slightly thickened.

4 Pour hot dressing over salad and toss well to coat.

Exchanges/Choices
1 Vegetable　　　　　1 Fat

Calories 55
　Calories from Fat 35
Total Fat . . . . .4.0 g
　Saturated Fat . . . . .0.8 g
　Trans Fat . . . . .0.0 g
Cholesterol. . . . . 5 mg
Sodium . . . . 145 mg
Potassium. . . . . 190 mg
Total Carbohydrate . . . . 2 g
　Dietary Fiber . . . . 1 g
　Sugars . . . . 1 g
Protein . . . . 3 g
Phosphorus . . . . 50 mg

Chef's Tip

Most people think wilted lettuce is a bad thing, but try this delicious salad!

MAY

WEEK 2

DAY 1
Smokin' Turkey
   Sandwich   156

DAY 2
Mexican Meatloaf   157
Spicy Sweet Potato
   Fries   158

DAY 3
Chicken Tostadas   159

DAY 4
Sweet Onion
   Salmon   160
Melon Salad   161

DAY 5
Chicken with Broccoli
   and Cheese   162

GROCERY LIST

Fresh Produce
Broccoli—2 heads
Cantaloupe—1
Garlic—1 clove
Greens, field, mixed—2 cups
Lettuce—1 head
Melon, honeydew—1
Mint leaves—1 bunch
Onions, yellow or white—4
Potatoes, sweet, large—2
Tomatoes—2

Meat, Poultry, & Fish
Beef, ground, 95% lean—
   1 pound
Chicken breasts, boneless,
   skinless—2 pounds
Salmon fillets, 4 ounces
   each—4
Turkey breast, deli style,
   roasted, no-added-salt,
   thinly sliced—8 ounces

Grains, Bread, & Pasta
Oatmeal—1/2 cup
Sandwich thins,
   whole-wheat—4

Dairy & Cheese
Cheese, cheddar, 75%
   reduced-fat, shredded—
   1 bag
Cheese, Mexican, reduced-
   fat, shredded—2 ounces
Egg
Milk, fat-free

Canned Goods & Sauces
Beans, black, canned—1 cup
Beans, refried, fat-free,
   16-ounce can—1
Peppers, chipotle, packed
   in adobe sauce—1
Preserves, apricot,
   sugar-free—1 jar
Tomatoes, crushed, 15-ounce
   can—1

Frozen Foods
Corn—1 small bag

Staples, Seasonings, & Baking Needs
Black pepper, ground
Cayenne pepper
Chili powder
Cornstarch
Cumin
Garlic salt
Honey
Lemon juice
Mayonnaise, light
Nonstick cooking spray
Oil, olive
Salt
Vinegar, rice wine

Miscellaneous
Salsa
Tostada shells

Smokin' Turkey Sandwich

Makes: 4 servings   *Serving Size: 1 sandwich*   *Prep Time: 10 minutes*

1/4 cup light mayonnaise

2 tsp canned chipotle peppers packed in adobe sauce

1 garlic clove, sliced

4 whole-wheat sandwich thins

8 ounces thinly sliced, no-added-salt, roasted deli turkey breast

2 ounces shredded reduced-fat Mexican cheese

1 medium onion, thinly sliced

2 cups mixed field greens

1 Blend the first three ingredients in a blender or food processor until smooth.

2 Spread 1 Tbsp mayonnaise mixture onto 1 sandwich thin half. Add 2 ounces turkey breast, 1/2 ounce cheese, onion, and lettuce. Top with another sandwich thin half.

3 Repeat procedure for remaining three sandwiches.

National Women's Health Week is in May. Find out where you can get free health screenings in your neighborhood!

Exchanges/Choices
1 1/2 Starch	1 Vegetable
2 Lean Meat	1 Fat

Calories 270
  Calories from Fat 80
Total Fat . . . . 9.0 g
  Saturated Fat . . . . 2.2 g
  Trans Fat . . . . 0.0 g
Cholesterol . . . . 55 mg
Sodium . . . . 470 mg
Potassium . . . . 445 mg
Total Carbohydrate . . . . . . 28 g
  Dietary Fiber . . . . 6 g
  Sugars . . . . 5 g
Protein . . . . 24 g
Phosphorus . . . . 310 mg

Chef's Tip

Chipotle peppers have a great smoky flavor that complements roasted turkey well.

Mexican Meatloaf

Makes: 6 servings   *Serving Size: 1/6 recipe*   *Prep Time: 10 minutes*

1	pound 95% lean ground beef
1	cup canned black beans, rinsed and drained
1	cup salsa, divided
1/2	cup frozen corn
1	egg
1/2	cup oatmeal
	nonstick cooking spray

1 Preheat oven to 400°F.

2 In a medium bowl, add all ingredients except cooking spray, using 3/4 cup salsa, and mix well. Coat a 5 × 9-inch loaf pan with cooking spray. Spread mixture evenly in a loaf pan.

3 Bake for 50–60 minutes. Remove from oven and let sit for 15 minutes. Top with 1/4 cup salsa.

Exchanges/Choices

1 Starch   3 Lean Meat

Calories	200
Calories from Fat	45
Total Fat	5.0 g
Saturated Fat	2.1 g
Trans Fat	0.3 g
Cholesterol	75 mg
Sodium	355 mg
Potassium	550 mg
Total Carbohydrate	16 g
Dietary Fiber	4 g
Sugars	2 g
Protein	21 g
Phosphorus	255 mg

Chef's Tip

Meatloaf certainly doesn't have to be boring, as this recipe proves. You can have fun inventing your own meatloaf recipes. Try adding roasted red peppers, chopped garbanzo beans, and fresh oregano to ground turkey to make a Mediterranean-style meatloaf. It's easy and fun to create your own recipes!

Spicy Sweet Potato Fries GF

Makes: 4 servings   *Serving Size: 1/4 recipe*   *Prep Time: 20 minutes*

2 large sweet potatoes, peeled and cut into 2-inch wedges
1 Tbsp olive oil
1/2 tsp cayenne pepper
1 tsp cumin
1 tsp chili powder
1 tsp garlic salt

1 Preheat oven to 400°F.

2 Place potato wedges in a bowl and add oil; toss to coat.

3 In a small bowl, combine remaining ingredients.

4 Sprinkle spice mixture over potatoes and toss to coat.

5 Place on a baking sheet and bake for 30 minutes or until potatoes are soft.

May is Older Americans Month. Pay tribute to an older American in your community today!

Exchanges/Choices
1 Starch   1/2 Fat

Calories 115
   Calories from Fat 30
Total Fat . . . . 3.5 g
   Saturated Fat . . . . 0.5 g
   Trans Fat . . . . 0.0 g
Cholesterol . . . . 0 mg
Sodium . . . . 360 mg
Potassium . . . . 450 mg
Total Carbohydrate . . . . . . 19 g
   Dietary Fiber . . . . 3 g
   Sugars . . . . 6 g
Protein . . . . 2 g
Phosphorus . . . . 55 mg

Chef's Tip

If you prefer sweeter sweet potato fries, omit the cayenne pepper, cumin, and chili powder from this recipe. It'll still taste great!

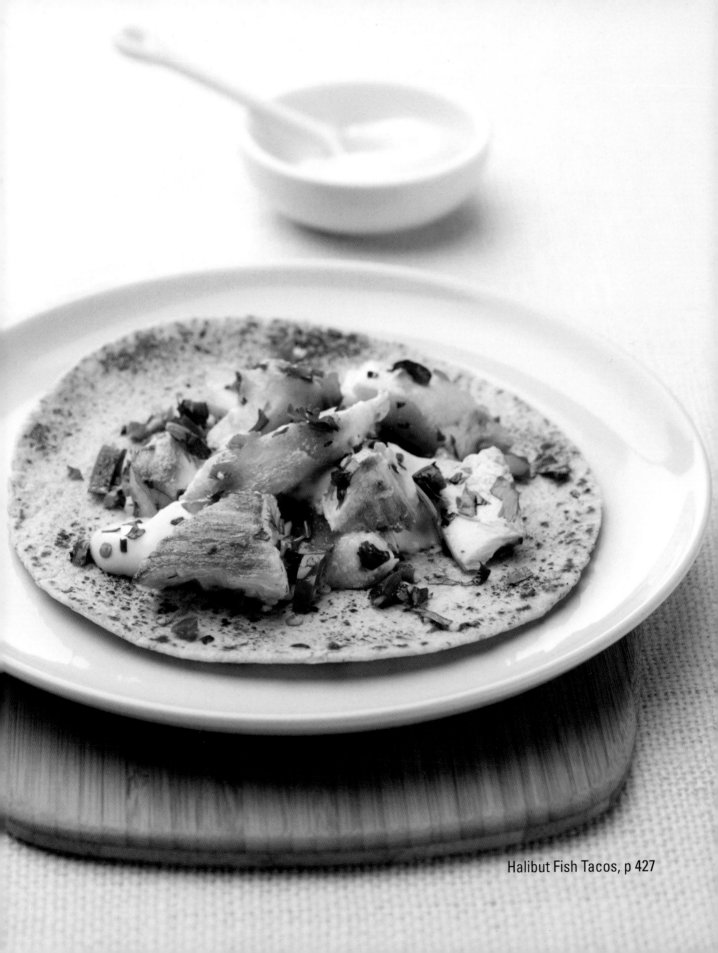

Halibut Fish Tacos, p 427

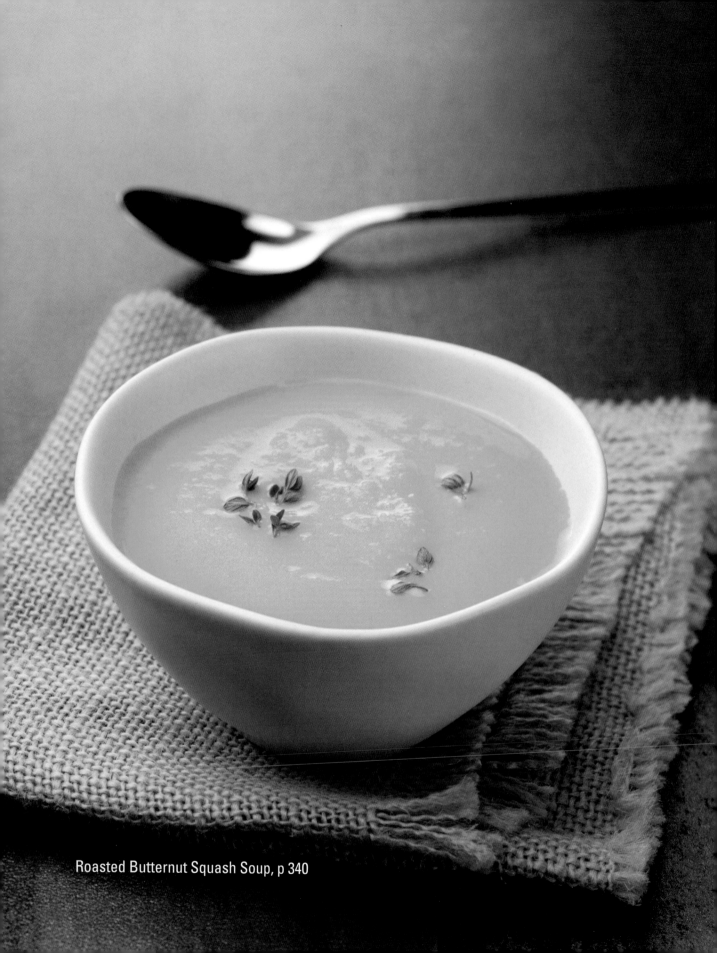

Roasted Butternut Squash Soup, p 340

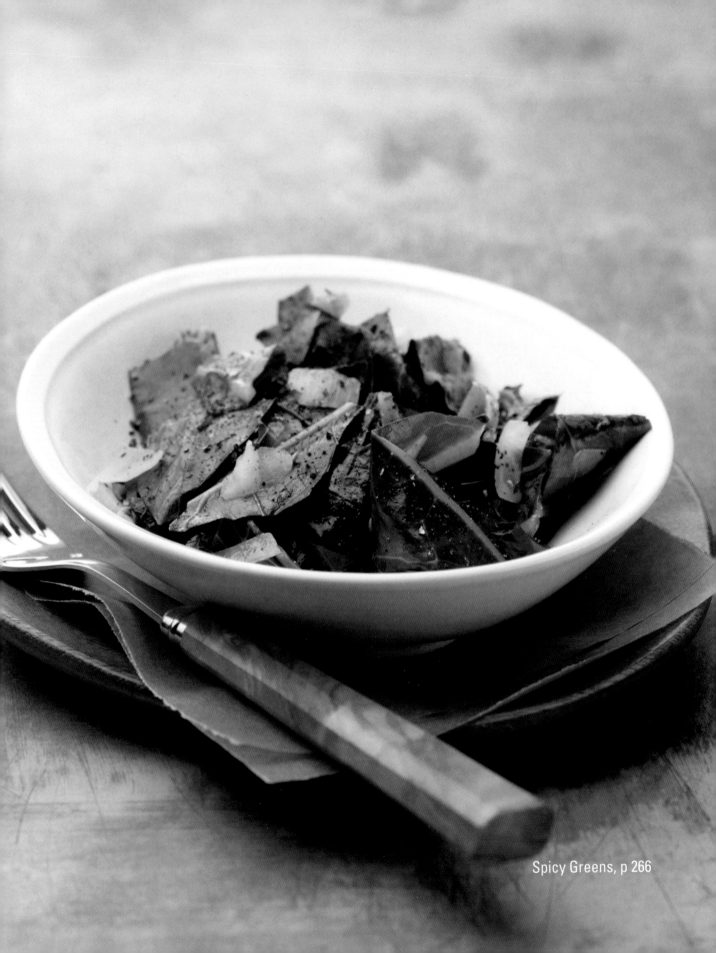

Spicy Greens, p 266

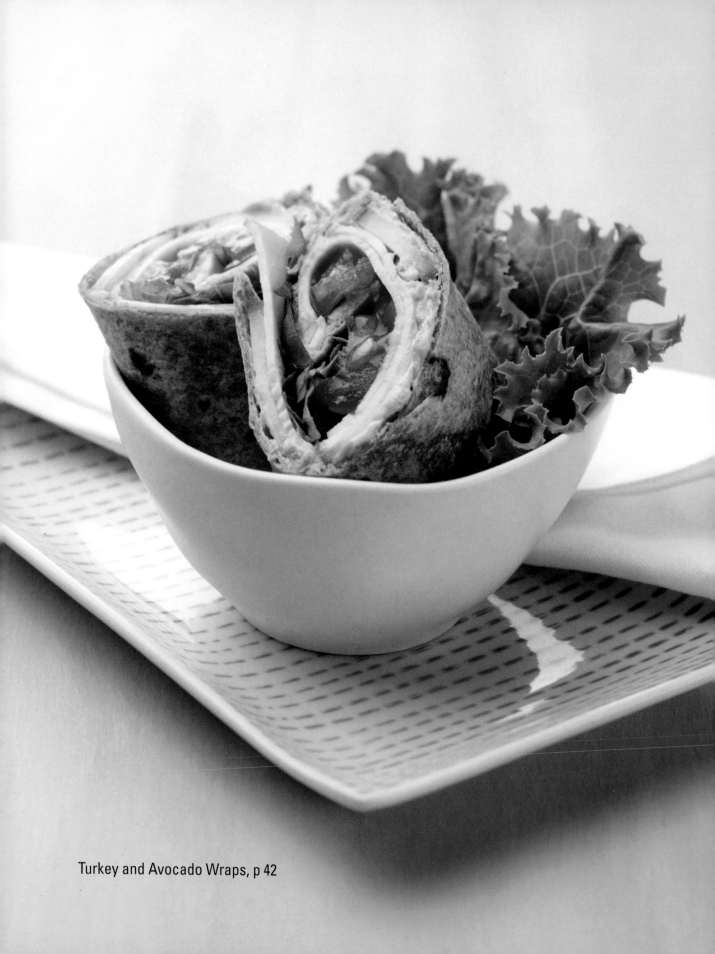

Turkey and Avocado Wraps, p 42

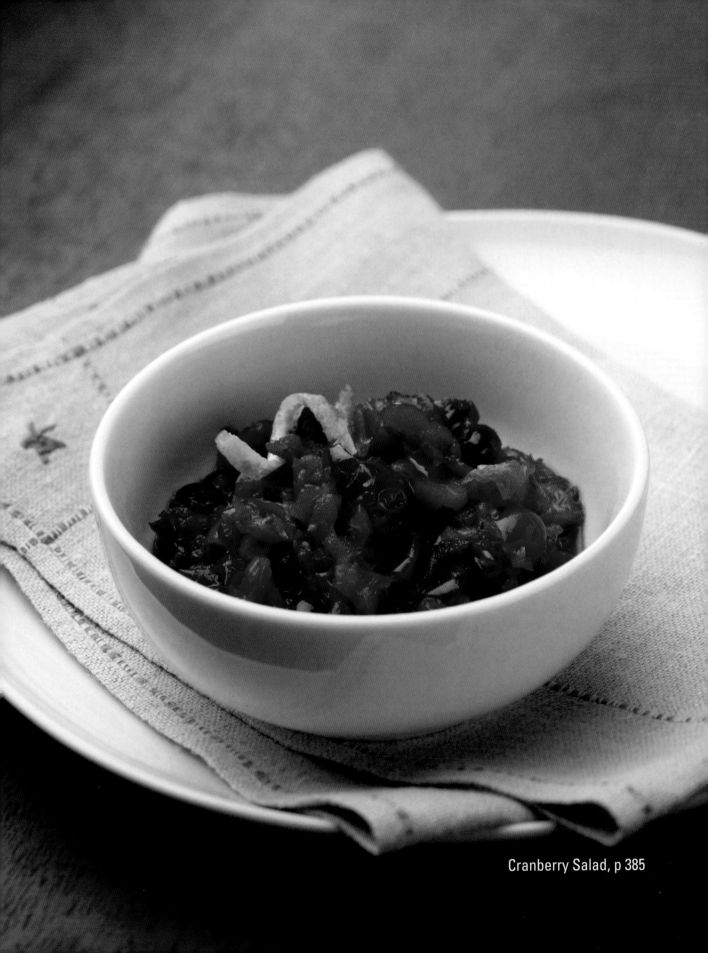

Cranberry Salad, p 385

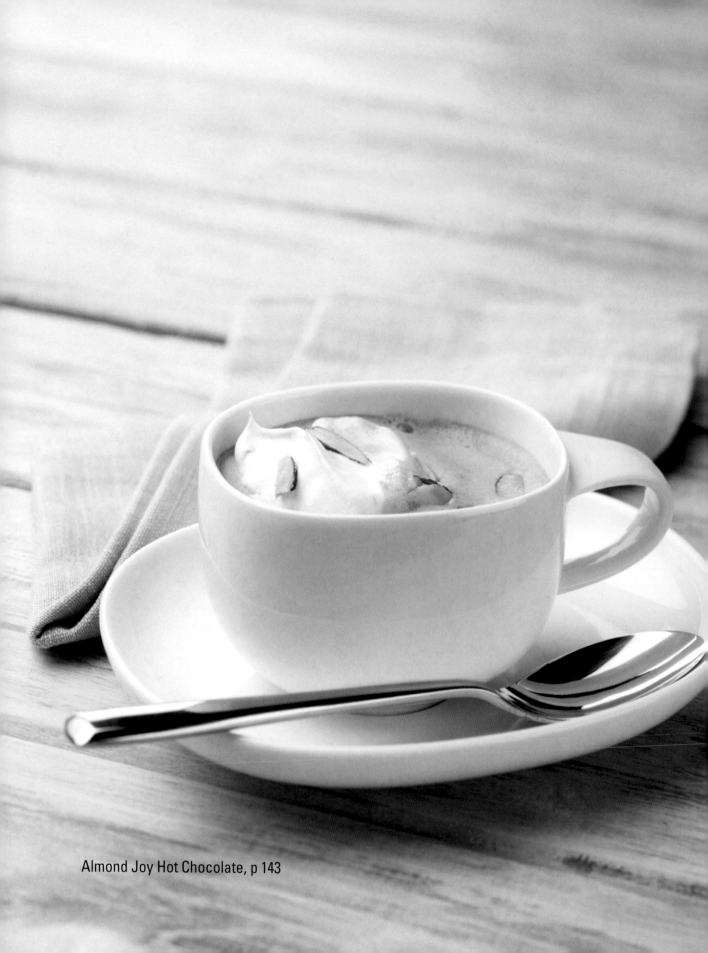

Almond Joy Hot Chocolate, p 143

Chicken Tostadas GF

Makes: 8 servings   *Serving Size: 1 tostada*   *Prep Time: 15 minutes*

1	pound boneless, skinless chicken breasts, cooked and shredded
1	15-ounce can crushed tomatoes
1/2	Tbsp chili powder
1	tsp cumin
1/4	tsp cayenne pepper
8	tostada shells
1	16-ounce can fat-free refried beans
3/4	cup reduced-fat shredded cheddar cheese
1	cup shredded lettuce
2	tomatoes, diced

1 Preheat oven to 350°F.

2 In a medium bowl, combine shredded chicken, tomatoes, chili powder, cumin, and cayenne pepper.

3 Place tostada shells on a large baking sheet. Spread 1/4 cup refried beans on each tostada, top with 1/4 cup chicken mixture, and sprinkle with 2 Tbsp cheese.

4 Bake for 15–20 minutes or until heated through and cheese is melted. Remove from oven and top with lettuce and tomato.

Exchanges/Choices

1 Starch	1 Vegetable
2 Lean Meat	1/2 Fat

Calories 215
 Calories from Fat 65
Total Fat . . . . .7.0 g
 Saturated Fat . . . . .2.3 g
 Trans Fat . . . . .0.0 g
Cholesterol. . . . . 40 mg
Sodium . . . . 485 mg
Potassium. . . . . 570 mg
Total Carbohydrate . . . . . . 20 g
 Dietary Fiber . . . . 5 g
 Sugars . . . . 4 g
Protein . . . . 20 g
Phosphorus . . . . 275 mg

Chef's Tip

To cook shredded chicken, place chicken breasts in a shallow baking dish and bake in a 350°F oven for 30–35 minutes. Remove the chicken from the oven and shred the meat with a fork.

Sweet Onion Salmon GF LC

Makes: 4 servings   *Serving Size: 1 fillet*   *Prep Time: 5 minutes*

4 4-ounce salmon fillets
1 Tbsp olive oil
3 small onions, sliced into thin rings
1 Tbsp honey
1/4 cup rice wine vinegar
1 Tbsp sugar-free apricot preserves

1 Preheat oven to 350°F.

2 Place salmon fillets on a medium baking sheet and bake for 10–12 minutes.

3 Meanwhile, heat oil in a medium nonstick skillet over medium-high heat. Add onions and sauté 7–10 minutes or until onions are caramelized.

4 In a small bowl, whisk together honey, vinegar, and apricot preserves. Pour over onions in pan and sauté for 2 more minutes. Serve onions over fillets.

Exchanges/Choices
1/2 Carbohydrate   1 Vegetable
3 Lean Meat   1 1/2 Fat

Calories 280
  Calories from Fat 125
Total Fat . . . . 14.0 g
  Saturated Fat . . . . 2.3 g
  Trans Fat . . . . 0.0 g
Cholesterol . . . . 80 mg
Sodium . . . . 65 mg
Potassium . . . . 470 mg
Total Carbohydrate . . . . . . 13 g
  Dietary Fiber . . . . 1 g
  Sugars . . . . 8 g
Protein . . . . 26 g
Phosphorus . . . . 280 mg

Chef's Tip

The slight sweetness of the onion is a nice complement to the rich flavor of salmon.

Melon Salad GF

Makes: 6 servings *Serving Size: 1 cup* *Prep Time: 15 minutes*

3 cups cubed cantaloupe
3 cups cubed honeydew melon
1 Tbsp chopped mint leaves
1 Tbsp honey

1 Place melons in a medium bowl.

2 Sprinkle with mint leaves and honey and toss gently to coat.

Exchanges/Choices
1 Fruit

Calories	70
Calories from Fat	0
Total Fat	0.0 g
Saturated Fat	0.1 g
Trans Fat	0.0 g
Cholesterol	0 mg
Sodium	30 mg
Potassium	410 mg
Total Carbohydrate	17 g
Dietary Fiber	1 g
Sugars	16 g
Protein	1 g
Phosphorus	20 mg

Chef's Tip

This is a quick, delicious summer dessert.

Chicken with Broccoli and Cheese GF LC NEW

Makes: 4 servings   *Serving Size: 1 chicken breast and 1/2 cup broccoli*   *Prep Time: 20 minutes*

4	4-ounce boneless, skinless chicken breasts
1/4	cup fresh lemon juice
4	cups broccoli florets
1	cup fat-free milk
1	Tbsp cornstarch
1	cup 75% reduced-fat shredded cheddar cheese
1/2	tsp salt (optional)
1/4	tsp ground black pepper

1 Preheat oven to 350°F.

2 In a medium bowl marinate chicken breasts in lemon juice for 15–30 minutes.

3 Coat a shallow baking dish with cooking spray. Arrange chicken breasts in bottom of pan. Bake for 25–30 minutes or until done.

4 Steam broccoli until tender-crisp; set aside.

5 In a small bowl, whisk together milk and cornstarch until the cornstarch is dissolved.

6 In a medium saucepan, bring milk and cornstarch to a boil. Reduce heat to a simmer. Add cheese, salt (optional), and pepper. Stirring constantly, simmer until all cheese is melted.

7 Pour cheese sauce over broccoli and toss gently to coat. Serve 1/2 cup broccoli over each cooked chicken breast.

May is National Osteoporosis Awareness and Prevention Month. Make sure you get enough calcium and weight-bearing exercise every day!

Exchanges/Choices
2 Vegetable   2 Lean Meat

Calories	140
Calories from Fat	30
Total Fat	3.5 g
Saturated Fat	1.7 g
Trans Fat	0.0 g
Cholesterol	25 mg
Sodium	260 mg
Potassium	425 mg
Total Carbohydrate	10 g
Dietary Fiber	2 g
Sugars	5 g
Protein	19 g
Phosphorus	290 mg

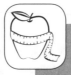

Dietitian's Tip

You can add protein to this meal by stirring in tuna or low-fat cottage cheese with the broccoli mixture.

MAY
WEEK 3

DAY 1
Pork and Apple
  Salad   164

DAY 2
Black Bean Salsa
  Chicken   165

DAY 3
Sirloin Steak with
  Chipotle Cream
  Sauce   166
Smashed Potatoes
  167

DAY 4
Turkey and Apple
  Grilled Cheese   168
Honey Tarragon
  Carrots   169

DAY 5
Chicken Tacos   170

GROCERY LIST

Fresh Produce
Apples, Granny Smith—3
Bell pepper, red—1
Carrots, baby—1 pound
Garlic—1 head
Greens, field—4 cups
Lettuce, shredded—2 cups
Potatoes, red, new—1 pound
Tomatoes—2

Meat, Poultry, & Fish
Beef, sirloin steak—1 pound
Chicken breasts, boneless,
  skinless—2 pounds
Pork tenderloin—1 pound
Turkey breast, deli style,
  roasted, no-salt-added,
  thinly sliced—4 ounces

Grains, Bread, & Pasta
Bread, whole-wheat,
  light—4 slices
Tortillas, whole-wheat,
  low-carb—8

Dairy & Cheese
Cheese, bleu—1 Tbsp
Cheese, cheddar, reduced-fat,
  shredded—1 cup
Cheese, Swiss, Laughing Cow
  brand, light—2 wedges
Half-and-half, fat-free—1 cup

Canned Goods & Sauces
Beans, black, canned—1 cup
Beans, refried, fat-free,
  8-ounce can—1
Peppers, chipotle, canned—
  1 Tbsp

Staples, Seasonings,
& Baking Needs
Black pepper, ground
Cayenne pepper
Chili powder
Cornstarch
Cumin
Honey
Mustard, Dijon
Nonstick cooking spray
Oil, olive
Sage
Salt
Tarragon
Vinegar, apple cider

Miscellaneous
Salsa

Pork and Apple Salad

Makes: 6 servings   *Serving Size: 1/6 recipe*   *Prep Time: 15 minutes*

Salad
- **1** Tbsp Dijon mustard
- **2** Tbsp apple cider vinegar
- **1** Tbsp honey
- **1** Tbsp dried sage
- **1** pound pork tenderloin
- **2** medium Granny Smith apples, cored and sliced into rings (1/4 inch thick)
- **1** large red bell pepper, sliced into thin strips
- **4** cups field greens
- **1** Tbsp bleu cheese

Dressing
- **2** tsp olive oil
- **2** Tbsp apple cider vinegar
- **1** Tbsp honey
- **1/4** tsp salt (optional)

1 Preheat broiler.

2 In a medium bowl, whisk together mustard, vinegar, honey, and sage. Reserve 2 Tbsp of this mixture. Add pork tenderloin to bowl and marinate in the refrigerator for 15 minutes.

3 Arrange apples on a baking sheet and brush all sides of apples with reserved Dijon mixture. Place apples under broiler for 2 minutes. Turn apples and return to broiler for 2 more minutes. Remove from broiler and set aside to cool.

4 Remove tenderloin from marinade and broil for 12–15 minutes, turning once. Remove from broiler and slice into thin pieces.

5 In a large salad bowl, toss together red pepper, field greens, and bleu cheese.

6 Whisk dressing ingredients in a small bowl and drizzle over salad; toss to coat. Arrange salad greens on a plate. Lay apple slices and pork slices over top of salad (pork should still be warm).

Exchanges/Choices
1/2 Fruit   1/2 Carbohydrate
2 Lean Meat

Calories	165
Calories from Fat	35
Total Fat	4.0 g
Saturated Fat	1.2 g
Trans Fat	0.0 g
Cholesterol	40 mg
Sodium	115 mg
Potassium	440 mg
Total Carbohydrate	16 g
Dietary Fiber	3 g
Sugars	13 g
Protein	16 g
Phosphorus	160 mg

Chef's Tip

Pork and applesauce is a classic combination, but you've probably never had pork and apple salad before! Try it; it's great.

Black Bean Salsa Chicken GF LC

Makes: 4 servings   *Serving Size: 1 breast*   *Prep Time: 5 minutes*

nonstick cooking spray
4 4-ounce boneless, skinless chicken breasts
1 cup canned black beans, rinsed and drained
1 cup salsa
1/2 tsp salt (optional)
1/4 tsp ground black pepper

1 Preheat oven to 350°F.

2 Coat a shallow baking dish with cooking spray. Arrange chicken breasts in bottom of pan. Bake for 20–25 minutes or until done.

3 In a medium bowl, combine remaining ingredients.

4 Coat a medium nonstick skillet with cooking spray. Add beans and salsa mixture to pan and cook over medium-high heat. Sauté for 5–6 minutes. While sautéing, use a spoon or spatula to slightly mash beans.

5 Serve bean and salsa mixture over chicken breasts.

Exchanges/Choices
1 Starch   3 Lean Meat

Calories	200
Calories from Fat	25
Total Fat	3.0 g
Saturated Fat	0.9 g
Trans Fat	0.0 g
Cholesterol	65 mg
Sodium	495 mg
Potassium	545 mg
Total Carbohydrate	14 g
Dietary Fiber	5 g
Sugars	3 g
Protein	29 g
Phosphorus	255 mg

Chef's Tip

You can also grill the chicken breasts instead of baking them.

Sirloin Steak with Chipotle Cream Sauce LC

Makes: 4 servings   *Serving Size: 4 ounces*   *Prep Time: 5 minutes*

1	pound sirloin steak
1/2	tsp salt (optional)
1/4	tsp ground black pepper
1/2	cup fat-free half-and-half
1 1/2	Tbsp cornstarch
1	garlic clove, minced
1	Tbsp canned chipotle peppers, puréed

1 Preheat broiler.

2 Season steaks with salt (optional) and pepper. Place in broiler and broil for 10–12 minutes, turning once.

3 In a small bowl, whisk together half-and-half and cornstarch until cornstarch is dissolved. Add mixture to a small saucepan and bring to a boil.

4 Reduce heat to a simmer and add garlic and chipotle pepper purée. Simmer for 5 minutes and serve sauce over each steak.

Exchanges/Choices
1/2 Carbohydrate   3 Lean Meat

Calories	165
Calories from Fat	45
Total Fat	5.0 g
Saturated Fat	1.9 g
Trans Fat	0.1 g
Cholesterol	45 mg
Sodium	100 mg
Potassium	360 mg
Total Carbohydrate	6 g
Dietary Fiber	0 g
Sugars	2 g
Protein	23 g
Phosphorus	225 mg

National Women's Checkup Day is in May . . . be sure to get yours!

Chef's Tip

Using canned chili peppers reduces the chances of burning your eyes with raw peppers!

Smashed Potatoes `GF`

Makes: 4 servings   *Serving Size: 1/4 recipe*   *Prep Time: 10 minutes*

1   pound red new potatoes, washed and quartered
4   garlic cloves, peeled
1/2   cup fat-free half-and-half, heated
1/2   tsp salt (optional)
1/4   tsp ground black pepper

1 Add potatoes and garlic cloves to a large soup pot. Cover with cold water and bring to a boil. Cook for 20 minutes or until potatoes are soft. Drain and return to pot.

2 Add remaining ingredients, and using a potato masher or sturdy whisk, smash potatoes and garlic until blended but still lumpy.

Exchanges/Choices
2 Starch

Calories 135
  Calories from Fat 5
Total Fat . . . . 0.5 g
  Saturated Fat . . . . 0.3 g
  Trans Fat . . . . 0.0 g
Cholesterol . . . . 0 mg
Sodium . . . . 40 mg
Potassium . . . . 555 mg
Total Carbohydrate . . . . . . 30 g
  Dietary Fiber . . . . 3 g
  Sugars . . . . 3 g
Protein . . . . 4 g
Phosphorus . . . . 160 mg

Dietitian's Tip

Leaving the skin on these potatoes increases the fiber content of the dish.

Turkey and Apple Grilled Cheese

Makes: 2 servings   *Serving Size: 1 sandwich*   *Prep Time: 5 minutes*

nonstick cooking spray

2   wedges light Laughing Cow Swiss cheese

4   slices light whole-wheat bread

4   ounces thinly sliced, no-salt-added, deli turkey breast

1/2 Granny Smith apple, sliced

1 Coat a large nonstick skillet with cooking spray over medium heat.

2 Spread 1 wedge of cheese on 1 slice of bread. Top with 2 ounces turkey and half of the apple slices and 1 slice bread. Repeat procedure for the other sandwich.

3 Place sandwiches on skillet. Brown on one side until cheese begins to melt and then flip and grill on other side for about 2 minutes.

Exchanges/Choices

1 Starch   1/2 Fruit

2 Lean Meat

Calories 220
  Calories from Fat 25
Total Fat . . . . .3.0 g
  Saturated Fat . . . . .1.3 g
  Trans Fat . . . . .0.0 g
Cholesterol . . . . 45 mg
Sodium . . . . 430 mg
Potassium . . . . 265 mg
Total Carbohydrate . . . . . . 24 g
  Dietary Fiber . . . . 9 g
  Sugars . . . . 7 g
Protein . . . . 21 g
Phosphorus . . . . 305 mg

Dietitian's Tip

This sandwich includes a variety of food groups—fruit, protein, and whole grains—in one easy and delicious recipe. It would go great served with a green salad with vegetables.

Honey Tarragon Carrots GF

Makes: 4 servings *Serving Size: 1/2 cup* *Prep Time: 3 minutes*

1 pound baby carrots
1 cup water
2 Tbsp honey
1 tsp dried tarragon
1/4 tsp salt (optional)
1/4 tsp ground black pepper

1 In a medium sauté pan, simmer carrots in water, covered, for 10 minutes.

2 Remove lid and add remaining ingredients.

3 Turn flame to high and cook until all liquid is reduced.

4 Sauté carrots until caramelized (golden brown).

Exchanges/Choices
1/2 Carbohydrate   2 Vegetable

Calories 80
 Calories from Fat 0
Total Fat . . . . 0.0 g
 Saturated Fat . . . . 0.0 g
 Trans Fat . . . . 0.0 g
Cholesterol . . . . 0 mg
Sodium . . . . 80 mg
Potassium . . . . 375 mg
Total Carbohydrate . . . . . . 20 g
 Dietary Fiber . . . . 3 g
 Sugars . . . . 14 g
Protein . . . . 1 g
Phosphorus . . . . 40 mg

Chef's Tip

This is an excellent and quick side dish that can be served with a variety of entrées.

Chicken Tacos

Makes: 8 servings   *Serving Size: 1 taco*   *Prep Time: 10 minutes*

1	Tbsp olive oil
	nonstick cooking spray
1	pound boneless, skinless chicken breasts, sliced into 2-inch strips
1	Tbsp chili powder
1	tsp cumin
1/4	tsp cayenne pepper
3	Tbsp water
8	whole-wheat, low-carb tortillas, heated
8	ounces fat-free refried beans, heated
2	cups shredded lettuce
2	cups diced tomatoes
1	cup reduced-fat shredded cheddar cheese

1 Add oil and a generous amount of cooking spray to a large nonstick skillet over high heat. Add chicken and sauté until beginning to brown. Stir in chili powder, cumin, cayenne pepper, and water. Sauté until all liquid evaporates.

2 Fill each tortilla with 2 Tbsp refried beans, 1/4 cup chicken, 1/4 cup lettuce, 1/4 cup tomatoes, and 2 Tbsp cheese.

May is National High Blood Pressure Education Month. Make sure you're taking your medication and watching your sodium intake if you have high blood pressure.

Exchanges/Choices
1 Starch   3 Lean Meat

Calories	205
Calories from Fat	80
Total Fat	9.0 g
Saturated Fat	2.5 g
Trans Fat	0.0 g
Cholesterol	40 mg
Sodium	495 mg
Potassium	375 mg
Total Carbohydrate	17 g
Dietary Fiber	9 g
Sugars	2 g
Protein	23 g
Phosphorus	260 mg

Chef's Tip

To make this dish a little spicier, stir in 1/2 cup salsa with the rest of the spices.

MAY
WEEK 4

DAY 1
Chicken Hash   172
Spanish Rice   173

DAY 2
Black Bean Burrito
    Bowl   174

DAY 3
Asian Tuna Salad   175

DAY 4
Spicy Shrimp
    Tacos   177
Fried Corn   178

DAY 5
Beef Barley Soup   179

**DESSERT OF
THE MONTH**
Pretzel and Strawberry
    Delight   180

GROCERY LIST

Fresh Produce
Asparagus—1 pound
Bell pepper, green—1
Bell peppers, red—2
Carrots—2
Celery—3 stalks
Cucumber, medium—1
Garlic—2 cloves
Lettuce, mixed, or mesclun
    mix—6 cups
Mushrooms, button—8 ounces
Onions, yellow or white—5
Strawberries—3 cups
Tomatoes—2 small
Lettuce—1 small head

Meat, Poultry, & Fish
Beef, top round steak—
    1/2 pound
Chicken breasts, boneless,
    skinless—1/2 pound
Shrimp—1 pound
Tuna, albacore, fresh—
    1 pound

Grains, Bread, & Pasta
Barley—1 bag
Rice, brown—1 bag
Tortillas, corn—8

Dairy & Cheese
Cheese, cheddar, reduced-fat,
    shredded—1 1/2 cups
Cream cheese, light—7 ounces
Margarine, trans-fat-free

Canned Goods & Sauces
Beans, black, 16-ounce
    can—1
Broth, beef, fat-free, low-
    sodium, 14.5-ounce cans—3

Broth, chicken, fat-free, low-
    sodium, 14.5-ounce can—1
Hot pepper sauce
Peppers, chipotle, canned—2 Tbsp
Soy sauce, lite
Sriracha sauce (Asian hot
    sauce)—1 bottle
Tomato sauce—1/2 cup
Tomatoes, diced, no-salt-
    added, 15-ounce can—1

Frozen Foods
Corn—1-pound bag
Hash browns—1-pound bag
Whipped topping, fat-free,
    8-ounce container—1

Staples, Seasonings,
& Baking Needs
Bay leaf
Black pepper, ground
Cayenne pepper
Chili powder
Cumin
Flour, all-purpose
Garlic salt
Nonstick cooking spray
Oil canola
Oil, olive
Oil, toasted sesame
Paprika
Red pepper flakes
Salt
Sesame seeds
Splenda Brown Sugar Blend
Splenda Sugar Blend
Vinegar, rice wine

Miscellaneous
Gelatin mix, strawberry, sugar-
    free, 0.6-ounce package—1
Pretzels, thin—1 bag

Chicken Hash

Makes: 7 servings   *Serving Size: 1 cup*   *Prep Time: 10 minutes*

nonstick cooking spray
2   tsp olive oil
1/2   pound boneless, skinless chicken breasts, cubed
1   medium onion, chopped
1   medium green bell pepper, chopped
1   medium red bell pepper, chopped
1   1-pound bag frozen or refrigerated hash browns

1   cup fat-free, low-sodium chicken broth
1/2   tsp hot pepper sauce
1/4   tsp ground black pepper
1/2   tsp cumin
1/2   tsp garlic salt
1   tsp paprika
1   cup reduced-fat shredded cheddar cheese

1 Preheat oven to 375°F. Coat a 9 × 13-inch baking dish with cooking spray.

2 Add oil to a large nonstick skillet and heat over high heat. Add chicken and sauté for 3–4 minutes. Add onion and bell peppers and sauté another 4 minutes or until onion begins to turn clear. Stir in hash browns; set aside.

3 In a small bowl, combine broth, hot pepper sauce, black pepper, cumin, garlic salt, and paprika.

4 Pour chicken-hash brown mixture into baking dish. Pour broth mixture over the chicken and bake for 20 minutes. Sprinkle the cheese over the top and bake for 5 more minutes or until cheese is melted.

Exchanges/Choices
1 Starch   1 Vegetable
1 Med-Fat Meat

Calories	170
Calories from Fat	55
Total Fat	6.0 g
Saturated Fat	2.5 g
Trans Fat	0.0 g
Cholesterol	30 mg
Sodium	330 mg
Potassium	430 mg
Total Carbohydrate	17 g
Dietary Fiber	2 g
Sugars	3 g
Protein	13 g
Phosphorus	195 mg

Dietitian's Tip

Hash is traditionally made with high-fat corned beef, but this recipe uses chicken for a healthy and tasty twist on this old diner favorite.

Spanish Rice

Makes: 6 servings   *Serving Size: 1/2 cup*   *Prep Time: 10 minutes*

nonstick cooking spray
1 Tbsp olive oil
1 small onion, finely diced
1 cup uncooked brown rice
1 cup canned crushed tomatoes
3/4 cup fat-free, low-sodium chicken broth
1/2 tsp salt (optional)
1/4 tsp ground black pepper
1/8 tsp cayenne pepper

1 Coat a large saucepan with cooking spray and heat oil over medium-high heat. Add onion and sauté until onion turns clear. Add rice and sauté 2 more minutes.

2 Add remaining ingredients and bring to a boil. Reduce heat and simmer, covered, for 40 minutes (or according to rice package directions). Fluff with a fork and serve.

National Senior Health & Fitness Day is in May. Go to www.fitnessday.com to find out when. Start by taking a walk this morning to wake yourself up!

Exchanges/Choices
1 1/2 Starch   1 Vegetable
1/2 Fat

Calories 155
Calories from Fat 30
Total Fat . . . . .3.5 g
Saturated Fat . . . . .0.5 g
Trans Fat . . . . .0.0 g
Cholesterol. . . . . 0 mg
Sodium . . . . 120 mg
Potassium. . . . . 235 mg
Total Carbohydrate . . . . . . 29 g
Dietary Fiber . . . . 2 g
Sugars . . . . 3 g
Protein . . . . 4 g
Phosphorus . . . . 125 mg

Chef's Tip

Serve this zesty rice with other dishes as well. It goes great with fish, chicken, and steak.

Black Bean Burrito Bowl

Makes: 4 servings   *Serving Size: 1 burrito*   *Prep Time: 10 minutes*

nonstick cooking spray
1 Tbsp canola oil
1 medium onion, finely diced
2 garlic cloves, minced
1 15.5-ounce can black beans, rinsed and drained
1/2 cup tomato sauce
1 tsp chili powder
1/2 tsp cumin
1/4 tsp crushed red pepper flakes
1/2 tsp salt (optional)
1/4 tsp ground black pepper

1 cup cooked brown rice
1 cup diced tomatoes
2 cups shredded lettuce
1/2 cup reduced-fat shredded cheddar cheese

1 Coat a large nonstick skillet with cooking spray. Add oil and heat over medium-high heat. Add onion and sauté about 4–5 minutes, or until onion turns clear. Add all ingredients except rice, tomatoes, lettuce, and cheese and bring to a boil. Reduce heat and simmer 10 minutes.

2 In a small bowl, add 1/4 cup rice and 1/4 of the bean mixture. Top with 1/4 cup tomatoes, 1/2 cup lettuce, and 2 Tbsp cheese. Repeat for remaining three bowls.

Exchanges/Choices

1 1/2 Starch	2 Vegetable
1 Lean Meat	1 Fat

Calories 250
   Calories from Fat 70
Total Fat . . . . 8.0 g
   Saturated Fat . . . . 2.3 g
   Trans Fat . . . . 0.0 g
Cholesterol . . . . 10 mg
Sodium . . . . 375 mg
Potassium . . . . 590 mg
Total Carbohydrate . . . . . . 35 g
   Dietary Fiber . . . . 9 g
   Sugars . . . . 6 g
Protein . . . . 12 g
Phosphorus . . . . 255 mg

Dietitian's Tip

Who says you need to go out to eat for a burrito bowl? Make your own quick, healthy version at home.

Asian Tuna Salad `NEW`

Makes: 4 servings   Serving Size: 1 1/2 cups salad and about 4 ounces fish   Prep Time: 20 minutes

Salad

2	Tbsp lite soy sauce
1 1/2	Tbsp Splenda Brown Sugar Blend
1	tsp sriracha (Asian hot sauce) (optional)
1/4	tsp ground black pepper nonstick cooking spray
1	pound fresh albacore tuna
1	pound asparagus, trimmed
1	tsp sesame seeds
6	cups mixed baby lettuces or mesclun mix, washed and dried (or spun in a salad spinner)
1	large red bell pepper, julienned
1	medium cucumber, seeded and julienned

Dressing

1/4	cup rice wine vinegar
1	Tbsp Splenda Brown Sugar Blend
1	Tbsp toasted sesame oil
1/8	tsp ground black pepper

Exchanges/Choices

1/2 Carbohydrate   2 Vegetable
4 Lean Meat

Calories	270
Calories from Fat	55
Total Fat	6.0 g
Saturated Fat	0.8 g
Trans Fat	0.0 g
Cholesterol	60 mg
Sodium	350 mg
Potassium	800 mg
Total Carbohydrate	19 g
Dietary Fiber	4 g
Sugars	8 g
Protein	34 g
Phosphorus	405 mg

1 Preheat an indoor or outdoor grill.

2 In a small bowl, whisk together the soy sauce, brown sugar, sriracha sauce (optional), and black pepper. Set aside.

3 Spray the grill with cooking spray. Or, if using an outdoor grill, ensure that the grates are cleaned and lightly oiled.

4 Brush tuna and asparagus with the soy sauce marinade. Place onto grill. Grill the tuna for 3 minutes on each side. Grill asparagus, turning often, until beginning to soften (about 6–8 minutes). Remove tuna and asparagus from grill, sprinkle with sesame seeds and set aside to cool. Tuna should be slightly pink in the center but not raw.

(continued on next page)

Asian Tuna Salad (Continued)

5 Toss the lettuce, bell pepper, and cucumber in a salad bowl.

6 In a small bowl, whisk together dressing ingredients. Pour over salad and toss gently to coat. Divide the salad equally among four plates.

7 Once tuna and asparagus are room temperature or slightly warmer, slice the tuna and divide equally among the four salads (just under 4 ounces of tuna per salad). Lay it gently on top of the salad. Cut the asparagus spears in half and lay them around the edge of the salad.

Chef's Tip

If your grocer does not carry fresh tuna in the seafood department, fresh-frozen tuna is also great to use for this recipe. Just be sure to thaw it overnight in the refrigerator, NOT on the counter or in the microwave. The tuna is so delicate that thawing it in the microwave will start to cook it and cause it to get tough. Thawing raw fish, meat, or poultry on the counter is unsafe, no matter what you've heard!

▲ American Diabetes Association.
My Food Advisor

This is an original recipe from the American Diabetes Association's online nutrition resource, **Recipes for Healthy Living**—your one-stop shop for diabetes-friendly recipes, meal plans, and other nutrition tips. Sign up today for the FREE *Recipes for Healthy Living* newsletter and to get access to the website by visiting **www.diabetes.org/recipes**.

Spicy Shrimp Tacos GF LC

Makes: 8 servings   *Serving Size: 1 taco*   *Prep Time: 10 minutes*

2 tsp olive oil
2 small onions, thinly sliced
2 Tbsp canned chipotle peppers, chopped
1 15-ounce can no-salt-added diced tomatoes, drained
2 Tbsp water
1 pound shrimp, peeled and deveined
1/2 tsp salt (optional)
8 corn tortillas, warmed

1 Add oil to a large nonstick skillet over medium heat. Sauté onion for 4 minutes or until onion is clear. Stir in peppers, tomatoes, and water and bring to a simmer for 10 minutes.

2 Add shrimp and cook, covered, for an additional 4 minutes or until shrimp are done. Season with salt (optional).

3 Serve equal portions of shrimp mixture on each tortilla.

Exchanges/Choices
1/2 Starch   1 Vegetable
1 Lean Meat

Calories 125
    Calories from Fat 20
Total Fat . . . . .2.5 g
    Saturated Fat . . . . .0.5 g
    Trans Fat . . . . .0.0 g
Cholesterol. . . . . 75 mg
Sodium . . . . 390 mg
Potassium. . . . . 210 mg
Total Carbohydrate . . . . . . 15 g
    Dietary Fiber . . . . 2 g
    Sugars . . . . 2 g
Protein . . . . 10 g
Phosphorus . . . . 200 mg

Chef's Tip

If you want to add even more kick to this spicy dish, add another tablespoon of chopped chipotle peppers.

Fried Corn

Makes: 6 servings   *Serving Size: 1/4 cup*   *Prep Time: 5 minutes*

1/2 cup water
  1 Tbsp all-purpose flour
1/2 tsp salt (optional)
     Dash pepper
  3 cups frozen corn, thawed
     nonstick cooking spray
  1 Tbsp trans-fat-free margarine

1 In a medium bowl, whisk together water, flour, salt (optional), and pepper. Add corn and toss to coat. Set aside.

2 Coat a medium nonstick skillet with cooking spray; add margarine and melt over high heat. Add corn and fry for 10–12 minutes.

World No Tobacco Day is May 31.

If you smoke, quit—today!

Exchanges/Choices
1 Starch

Calories 75
  Calories from Fat 20
Total Fat . . . . .2.0 g
  Saturated Fat . . . . .0.5 g
  Trans Fat . . . . .0.0 g
Cholesterol. . . . . 0 mg
Sodium . . . . 15 mg
Potassium. . . . . 160 mg
Total Carbohydrate . . . . . . 14 g
  Dietary Fiber . . . . 2 g
  Sugars . . . . 2 g
Protein . . . . 2 g
Phosphorus . . . . 55 mg

Dietitian's Tip

Work the carb in this corn dish into your daily meal plan along with any other starchy vegetables, bread, pasta, or sweets.

Beef Barley Soup

Makes: 6 servings   *Serving Size: 1 cup*   *Prep Time: 10 minutes*

2	tsp canola oil
1/2	pound top round steak, finely diced
3	medium celery stalks, finely diced
2	medium carrots, finely diced
1	small onion, finely diced
8	ounces button mushrooms, sliced
3	14.5-ounce cans fat-free, reduced-sodium beef broth
1/2	tsp salt (optional)
1/4	tsp ground black pepper
	bay leaf
1/2	cup uncooked barley

1 Add oil to a large soup pot and heat over high heat. Add beef and sauté for 7–8 minutes; brown well. Stir in celery, carrots, and onion and sauté an additional 7–8 minutes or until vegetables begin to caramelize.

2 Add mushrooms and sauté for 5 more minutes. Add remaining ingredients and bring to a boil. Reduce heat and simmer for 45 minutes. Remove bay leaf and serve.

Exchanges/Choices

1 Starch   1 Vegetable
1 Lean Meat

Calories	155
Calories from Fat	25
Total Fat	3.0 g
Saturated Fat	0.6 g
Trans Fat	0.0 g
Cholesterol	20 mg
Sodium	425 mg
Potassium	540 mg
Total Carbohydrate	19 g
Dietary Fiber	5 g
Sugars	4 g
Protein	14 g
Phosphorus	170 mg

Chef's Tip

Barley, a heartier grain than rice, is very filling and helps make this soup a satisfying meal.

Pretzel and Strawberry Delight LC

Makes: 16 servings   *Serving Size: 1/16 recipe*   *Prep Time: 40 minutes*

2	cups thin pretzels, crushed
2	Tbsp trans-fat-free margarine, melted
1/4	cup plus 1 tsp Splenda Sugar Blend
7	ounces light cream cheese, softened
1	8-ounce container fat-free whipped topping, thawed
1	0.6-ounce package sugar-free strawberry gelatin mix
3	cups fresh strawberries, thinly sliced

1 Preheat oven to 400°F.

2 In a medium bowl, mix together pretzels, margarine, and 1 tsp Splenda. Pour mixture into a 9 × 13-inch glass baking dish and press to cover bottom of pan. Bake 8–10 minutes. Remove from oven and let cool.

3 In a medium bowl, beat 1/4 cup Splenda and cream cheese with electric mixer on high until creamy and smooth. Fold in whipped topping. Pour cream cheese mixture around edge of pretzel layer in baking dish and use a flat spatula to spread mixture evenly and gently toward the center. Refrigerate.

4 In a large bowl, add 2 cups boiling water to gelatin mix and stir constantly for 2 minutes or until dissolved. Stir in 1 cup cold water and refrigerate 30 minutes. Remove gelatin from refrigerator and stir in strawberries; refrigerate another 30 minutes.

5 Pour gelatin over cream cheese layer and refrigerate dessert 2–3 hours.

Exchanges/Choices

1 Carbohydrate   1 Fat

Calories 115
Calories from Fat 35
Total Fat . . . . .4.0 g
Saturated Fat . . . . .1.9 g
Trans Fat . . . . .0.0 g
Cholesterol. . . . . 10 mg
Sodium . . . . 180 mg
Potassium. . . . . 90 mg
Total Carbohydrate . . . . . . 15 g
Dietary Fiber . . . . 1 g
Sugars . . . . 10 g
Protein . . . . 3 g
Phosphorus . . . . 60 mg

Chef's Tip

When you spread the cream cheese mixture over the pretzel layer, be sure to use a flat spatula and slowly spread the mixture toward the center. This will prevent the pretzel layer from mixing in with the cream cheese layer.

JUNE

Fruits of the Harvest

June is the official start of summer. Take advantage of the abundant fruits and low-carb vegetables of the season. Fruits and low-carb vegetables provide many vitamins, minerals, antioxidants, and fiber—you should aim to eat 5 servings every day. Choose fruits and low-carb vegetables over other snack foods and try to incorporate more at meal times. This month, look for exciting side dishes that will liven up any meal, such as Grilled Eggplant or Broccoli Salad with Raisins. Fruit can be a great-tasting addition to the Mango Salsa Chicken or Shrimp Skewers with Pineapple and Peppers.

Sesame-Crusted Salmon (page 204)

Searing this fish on both sides seals in its natural juices and enhances the flavor of the sesame seeds. It's delicious with broccoli and steamed rice.

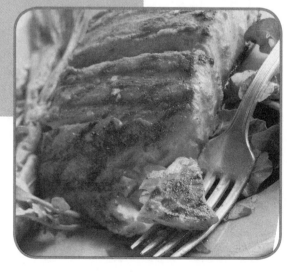

GF gluten-free recipe, but always check ingredients for gluten.

LC these recipes contain 15 grams of carbohydrate or less per serving.

NEW new recipe for the second edition.

JUNE
WEEK 1

DAY 1
Pesto Pasta Salad   184

DAY 2
Curry Turkey and
    Chickpea Burgers   185
Tortellini Salad   186

DAY 3
Grilled Pork Chops with
    Peach Compote   187

DAY 4
Grilled Halibut   188
Grilled Eggplant   189

DAY 5
Mango Salsa Chicken
    over Rice   190

GROCERY LIST

Fresh Produce
Basil—1 bunch
Bell pepper, green—1
Bell pepper, yellow—1
Broccoli—1 head
Eggplant, medium—1 (about
    1 pound)
Garlic—1 head
Ginger—1 small root
Lettuce, butter (Bibb)—
    12 leaves
Mango—1
Marjoram—1 bunch
Onion, red—1
Orange—1
Parsley—1 bunch
Peaches, large—4
Tomato—1
Tomatoes, grape—3/4 cup

Meat, Poultry, & Fish
Chicken breasts, boneless,
    skinless—1 pound
Halibut fillets, 4 ounces
    each—4
Pork chops, bone-in, center-
    cut, 5 ounces each—4
Turkey, ground, 93% lean—
    1 pound

Grains, Bread, & Pasta
Pasta, farfalle, whole-
    wheat—12 ounces
Pasta, tortellini, whole-wheat,
    three-cheese, 9-ounce
    package—1
Rice, brown—1 bag

Dairy & Cheese
Cheese, Parmesan—1 block
Yogurt, fat-free, plain—
    1/3 cup

Canned Goods & Sauces
Chickpeas (garbanzo beans),
    15-ounce can—1
Hot pepper sauce
Preserves, apricot, reduced-
    sugar—1 jar

Staples, Seasonings, & Baking Needs
Black pepper, ground
Garam masala
Garlic salt
Honey
Mayonnaise, light
Nonstick cooking spray
Oil, olive
Sage
Salt
Vinegar, balsamic
Vinegar, rice wine

Miscellaneous
Pine nuts
Salad dressing, Italian,
    fat-free

Pesto Pasta Salad

Makes: 6 servings   *Serving Size: 1 cup*   *Prep Time: 13 minutes*

12	ounces uncooked whole-wheat farfalle pasta
1	cup fresh basil leaves
2	Tbsp pine nuts
1/3	cup light mayonnaise
1/3	cup fat-free plain yogurt
1/2	tsp garlic salt (optional)
1	Tbsp red wine vinegar
3	Tbsp freshly grated Parmesan cheese

1 Cook pasta according to package directions, omitting salt. Rinse under cold water to cool.

2 In a food processor, purée basil and pine nuts.

3 In a large mixing bowl, whisk together mayonnaise, yogurt, garlic salt, red wine vinegar, and Parmesan cheese. Add basil and pine nuts and mix well.

4 Add cooled pasta to bowl; toss lightly to coat. Refrigerate.

Exchanges/Choices

3 Starch	1 Fat

Calories	270
Calories from Fat	65
Total Fat	7.0 g
Saturated Fat	1.1 g
Trans Fat	0.0 g
Cholesterol	5 mg
Sodium	155 mg
Potassium	210 mg
Total Carbohydrate	46 g
Dietary Fiber	5 g
Sugars	4 g
Protein	10 g
Phosphorus	210 mg

Dietitian's Tip

The fat-free yogurt in this recipe provides creaminess without changing the flavor of the salad. Try using fat-free plain yogurt mixed with light mayonnaise in many mayonnaise-based salads, such as tuna or chicken salad.

Curry Turkey and Chickpea Burgers

Makes: 6 servings   *Serving Size: 1 burger*   *Prep Time: 10 minutes*

1 pound 93% lean ground turkey
1 tsp orange zest (from 1 medium orange)
1 tsp garam masala (or use 1/2 tsp cumin, 1/2 tsp ground coriander, 1/4 tsp cayenne pepper)
1 Tbsp minced fresh parsley
1 tsp fresh grated ginger
2 garlic cloves, minced
2 Tbsp lite mayonnaise
1/2 tsp salt (optional)
1/2 tsp ground black pepper
1 15-ounce can chickpeas (garbanzo beans), drained and rinsed

1/3 cup reduced-sugar apricot preserves
1 Tbsp hot pepper sauce
12 large butter (Bibb) lettuce leaves
6 slices tomato

1 Prepare an indoor or outdoor grill.

2 In a medium bowl, combine turkey, orange zest, garam masala, parsley, ginger, garlic, mayonnaise, salt (optional), black pepper, and chickpeas.

3 Divide mixture into six equal portions and form into patties. Grill each patty for a total of 8–10 minutes (4–5 minutes each side) or until burger reaches an internal temperature of 165°F.

4 In a small bowl, mix together apricot preserves and hot sauce.

5 Place burger on top of one lettuce leaf. Top with a heaping tablespoon of apricot sauce, tomato slice, and the other piece of lettuce.

Exchanges/Choices

1 Starch	1/2 Carbohydrate
2 Lean Meat	1 Fat

Calories	230
Calories from Fat	80
Total Fat	9.0 g
Saturated Fat	1.9 g
Trans Fat	0.1 g
Cholesterol	60 mg
Sodium	180 mg
Potassium	465 mg
Total Carbohydrate	20 g
Dietary Fiber	4 g
Sugars	8 g
Protein	19 g
Phosphorus	235 mg

Chef's Tip

Garam masala is an Indian spice mixture that literally translates to "hot mix." It doesn't have to be spicy hot, though. There are many versions of garam masala on the market. You can make your own by combining your favorite spices, like cumin, coriander, ground mustard, cayenne pepper, turmeric, dried chilies, ground ginger, granulated garlic, and fenugreek, to name a few. For this recipe, if you don't have (or want to buy) garam masala, simply combine ground cumin, ground coriander, and cayenne pepper to taste. Make it as spicy (or mild) as you prefer.

Tortellini Salad

Makes: 6 servings   *Serving Size: 1 cup*   *Prep Time: 8 minutes*

1 9-ounce package three-cheese whole-wheat tortellini
1 cup broccoli florets
3/4 cup grape tomatoes, halved
1/2 cup yellow bell pepper strips
1/2 cup fat-free Italian dressing

1 Cook tortellini according to package directions; drain.

2 Toss all ingredients in a large salad bowl. Serve immediately or refrigerate until ready to serve.

Exchanges/Choices
1 1/2 Carbohydrate   1/2 Fat

Calories	150
Calories from Fat	40
Total Fat	4.5 g
Saturated Fat	1.3 g
Trans Fat	0.0 g
Cholesterol	25 mg
Sodium	440 mg
Potassium	170 mg
Total Carbohydrate	22 g
Dietary Fiber	3 g
Sugars	4 g
Protein	7 g
Phosphorus	130 mg

Chef's Tip

Feel free to experiment with this recipe by adding more of your favorite vegetables.

Grilled Pork Chops with Peach Compote GF

Makes: 4 servings   *Serving Size: 1 pork chop and 1/4 cup compote*   *Prep Time: 10 minutes*

4	5-ounce bone-in, center-cut pork chops
1/2	tsp salt (optional)
1/4	tsp ground black pepper
3	cups peaches, peeled, pitted, and chopped (about 4 large peaches)
1	tsp olive oil
1	tsp honey
3	tsp balsamic vinegar
1/4	tsp dried sage

1 Prepare an indoor or outdoor grill. Season pork chops with salt (optional) and pepper on both sides. Grill pork chops over medium heat until done.

2 Meanwhile, in a medium nonstick skillet, sauté peaches in olive oil and honey over medium heat for 7 minutes. Add balsamic vinegar and sage; sauté for another 2 minutes.

3 Serve 1/4 cup peach compote over each pork chop.

Exchanges/Choices

1 Fruit   3 Lean Meat

Calories 220
  Calories from Fat 65
Total Fat . . . . 7.0 g
  Saturated Fat . . . . 2.3 g
  Trans Fat . . . . 0.0 g
Cholesterol . . . . 60 mg
Sodium . . . . 45 mg
Potassium . . . . 560 mg
Total Carbohydrate . . . . . . 17 g
  Dietary Fiber . . . . 2 g
  Sugars . . . . 15 g
Protein . . . . 22 g
Phosphorus . . . . 160 mg

Chef's Tip

June is the best month to buy peaches. Check out your local farmer's market for the best selection. And make sure the peaches are very ripe for this recipe.

Grilled Halibut GF LC

Makes: 4 servings   *Serving Size: 1 fillet*   *Prep Time: 10 minutes*

1/2	cup finely chopped fresh marjoram (or 2 Tbsp dried marjoram)
4	garlic cloves, minced
1	tsp olive oil
1/2	tsp salt (optional)
1/4	tsp ground black pepper
4	4-ounce halibut fillets

1 Prepare an indoor or outdoor grill.

2 In a small bowl, combine marjoram, garlic, olive oil, salt (optional), and pepper.

3 Rub 2 Tbsp marjoram mixture on non-skin side of fillet.

4 Grill fillets over medium heat for 3 minutes on each side.

Exchanges/Choices
3 Lean Meat

Calories 140
  Calories from Fat 35
Total Fat . . . . 4.0 g
  Saturated Fat . . . . 0.5 g
  Trans Fat . . . . 0.0 g
Cholesterol . . . . 35 mg
Sodium . . . . 60 mg
Potassium . . . . 535 mg
Total Carbohydrate . . . . 2 g
  Dietary Fiber . . . . 0 g
  Sugars . . . . 0 g
Protein . . . . 24 g
Phosphorus . . . . 260 mg

Chef's Tip

If you can't find halibut, try flounder, haddock, or perch in this recipe instead.

Grilled Eggplant GF LC

Makes: 4 servings   *Serving Size: 2 slices*   *Prep Time: 3 minutes*

1   Tbsp olive oil
1   medium eggplant (about 1 pound)
1/2   tsp salt (optional)
1/4   tsp ground black pepper

1 Prepare an indoor or outdoor grill.

2 Cut the ends off eggplant and thinly slice lengthwise. Brush eggplant slices with olive oil. Sprinkle with salt (optional) and pepper.

3 Grill eggplant slices over medium-high heat for about 3 minutes for each side.

Exchanges/Choices
2 Vegetable   1/2 Fat

Calories 65
  Calories from Fat 30
Total Fat . . . . 3.5 g
  Saturated Fat . . . . 0.5 g
  Trans Fat . . . . 0.0 g
Cholesterol . . . . 0 mg
Sodium . . . . 0 mg
Potassium . . . . 130 mg
Total Carbohydrate . . . . 9 g
  Dietary Fiber . . . . 3 g
  Sugars . . . . 3 g
Protein . . . . 1 g
Phosphorus . . . . 15 mg

Chef's Tip

The best time to buy eggplant is in the summer. Stop by your local farmer's market and pick up the plumpest eggplant you can find.

Mango Salsa Chicken over Rice GF

Makes: 4 servings

Serving Size: 1 chicken breast and 1/2 cup brown rice

Prep Time: 10 minutes

4	4-ounce boneless, skinless chicken breasts
1/2	tsp salt (optional)
1/4	tsp ground black pepper
1	tsp olive oil
1	Tbsp rice wine vinegar
1	mango, finely diced (1 cup)
1/2	cup finely diced red onion
1	green bell pepper, finely diced
2	cups brown rice, cooked

1 Prepare an indoor or outdoor grill.

2 Season chicken breasts with salt (optional) and pepper on both sides. Grill chicken breasts over medium heat for about 5 minutes on each side or until juices run clear.

3 In a small bowl, whisk olive oil and vinegar. Add remaining ingredients except rice and toss to coat.

4 Pour mango salsa over grilled chicken breasts. Serve each chicken breast over 1/2 cup brown rice.

Exchanges/Choices

1 1/2 Starch	1/2 Fruit
1 Vegetable	3 Lean Meat

Calories	295
Calories from Fat	45
Total Fat	5.0 g
Saturated Fat	1.2 g
Trans Fat	0.0 g
Cholesterol	65 mg
Sodium	65 mg
Potassium	415 mg
Total Carbohydrate	35 g
Dietary Fiber	3 g
Sugars	9 g
Protein	27 g
Phosphorus	275 mg

Dietitian's Tip

Mangoes are a good source of vitamin C. They taste great in smoothies, too!

JUNE
WEEK 2

DAY 1

Marinated Grilled
    Chicken   192
Broccoli Salad with
    Raisins   193

DAY 2

Turkey and Artichoke
    Sandwich   194

DAY 3

Asian Noodle Salad
    with Shredded
    Pork   195

DAY 4

Italian Garden
    Frittata   196

DAY 5

Beef Kabobs   197
Herb-Grilled
    Potatoes   198

GROCERY LIST

Fresh Produce

Basil—1 bunch
Bell peppers, red—3
Broccoli—2 heads
Cabbage, Napa—1 small
    head
Carrot—1
Garlic—1 head
Mushrooms, button—1 pint
Onion, red—1
Onion, yellow or white—1
Potatoes, red, small—12
Scallions—2
Squash, yellow, large—1
Sugar snap peas—2 cups
Tomatoes—2
Zucchini—3

Meat, Poultry, & Fish

Beef tenderloin—1 pound
Chicken breasts, boneless,
    skinless—1 pound
Pork tenderloin—1 pound
Turkey bacon—8 slices
Turkey breast, deli style,
    roasted, no-added-salt,
    thinly sliced—1 1/2
    pounds

Grains, Bread, & Pasta

Pasta, angel hair, whole-
    wheat—8 ounces
Sandwich thins, whole-
    wheat—8

Dairy & Cheese

Cheese, mozzarella, part-
    skim, shredded—1/2 cup
Egg substitute—12 ounces
Yogurt, plain, fat-free—
    1/4 cup

Canned Goods & Sauces

Artichoke hearts, 14-ounce
    cans—2
Hot pepper sauce
Soy sauce, lite
Teriyaki sauce
Tomatoes, diced, no-salt-
    added, 15-ounce can—1

Staples, Seasonings, & Baking Needs

Basil
Black pepper, ground
Garlic powder
Honey
Mayonnaise, light
Nonstick cooking spray
Oil, olive
Oil, sesame
Rosemary
Salt
Sugar
Vinegar, apple cider
Vinegar, balsamic
Vinegar, rice wine

Miscellaneous

Bamboo skewers—8
Raisins, golden—1/3 cup
Ramen-style noodles,
    3-ounce packages—2
Salad dressing, Italian,
    fat-free—1/2 cup

Marinated Grilled Chicken GF LC

Makes: 4 servings   *Serving Size: 1 chicken breast*   *Prep Time: 5 minutes*

1   Tbsp olive oil
1/4   cup balsamic vinegar
1   Tbsp honey
3   Tbsp fresh basil, coarsely chopped
3   garlic cloves, minced
4   4-ounce boneless, skinless chicken breasts

1 Prepare an indoor or outdoor grill.

2 In a large bowl, whisk together oil, balsamic vinegar, honey, basil, and garlic. Add chicken breasts and coat well. Marinate in the refrigerator for 15–30 minutes.

3 Grill chicken breasts over medium heat for about 5 minutes on each side or until juices run clear.

Exchanges/Choices
1/2 Carbohydrate   3 Lean Meat

Calories 175
   Calories from Fat 45
Total Fat . . . . 5.0 g
   Saturated Fat . . . . 1.1 g
   Trans Fat . . . . 0.0 g
Cholesterol . . . . 65 mg
Sodium . . . . 60 mg
Potassium . . . . 225 mg
Total Carbohydrate . . . . 6 g
   Dietary Fiber . . . . 0 g
   Sugars . . . . 5 g
Protein . . . . 24 g
Phosphorus . . . . 185 mg

Dietitian's Tip

Marinating meats and vegetables can be a great way to add flavor without adding fat.

Broccoli Salad with Raisins GF LC

Makes: 7 servings　　　　*Serving Size: 1 cup*　　　　*Prep Time: 15 minutes*

Salad

8	slices cooked turkey bacon, cut into 1-inch pieces
6	cups broccoli florets
1/3	cup finely diced red onion
1/3	cup golden raisins

Dressing

1/3	cup light mayonnaise
1/4	cup fat-free plain yogurt
1	Tbsp sugar
1	Tbsp apple cider vinegar

1 In a large salad bowl, toss together salad ingredients.

2 In a small bowl, whisk together dressing ingredients.

3 Drizzle dressing over broccoli salad and toss well to coat.

June is National Dairy Month. Try some of the delicious fat-free and reduced-fat dairy products on the market today! Your family recipes will taste just as delicious as they used to and will be healthier for you, too.

Exchanges/Choices

1/2 Fruit	1 Vegetable
1 Fat	

Calories	120
Calories from Fat	55
Total Fat	6.0 g
Saturated Fat	1.2 g
Trans Fat	0.0 g
Cholesterol	10 mg
Sodium	320 mg
Potassium	325 mg
Total Carbohydrate	14 g
Dietary Fiber	2 g
Sugars	9 g
Protein	5 g
Phosphorus	110 mg

Chef's Tip

To quickly cook the bacon pieces, microwave them on high for 2 minutes.

Turkey and Artichoke Sandwich

Makes: 4 servings   *Serving Size: 1 sandwich*   *Prep Time: 10 minutes*

1	14-ounce can artichoke hearts, drained
1/3	cup light mayonnaise
1	tsp garlic powder
4	whole-wheat sandwich thins
12	ounces thinly sliced no-added-salt deli turkey
1	large tomato, sliced

1 In a food processor or blender, purée artichoke hearts, mayonnaise, and garlic powder to form a spread.

2 Spread 2 1/2 Tbsp of artichoke mixture on half of a whole-wheat sandwich thin. Add 3 ounces turkey breast and 1–2 tomato slices. Top with other half of whole-wheat sandwich thin.

3 Repeat procedure for remaining three sandwiches.

Exchanges/Choices

1 1/2 Starch   1 Vegetable
3 Lean Meat   1/2 Fat

Calories	305
Calories from Fat	70
Total Fat	8.0 g
Saturated Fat	0.9 g
Trans Fat	0.0 g
Cholesterol	65 mg
Sodium	580 mg
Potassium	675 mg
Total Carbohydrate	32 g
Dietary Fiber	9 g
Sugars	5 g
Protein	31 g
Phosphorus	340 mg

Chef's Tip

Don't be afraid to try this delicious flavor combination.

Asian Noodle Salad with Shredded Pork

Makes: 8 servings   *Serving Size: 1/8 recipe*   *Prep Time: 30 minutes*

Salad

- **2** Tbsp lite soy sauce
- **1** tsp hot pepper sauce
- **1** pound pork tenderloin
- **2** 3-ounce packages ramen-style noodles (discard seasoning packet)
- **1** red bell pepper, sliced into strips
- **1 1/2** cups Napa cabbage, shredded
- **2** scallions, chopped
- **2** cups sugar snap peas
- **1** cup shredded carrot

Dressing

- **1/4** cup rice wine vinegar
- **1** Tbsp olive oil
- **1** Tbsp sesame oil
- **1** Tbsp teriyaki sauce
- **1/2** tsp hot pepper sauce

1 Preheat oven to 400°F. In a small bowl, whisk together soy sauce and 1 tsp hot pepper sauce. Brush entire pork tenderloin with soy sauce mixture and place in a medium baking dish. Roast for 20–25 minutes or until done.

2 While pork is roasting, cook noodles according to package directions, omitting salt; drain and run under cold water to cool.

3 In a large salad bowl, toss together cooled noodles and all vegetables. In a small bowl, whisk together all dressing ingredients. Drizzle dressing over salad; toss to coat.

4 Remove pork from oven and shred the meat with a fork. Toss the shredded pork with the salad and serve.

Exchanges/Choices

1 Starch	1 Vegetable
1 Lean Meat	1 1/2 Fat

Calories	215
Calories from Fat	90
Total Fat	10.0 g
Saturated Fat	2.3 g
Trans Fat	0.0 g
Cholesterol	30 mg
Sodium	335 mg
Potassium	380 mg
Total Carbohydrate	19 g
Dietary Fiber	2 g
Sugars	3 g
Protein	14 g
Phosphorus	160 mg

Chef's Tip

If you can't find Napa (or Chinese) cabbage for this recipe, regular cabbage will work just fine.

Italian Garden Frittata

Makes: 8 servings   *Serving Size: 1/8 recipe*   *Prep Time: 15 minutes*

8 ounces uncooked whole-wheat angel hair pasta, broken in half
   nonstick cooking spray
2 zucchini, diced
1 15-ounce can no-salt-added diced tomatoes, drained
3 garlic cloves, minced
1 tsp dried basil
1/2 tsp salt (optional)
12 ounces egg substitute
1/2 cup shredded part-skim mozzarella cheese

1 Preheat oven to 300°F. Cook pasta according to package directions, omitting salt. Drain.

2 Coat a large oven-safe skillet with cooking spray and sauté zucchini over medium-high heat for about 8 minutes. Stir frequently.

3 Add diced tomatoes, garlic, basil, and salt (optional). Add cooked pasta and cook 1 minute, tossing to coat.

4 Add egg substitute and cheese and mix well to distribute eggs evenly. Cook 3–5 more minutes.

5 Place in oven and bake for 15 minutes

Exchanges/Choices
1 1/2 Starch   1 Vegetable
1 Lean Meat

Calories 160
  Calories from Fat 20
Total Fat . . . . 2.0 g
  Saturated Fat . . . . 0.8 g
  Trans Fat . . . . 0.0 g
Cholesterol . . . . 5 mg
Sodium . . . . 150 mg
Potassium . . . . 325 mg
Total Carbohydrate . . . . . . 25 g
  Dietary Fiber . . . . 4 g
  Sugars . . . . 3 g
Protein . . . . 12 g
Phosphorus . . . . 140 mg

Dietitian's Tip

Pasta is a delicious addition to this frittata.

Beef Kabobs GF LC

Makes: 4 servings   *Serving Size: 2 skewers*   *Prep Time: 20 minutes*

1   pint button mushrooms
1   large zucchini, sliced into
    1/2-inch-thick rounds
1   large yellow squash, sliced into
    1/2-inch-thick rounds
2   red bell peppers, sliced into 1-inch
    chunks
1   pound beef tenderloin, cut into
    1-inch cubes
1/2 cup fat-free Italian dressing
8   bamboo skewers, soaked in warm
    water

1 Prepare an indoor or outdoor grill.

2 Assemble kabobs by alternating mushrooms, zucchini, squash, peppers, and beef on each skewer.

3 Brush all sides of kabobs with Italian dressing. Grill over medium heat for 10 minutes, turning occasionally.

Exchanges/Choices
3 Vegetable   3 Lean Meat

Calories 210
  Calories from Fat 65
Total Fat . . . . 7.0 g
  Saturated Fat . . . . 2.4 g
  Trans Fat . . . . 0.0 g
Cholesterol . . . . 60 mg
Sodium . . . . 405 mg
Potassium . . . . 985 mg
Total Carbohydrate . . . . . . 14 g
  Dietary Fiber . . . . 4 g
  Sugars . . . . 9 g
Protein . . . . 25 g
Phosphorus . . . . 310 mg

Chef's Tip

If you don't soak these skewers before using them, they can catch fire on the grill!

Herb-Grilled Potatoes GF

Makes: 6 servings   *Serving Size: 2 potatoes (8 quarters)*   *Prep Time: 10 minutes*

12	small red potatoes, cut into quarters
1/2	tsp ground black pepper
3/4	tsp salt (optional)
1	small onion, thinly sliced
3	garlic cloves, minced
1	Tbsp olive oil
2	tsp dried rosemary nonstick cooking spray

1 Prepare an indoor or outdoor grill.

2 In a large bowl, toss together all ingredients.

3 Cut aluminum foil into six 8 × 8-inch pieces. Spray foil with cooking spray. Put 2 cups of potato mixture into one foil piece and fold together to create a packet.

4 Repeat procedure for remaining five aluminum foil pieces.

5 Place aluminum foil packets on grill and cook over medium-high heat for 30–40 minutes.

Exchanges/Choices
2 Starch

Calories 145
  Calories from Fat 20
Total Fat . . . . .2.5 g
  Saturated Fat . . . . .0.4 g
  Trans Fat . . . . .0.0 g
Cholesterol. . . . . 0 mg
Sodium . . . . 10 mg
Potassium. . . . . 530 mg
Total Carbohydrate . . . . . . 29 g
  Dietary Fiber . . . . 3 g
  Sugars . . . . 2 g
Protein . . . . 3 g
Phosphorus . . . . 125 mg

Chef's Tip

Cooking potatoes in a foil packet is a great way to enhance their flavor.

JUNE
WEEK 3

DAY 1
Harvest Beef
    Burrito   200

DAY 2
Lemon Chicken with
    Bell Peppers   201

DAY 3
Vegetable
    Quesadillas   202
Fruit with Dip   203

DAY 4
Sesame-Crusted
    Salmon   204
Stir-Fried
    Vegetables   205

DAY 5
Egg Salad
    Sandwich   206

GROCERY LIST

Fresh Produce
Apples—2
Avocado—1
Bananas—2
Bell peppers, green—2
Bell peppers, red—2
Broccoli—3 heads
Cantaloupe—1
Carrots, medium—2
Lemon—1
Melon, honeydew—1
Onion, yellow or white—1
Pea pods—2 cups
Strawberries—1 cup
Tomatoes, small—2
Watermelon—1

Meat, Poultry, & Fish
Beef, flank steak—1 pound
Chicken breasts, boneless,
    skinless, 4 ounces each—4
Salmon fillets, 4 ounces
    each—4

Grains, Bread, & Pasta
Bread, whole-wheat—8 slices
Tortillas, whole-wheat, low-
    carb, 10-inch—10

Dairy & Cheese
Cheese, mozzarella, reduced-
    fat, shredded—3/4 cup
Eggs

Canned Goods & Sauces
Beans, black, canned—1 cup
Broth, chicken, fat-free,
    low-sodium, 14.5-ounce
    can—1
Soy sauce, lite
Tomato paste, can—1

Frozen Foods
Whipped topping, sugar-
    free—4 ounces

Staples, Seasonings, & Baking Needs
Black pepper, ground
Cayenne pepper
Chili powder
Cumin
Flour, all-purpose
Lemon juice
Mayonnaise, light
Mustard, Dijon
Nonstick cooking spray
Oil, canola
Oil, olive
Oil, sesame
Oregano
Salt
Sesame seeds
Vanilla extract

Miscellaneous
Pudding, vanilla,
    sugar-free—1 cup
Salsa
Tofu, firm, silken—8 ounces

Harvest Beef Burrito

Makes: 6 servings   *Serving Size: 1 burrito*   *Prep Time: 15 minutes*

1 tsp olive oil
1 pound flank steak, sliced into 1-inch pieces
1 Tbsp chili powder
1 tsp cayenne pepper
1 tsp cumin
4 cups broccoli florets
1 cup canned black beans, rinsed and drained
1/2 tsp salt (optional)
6 10-inch whole-wheat, low-carb tortillas

1 Heat oil in a large sauté pan and sear beef over high heat. Reduce heat to medium.

2 Add chili powder, cayenne pepper, cumin, broccoli, beans, and salt (optional) and cook 5 more minutes. Remove from heat.

3 Place even amounts of meat and bean mixture in a tortilla and wrap.

4 Repeat for remaining five tortillas.

The American Diabetes Association recommends eating only a small amount of saturated fat every day. This recipe is higher in saturated fat, so try to balance it by eating foods low in saturated fat at your other meals today.

Exchanges/Choices
1 1/2 Starch   3 Lean Meat

Calories	245
Calories from Fat	70
Total Fat	8.0 g
Saturated Fat	2.0 g
Trans Fat	0.0 g
Cholesterol	25 mg
Sodium	395 mg
Potassium	515 mg
Total Carbohydrate	28 g
Dietary Fiber	16 g
Sugars	3 g
Protein	27 g
Phosphorus	320 mg

Dietitian's Tip

This dish can be made just as easily with chicken pieces, further reducing its fat content.

Lemon Chicken with Bell Peppers LC

Makes: 4 servings   *Serving Size: 1 chicken breast*   *Prep Time: 15 minutes*

4	4-ounce boneless, skinless chicken breasts
1 1/2	tsp dried oregano
1/2	tsp salt (optional)
1/4	tsp ground black pepper
1/4	tsp cayenne pepper
	nonstick cooking spray
1 1/2	cups red bell pepper strips
1 1/2	cups green bell pepper strips
1	Tbsp grated lemon rind
1/2	cup fresh lemon juice
1/2	cup fat-free, low-sodium chicken broth
1	Tbsp tomato paste

1 Season the chicken with oregano, salt (optional), black pepper, and cayenne pepper.

2 Heat a large sauté pan coated with cooking spray over medium-high heat. Add chicken and sear on one side for 3 minutes or until lightly browned.

3 Turn chicken over; top with bell peppers, lemon rind, and lemon juice.

4 Cover, reduce heat, and simmer 15 minutes or until chicken is done.

5 Combine broth and tomato paste in a small bowl. Stir tomato mixture into pan; bring to a boil. Serve pepper mixture with chicken.

Exchanges/Choices
1 Vegetable   3 Lean Meat

Calories	160
Calories from Fat	25
Total Fat	3.0 g
Saturated Fat	0.9 g
Trans Fat	0.0 g
Cholesterol	65 mg
Sodium	160 mg
Potassium	435 mg
Total Carbohydrate	7 g
Dietary Fiber	2 g
Sugars	4 g
Protein	25 g
Phosphorus	205 mg

Chef's Tip

Be sure to grate only the yellow rind (the zest) of the lemon. The white part, or pith, is bitter.

Vegetable Quesadillas

Makes: 4 servings   *Serving Size: 1 quesadilla*   *Prep Time: 8 minutes*

nonstick cooking spray
1 cup diced red bell pepper
1 cup diced green bell pepper
1/2 cup diced onion
2 small tomatoes, cut into 6 slices
4 10-inch whole-wheat, low-carb tortillas
1/2 cup + 2 Tbsp reduced-fat shredded mozzarella cheese
4 Tbsp mashed avocado
1/4 cup salsa

1 Spray a large nonstick skillet with cooking spray. Over medium-high heat, sauté bell peppers and onion for about 4 minutes. Add tomatoes and sauté for 1 more minute.

2 Remove vegetables from pan. Spray pan again with cooking spray and add one tortilla to pan. Top tortilla with 2 1/2 Tbsp mozzarella cheese. Add 2/3 cup veggie mixture over cheese. Fold tortilla in half. Grill about 2 minutes each side.

3 Top quesadilla with 1 Tbsp avocado and 1 Tbsp salsa.

4 Repeat procedure for remaining three quesadillas.

Exchanges/Choices
1 Starch   1 Vegetable
1 Med-Fat Meat

Calories 185
 Calories from Fat 70
Total Fat . . . . .8.0 g
 Saturated Fat . . . . .2.4 g
 Trans Fat . . . . .0.0 g
Cholesterol . . . . 10 mg
Sodium . . . . 515 mg
Potassium . . . . 445 mg
Total Carbohydrate . . . . . . 28 g
 Dietary Fiber . . . . 15 g
 Sugars . . . . 6 g
Protein . . . . 14 g
Phosphorus . . . . 255 mg

Chef's Tip

Feel free to experiment with this dish by adding more of your favorite vegetables.

Fruit with Dip GF

Makes: 10 servings   *Serving Size: 1/10 recipe*   *Prep Time: 15 minutes*

Dip
- **1** cup sugar-free vanilla pudding
- **4** ounces light whipped topping
- **1** tsp vanilla extract

Fruit
- **1** cup cubed watermelon
- **1** cup cubed cantaloupe
- **1** cup cubed honeydew
- **1** cup strawberries, stems cut off
- **2** bananas, sliced
- **2** apples, sliced with skin on

1 In a medium bowl, combine dip ingredients and mix well.

2 Arrange fruit on a platter with dip bowl in middle. Provide toothpicks.

Exchanges/Choices
1 Fruit   1/2 Carbohydrate

Calories	100
Calories from Fat	20
Total Fat	2.0 g
Saturated Fat	1.3 g
Trans Fat	0.0 g
Cholesterol	0 mg
Sodium	45 mg
Potassium	295 mg
Total Carbohydrate	21 g
Dietary Fiber	2 g
Sugars	16 g
Protein	2 g
Phosphorus	60 mg

Chef's Tip

This is a wonderful dish to serve at a picnic. It looks beautiful on a platter, and the dip tastes so great it's hard to believe it's low-fat.

Sesame-Crusted Salmon LC

Makes: 4 servings   *Serving Size: 1 fillet*   *Prep Time: 10 minutes*

1/4   cup all-purpose flour
1/4   cup sesame seeds
1/2   tsp salt (optional)
1/4   tsp ground black pepper
 4   4-ounce salmon fillets
 1   tsp sesame oil
      nonstick cooking spray
 2   tsp canola oil

1 In a medium bowl, combine flour, sesame seeds, salt (optional), and pepper. Brush one side of each fillet with sesame oil. Press oiled side of fish into sesame mixture.

2 Coat a medium nonstick skillet with cooking spray. Heat canola oil over medium-high heat. Place salmon fillets crust side down into the hot pan.

3 Cook on both sides for 3–4 minutes.

Exchanges/Choices
1/2 Carbohydrate
3 Lean Meat   2 Fat

Calories	290
Calories from Fat	155
Total Fat	17.0 g
Saturated Fat	2.6 g
Trans Fat	0.0 g
Cholesterol	80 mg
Sodium	60 mg
Potassium	385 mg
Total Carbohydrate	6 g
Dietary Fiber	1 g
Sugars	0 g
Protein	27 g
Phosphorus	305 mg

Chef's Tip

This recipe is also good with tuna or halibut.

Stir-Fried Vegetables LC

Makes: 4 servings   *Serving Size: 1/4 recipe*   *Prep Time: 10 minutes*

nonstick cooking spray
1 tsp sesame oil
3 cups broccoli florets
2 cups pea pods
2 medium carrots, sliced into thin sticks
2 Tbsp lite soy sauce

1 Coat a large nonstick skillet with cooking spray and heat oil over medium heat. Add the broccoli, pea pods, and carrots. Stir-fry for 6–7 minutes.

2 Drizzle soy sauce over vegetables and continue to stir-fry for 1 more minute.

Exchanges/Choices
2 Vegetable

Calories 60
　Calories from Fat 15
Total Fat . . . . 1.5 g
　Saturated Fat . . . . 0.2 g
　Trans Fat . . . . 0.0 g
Cholesterol . . . . 0 mg
Sodium . . . . 310 mg
Potassium . . . . 350 mg
Total Carbohydrate . . . . . . 9 g
　Dietary Fiber . . . . 3 g
　Sugars . . . . 4 g
Protein . . . . 3 g
Phosphorus . . . . 70 mg

Dietitian's Tip

You can make a meal out of these vegetables by adding chicken or beef and serving them over brown rice.

Egg Salad Sandwich

Makes: 4 servings   *Serving Size: 1 sandwich*   *Prep Time: 5 minutes*

4	hard-boiled eggs, peeled and mashed
2	egg whites
8	ounces silken firm tofu, patted dry
1	Tbsp Dijon mustard
2	Tbsp light mayonnaise
1/4	tsp salt (optional)
1/4	tsp ground black pepper
8	slices whole-wheat bread

1 In a medium bowl, combine all ingredients except bread and mix well.

2 Spoon 1/2 cup egg salad onto 1 slice whole-wheat bread and top with slice of whole-wheat bread.

3 Repeat for remaining three sandwiches.

Exchanges/Choices
2 Starch   2 Med-Fat Meat

Calories	280
Calories from Fat	90
Total Fat	10.0 g
Saturated Fat	2.5 g
Trans Fat	0.0 g
Cholesterol	185 mg
Sodium	530 mg
Potassium	355 mg
Total Carbohydrate	26 g
Dietary Fiber	4 g
Sugars	5 g
Protein	19 g
Phosphorus	270 mg

Chef's Tip

This a great recipe to try if you've never eaten tofu. The consistency of tofu is similar to that of hard-boiled egg whites. Tofu picks up the flavor of foods it's mixed with—you'll barely know it's there.

JUNE
WEEK 4

DAY 1
Shrimp Skewers with
Pineapple and
Peppers   208
Green Bean Tomato
Salad   209

DAY 2
Stir-Fried Beef and
Noodles   210

DAY 3
Pork Tenderloin with
Black Bean and Corn
Salsa   211

DAY 4
Chicken Guacamole
Salad   212

DAY 5
Broccoli Scallop
Pasta   213
Caprese Salad   214

**DESSERT OF THE
MONTH**
Banana Split
Cake   215

GROCERY LIST

Fresh Produce
Avocado, medium—1
Bananas, medium—4
Basil—1 bunch
Bell peppers, green—3
Broccoli—1 head
Cilantro—1 bunch
Garlic—2 cloves
Onion, red—1
Onion, yellow or white—1
Tomatoes—5
Tomatoes, cherry—1 pint

Meat, Poultry, & Fish
Bay scallops—1 pint
Beef, flank steak—1 pound
Chicken breasts, boneless,
  skinless—1 pound
Pork tenderloin—1 pound
Shrimp, peeled and
  deveined—10 ounces

Grains, Bread, & Pasta
Pasta, angel hair, whole-
  wheat—8 ounces
Pasta, rotini, whole-wheat—
  8 ounces

Dairy & Cheese
Cheese, mozzarella, fresh—3
  ounces
Cheese, Parmesan—1 small
  block
Cream cheese, light—8
  ounces
Milk, fat-free—2 cups
Sour cream, fat-free—2 Tbsp

Canned Goods & Sauces
Beans, black, canned—1 cup
Broth, chicken, fat-free, low-
  sodium, 14.5-ounce cans—2

Hot pepper sauce
Pineapple chunks, packed in
  juice, 16-ounce cans—2
Soy sauce, lite

Frozen Foods
Corn—1 cup
Green beans, cut—16-ounce
  bag
Whipped topping, fat-free,
  8-ounce container—1

Staples, Seasonings,
& Baking Needs
Basil
Black pepper, ground
Mustard, Dijon
Mustard, dry
Nonstick cooking spray
Oil, canola
Oil, olive
Red pepper flakes
Sage
Salt
Sugar
Tarragon
Thyme
Vinegar, apple cider
Vinegar, balsamic

Miscellaneous
Almonds, slivered—3 Tbsp
Bamboo skewers—10
Graham crackers
Peanut butter, creamy
Pecans
Pudding mix, instant, vanilla,
  sugar-free—1 ounce
Salad dressing, Italian, fat-
  free—3 Tbsp
Wine, white

Shrimp Skewers with Pineapple and Peppers GF

Makes: 5 servings   *Serving Size: 2 skewers*   *Prep Time: 10 minutes*

10 ounces peeled and deveined shrimp
 1 16-ounce can pineapple chunks packed in juice, drained (reserve 1/4 cup juice)
 3 green bell peppers, cut into 1-inch chunks
 3 Tbsp fat-free Italian dressing
10 bamboo skewers, soaked in warm water

1 Prepare an indoor or outdoor grill.

2 Assemble skewers by alternating shrimp, pineapple, and green pepper on each skewer.

3 In a small bowl, whisk together reserved 1/4 cup pineapple juice and Italian dressing.

4 Brush all sides of shrimp skewers with dressing. Sprinkle with salt (optional) and pepper. Grill over medium heat for 5 minutes, turning occasionally.

Exchanges/Choices
1 Fruit   1 Vegetable
1 Lean Meat

Calories 125
  Calories from Fat 10
Total Fat . . . . 1.0 g
  Saturated Fat . . . . 0.2 g
  Trans Fat . . . . 0.0 g
Cholesterol . . . . 90 mg
Sodium . . . . 590 mg
Potassium . . . . 370 mg
Total Carbohydrate . . . . . . 16 g
  Dietary Fiber . . . . 2 g
  Sugars . . . . 13 g
Protein . . . . 13 g
Phosphorus . . . . 155 mg

Chef's Tip

Make this dish even more beautiful by using different color bell peppers, such as red, yellow, and orange.

Green Bean Tomato Salad GF LC

Makes: 7 servings   *Serving Size: 1/7 recipe*   *Prep Time: 20 minutes*

16	ounces frozen cut green beans
2	Tbsp olive oil
1/4	cup apple cider vinegar
1/2	tsp salt (optional)
2	tsp sugar
1/8	tsp dried basil
1	tsp Dijon mustard
3	Tbsp slivered almonds, toasted
2	cups cherry tomatoes, halved

1 Cook green beans according to package directions.

2 In a salad bowl, whisk together olive oil, vinegar, salt (optional), sugar, basil, and mustard. Add green beans, almonds, and tomatoes and toss well.

3 Serve warm or cover and chill 30 minutes.

Exchanges/Choices

2 Vegetable   1 Fat

Calories 85
  Calories from Fat 55
Total Fat . . . . 6.0 g
  Saturated Fat . . . . 0.7 g
  Trans Fat . . . . 0.0 g
Cholesterol . . . . 0 mg
Sodium . . . . 20 mg
Potassium . . . . 245 mg
Total Carbohydrate . . . . 8 g
  Dietary Fiber . . . . 3 g
  Sugars . . . . 4 g
Protein . . . . 2 g
Phosphorus . . . . 45 mg

Chef's Tip

You can use fresh green beans in this salad if you wish.

Stir-Fried Beef and Noodles

Makes: 6 servings   *Serving Size: 1/6 recipe*   *Prep Time: 15 minutes*

8   ounces uncooked whole-wheat angel hair pasta
2   Tbsp creamy peanut butter
1/4   cup canned fat-free, low-sodium chicken broth
1   Tbsp lite soy sauce
1/4   tsp hot pepper sauce
2   tsp canola oil
1   pound flank steak, sliced into thin strips against the grain

1 Cook pasta according to directions.

2 In a small bowl, whisk together peanut butter, chicken broth, soy sauce, and hot pepper sauce. Set aside.

3 Add oil to a medium sauté pan over high heat. Add beef strips and stir-fry for 4 minutes. Add peanut sauce to meat and stir-fry 2 more minutes.

4 Drain pasta and toss with the beef.

Exchanges/Choices
2 Starch   3 Lean Meat

Calories 285
  Calories from Fat 80
Total Fat . . . . .9.0 g
  Saturated Fat . . . . .2.4 g
  Trans Fat . . . . .0.0 g
Cholesterol . . . . 25 mg
Sodium . . . . 175 mg
Potassium . . . . 310 mg
Total Carbohydrate . . . . . . 29 g
  Dietary Fiber . . . . 4 g
  Sugars . . . . 1 g
Protein . . . . 23 g
Phosphorus . . . . 235 mg

Chef's Tip

Peanut butter is the secret ingredient in this recipe. It adds flavor, richness, and creaminess to the sauce.

Pork Tenderloin with Black Bean and Corn Salsa GF

Makes: 4 servings   *Serving Size: 4 ounces*   *Prep Time: 10 minutes*

1	cup canned black beans, drained and rinsed
1	cup frozen corn, thawed
1	cup diced tomato
1/2	cup chopped red onion
1	Tbsp dried thyme
1	Tbsp dried sage
1	Tbsp dried tarragon
2	tsp dry mustard
1/4	tsp salt (optional)
1/4	tsp ground black pepper
1	pound pork tenderloin, trimmed of fat

1 Preheat oven to 350°F. In a small bowl, toss together beans, corn, tomatoes, and onion.

2 Combine thyme, sage, tarragon, mustard, salt (optional), and pepper in a small bowl and transfer to a plate, spreading evenly.

3 Roll pork tenderloin in mixture and coat well.

4 Bake for 30 minutes or until juices run clear. Serve pork sliced with salsa.

Exchanges/Choices
1 Starch   3 Lean Meat

Calories	225
Calories from Fat	35
Total Fat	4.0 g
Saturated Fat	1.2 g
Trans Fat	0.0 g
Cholesterol	60 mg
Sodium	100 mg
Potassium	750 mg
Total Carbohydrate	22 g
Dietary Fiber	6 g
Sugars	4 g
Protein	28 g
Phosphorus	310 mg

Chef's Tip

This recipe is also great with beef tenderloin.

Chicken Guacamole Salad GF LC

Makes: 5 servings   *Serving Size: 1/5 recipe*   *Prep Time: 35 minutes*

1 14.5-ounce can fat-free, low-sodium chicken broth
1 can water
1 pound boneless, skinless chicken breasts
1 medium avocado, finely diced
1 small onion, finely diced (about 1/2 cup)
2 small tomatoes, diced
2 Tbsp chopped fresh cilantro
2 Tbsp fat-free sour cream
1/2 tsp salt (optional)
1/4 tsp ground black pepper

1 In a medium saucepan, bring broth and 1 can water to a boil. Add chicken breasts and simmer over low heat for about 20 minutes.

2 Remove chicken and chop into small chunks. Cool in a medium bowl for 10 minutes. Add remaining ingredients and mix well.

Exchanges/Choices
1 Vegetable   3 Lean Meat
1/2 Fat

Calories 170
 Calories from Fat 65
Total Fat . . . . 7.0 g
 Saturated Fat . . . . 1.3 g
 Trans Fat . . . . 0.0 g
Cholesterol . . . . 55 mg
Sodium . . . . 60 mg
Potassium . . . . 430 mg
Total Carbohydrate . . . . 7 g
 Dietary Fiber . . . . 3 g
 Sugars . . . . 2 g
Protein . . . . 21 g
Phosphorus . . . . 180 mg

Chef's Tip

You can serve this salad on toasted low-carb or gluten-free tortillas or pitas.

Broccoli Scallop Pasta [NEW]

Makes: 5 servings   *Serving Size: 1/5 of recipe*   *Prep Time: 15 minutes*

8	ounces whole-wheat rotini pasta
1	Tbsp olive oil
	nonstick cooking spray
12	ounces fresh or frozen broccoli florets (thawed if frozen)
2	Tbsp minced garlic
3/4	cup dry white wine
1/2	cup fat-free, low-sodium chicken broth
1	pound bay scallops, patted dry
1/2	tsp salt (optional)
1/2	tsp ground black pepper
1/4	tsp crushed red pepper flakes
1/4	cup freshly grated Parmesan cheese
2	Tbsp chopped fresh basil

1 Cook pasta according to package directions, omitting salt. Drain and set aside.

2 While pasta is cooking, heat olive oil and a generous amount of cooking spray in a large skillet over medium-high heat.

3 Add broccoli and sauté for 2–3 minutes. Add garlic and white wine and cook until wine in reduced by half, about 3 minutes.

4 Add chicken broth, scallops, salt (optional), pepper, and red pepper flakes and sauté until scallops are just cooked through, about 4 minutes.

5 Add cooked pasta to scallops. Stir in Parmesan cheese and fresh basil.

Exchanges/Choices

2 Starch   1 Vegetable
3 Lean Meat

Calories	325
Calories from Fat	55
Total Fat	6.0 g
Saturated Fat	1.3 g
Trans Fat	0.0 g
Cholesterol	30 mg
Sodium	270 mg
Potassium	540 mg
Total Carbohydrate	42 g
Dietary Fiber	7 g
Sugars	2 g
Protein	25 g
Phosphorus	470 mg

Chef's Tip

Frozen scallops work great for this recipe; just be sure to thaw them in the refrigerator or under cold running water before drying and sautéing.

Caprese Salad GF LC

Makes: 4 servings   *Serving Size: 1/4 recipe*   *Prep Time: 5 minutes*

3   ounces fresh mozzarella
2   medium tomatoes, sliced into 8 slices
8   fresh basil leaves
1/4 tsp salt (optional)
1/8 tsp ground black pepper
1   Tbsp balsamic vinegar

1 Slice mozzarella into eight 1/4-inch-thick slices. Layer tomato, basil leaves, and cheese into stacks, starting with tomato and ending with cheese (tomato, basil, cheese, tomato, basil, cheese), making 4 stacks.

2 Sprinkle each stack with salt (optional) and pepper. Drizzle balsamic vinegar lightly over each stack.

Exchanges/Choices
1 Med-Fat Meat

Calories 70
   Calories from Fat 40
Total Fat . . . . 4.5 g
   Saturated Fat . . . . 1.5 g
   Trans Fat . . . . 0.0 g
Cholesterol . . . . 5 mg
Sodium . . . . 20 mg
Potassium . . . . 205 mg
Total Carbohydrate . . . . 4 g
   Dietary Fiber . . . . 1 g
   Sugars . . . . 3 g
Protein . . . . 4 g
Phosphorus . . . . 100 mg

Chef's Tip

Fresh mozzarella cheese comes packed in water. You can usually find it in your grocer's deli or near the cheese aisle. Its texture is much different than the mozzarella you find on your pizza.

Banana Split Cake

Makes: 16 servings　　　*Serving Size: 1 slice*　　　*Prep Time: 15 minutes*

6 1/2　graham cracker sheets (two 1 1/2-inch squares per sheet)

1　ounce sugar-free, instant vanilla pudding mix

2　cups fat-free milk

8　ounces light cream cheese

10　ounces canned crushed pineapple packed in juice, drained

4　medium bananas, sliced 8-ounce container fat-free whipped topping

3　Tbsp pecans, chopped

1 Cover the bottom of a 9 × 13-inch pan with graham cracker sheets.

2 In a medium bowl, prepare pudding with fat-free milk according to package directions. Add cream cheese to pudding and whip together. Spread pudding mixture over graham crackers.

3 Spread the crushed pineapple over the pudding layer and top with bananas and then whipped topping. Sprinkle pecans on top.

The American Diabetes Association recommends eating only a small amount of saturated fat every day. This recipe is higher in saturated fat, so try to balance it by eating foods low in saturated fat at your other meals today.

Exchanges/Choices

1 1/2 Carbohydrate　　1 Fat

Calories 140
　Calories from Fat 45
Total Fat . . . . 5.0 g
　Saturated Fat . . . . 2.0 g
　Trans Fat . . . . 0.0 g
Cholesterol. . . . . 10 mg
Sodium . . . . 195 mg
Potassium. . . . . 220 mg
Total Carbohydrate . . . . . . 21 g
　Dietary Fiber . . . . 1 g
　Sugars . . . . 13 g
Protein . . . . 3 g
Phosphorus . . . . 120 mg

Chef's Tip

You can add sliced fresh strawberries on top of this cake if you like

JULY

Happy Birthday, America!

Fire up the grill and enjoy great summer cookouts with these nutritious backyard favorites. Grilling is a natural low-fat cooking method that allows fat to drip from foods rather than soak in. Grilling naturally boosts the flavor of foods without adding fat. Marinades can be a great way to add flavor. And don't be afraid to experiment with grilling new foods, like this month's grilled fruit recipe.

Also, kids and teenagers with diabetes love diabetes summer camps, where they can meet friends, have fun, and learn something along the way! To find a diabetes camp sponsored by the American Diabetes Association near you, visit the American Diabetes Association at www.diabetes.org.

Veggie Lasagna Roulades (page 240)
Cherry Tarts (page 251)

What's better than a great lasagna? You'll like this rolled pasta dish—it looks impressive, but is so easy to make! This month's festive dessert couldn't be any easier to make. These tarts look beautiful and taste even better, with a mixture of cream cheese, vanilla wafers, and cherries.

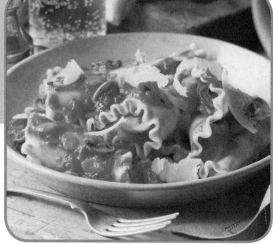

 gluten-free recipe, but always check ingredients for gluten.

 these recipes contain 15 grams of carbohydrate or less per serving.

 new recipe for the second edition.

JULY RECIPES

JULY
WEEK 1

DAY 1
Honey Lime
    Chicken   220
Grilled Fruit   221

DAY 2
Shrimp Salad   222

DAY 3
Grilled Pizza   223

DAY 4
Turkey Club   224

DAY 5
Apple and Raisin Stuffed
    Pork Chops   225
Grilled Tomatoes   226

GROCERY LIST

Fresh Produce
Apples, Granny Smith—3
Broccoli—2 heads
Carrots, medium—3
Garlic—1 head
Lettuce, romaine—1 large
    head
Mangoes, small—2
Onion, red—1
Spinach—1 bunch
Strawberries—1 pint
Tomato—1

Meat, Poultry, & Fish
Chicken breasts, boneless,
    skinless, 4 ounces each—4
Pork chops, center-cut,
    4 ounces each—4
Shrimp, medium, peeled,
    deveined, cooked—
    10 ounces
Turkey bacon—4 slices
Turkey breast, deli style,
    roasted, no-added-salt,
    thinly sliced—8 ounces

Grains, Bread, & Pasta
Pizza crust, whole-wheat,
    prepackaged, 12-inch—1
Sandwich thins, whole-
    wheat—4

Dairy & Cheese
Cheese, feta, reduced-
    fat—3/4 cup

Canned Goods & Sauces
Broth, chicken, fat-free,
    low-sodium, 14.5-ounce
    can—1
Hot pepper sauce
Pineapple chunks, packed in
    juice, 16-ounce can—1
Soy sauce, lite

Staples, Seasonings, & Baking Needs
Black pepper, ground
Cinnamon
Honey
Lime juice
Mayonnaise, light
Mustard, Dijon
Nonstick cooking spray
Nutmeg
Oil, canola
Oil, olive
Red pepper flakes
Sage
Salt
Vinegar, balsamic
Vinegar, red wine

Miscellaneous
Bamboo skewers—8
Brandy
Orange juice—1/2 cup
Raisins—2 Tbsp
Sun-dried tomatoes—small
    package, not packed in oil

Honey Lime Chicken GF LC

Makes: 4 servings   *Serving Size: 1 chicken breast*   *Prep Time: 5 minutes*

1/3   cup lime juice
3   Tbsp honey
3   garlic cloves, minced
1   Tbsp lite soy sauce
4   4-ounce boneless, skinless chicken breasts

1 In a medium bowl, whisk together lime juice, honey, garlic, and soy sauce. Place chicken in bowl and marinate in the refrigerator for at least 20 minutes (or longer, if possible).

2 Prepare an indoor or outdoor grill. Remove chicken from marinade and cook over medium heat until done.

Exchanges/Choices
1/2 Carbohydrate   3 Lean Meat

Calories 160
  Calories from Fat 25
Total Fat . . . . .3.0 g
  Saturated Fat . . . . .0.8 g
  Trans Fat . . . . .0.0 g
Cholesterol. . . . . 65 mg
Sodium . . . . 130 mg
Potassium. . . . . 220 mg
Total Carbohydrate . . . . 8 g
  Dietary Fiber . . . . 0 g
  Sugars . . . . 7 g
Protein . . . . 24 g
Phosphorus . . . . 180 mg

Chef's Tip

You can substitute lemon juice for lime juice if you prefer.

Grilled Fruit `GF`

Makes: 8 servings   *Serving Size: 1 skewer*   *Prep Time: 20 minutes*

1 pint strawberries, stemmed and halved

2 small mangoes, peeled and cut into 1-inch chunks

1 16-ounce can pineapple chunks packed in juice, drained

2 Granny Smith apples, peeled, cored, and sliced into eighths

8 bamboo skewers, soaked in warm water
nonstick cooking spray

1 Prepare an indoor or outdoor grill.

2 Assemble kabobs by alternating strawberries, mango, pineapple, and apple on each skewer.

3 Lightly spray all sides of kabobs with cooking spray. Grill over medium heat for 6 minutes, turning occasionally.

Exchanges/Choices
1 1/2 Fruit

Calories 85
  Calories from Fat 0
Total Fat . . . . .0.0 g
  Saturated Fat . . . . .0.1 g
  Trans Fat . . . . .0.0 g
Cholesterol. . . . . 0 mg
Sodium . . . . 0 mg
Potassium. . . . . 215 mg
Total Carbohydrate . . . . . . 21 g
  Dietary Fiber . . . . 3 g
  Sugars . . . . 18 g
Protein . . . . 1 g
Phosphorus . . . . 20 mg

Chef's Tip

Grilling fruit is a unique way to bring out its natural sweetness.

Shrimp Salad GF LC

Makes: 6 servings   *Serving Size: 2 cups*   *Prep Time: 15 minutes*

Salad

10	ounces peeled, deveined, and cooked medium shrimp (about 3 cups)
1/4	cup crumbled reduced-fat feta cheese
1/4	cup chopped sun-dried tomatoes
4	cups broccoli florets
1 1/2	cups carrots, sliced into rounds (about 3 medium carrots)
1	large head romaine lettuce, chopped

Dressing

1/2	cup orange juice
2	Tbsp rice wine vinegar
2	Tbsp olive oil
1/2	tsp hot pepper sauce
1/4	tsp salt (optional)
1/4	tsp ground black pepper

1 In a large salad bowl, toss together all salad ingredients.

2 In a medium bowl, whisk together all dressing ingredients.

3 Drizzle dressing over salad and toss well to coat.

Exchanges/Choices

2 Vegetable   2 Lean Meat
1/2 Fat

Calories	165
Calories from Fat	65
Total Fat	7.0 g
Saturated Fat	1.5 g
Trans Fat	0.0 g
Cholesterol	100 mg
Sodium	615 mg
Potassium	695 mg
Total Carbohydrate	13 g
Dietary Fiber	5 g
Sugars	6 g
Protein	15 g
Phosphorus	245 mg

Chef's Tip

This recipe has a lot of ingredients, but it's so easy to make!

Grilled Pizza

Makes: 6 servings   *Serving Size: 1 slice*   *Prep Time: 10 minutes*

Sauce
- 1/4   cup balsamic vinegar
- 1   Tbsp Dijon mustard
- 1/2   Tbsp honey
- 1/4   tsp crushed red pepper flakes

Topping
- 1   tsp olive oil
- 1/4   cup chopped sun-dried tomatoes
- 4   cups chopped fresh spinach
- 2   garlic cloves, minced
- 1/4   tsp salt (optional)
- 1/4   tsp ground black pepper
- 1   12-inch prepackaged whole-wheat pizza crust
- 2   Tbsp crumbled reduced-fat feta cheese

1 Prepare an indoor or outdoor grill and spray grill with cooking spray. In a small bowl, whisk together sauce ingredients.

2 Heat oil in a large nonstick skillet over medium-high heat. Add sun-dried tomatoes and cook for about 2 minutes. Add spinach and garlic and cook 2 more minutes.

3 Add sauce to pan and cook 3 minutes until sauce begins to reduce. Add salt (optional) and pepper.

4 Place pizza crust on top of grill. Spread spinach mixture on top of crust. Sprinkle with cheese and grill 5–7 minutes or until cheese begins to melt.

Exchanges/Choices
1 1/2 Starch   1/2 Carbohydrate
1/2 Fat

Calories	160
Calories from Fat	35
Total Fat	4.0 g
Saturated Fat	1.4 g
Trans Fat	0.0 g
Cholesterol	0 mg
Sodium	390 mg
Potassium	340 mg
Total Carbohydrate	28 g
Dietary Fiber	5 g
Sugars	6 g
Protein	7 g
Phosphorus	140 mg

Chef's Tip

Grilled pizza isn't your traditional pizza, but it's delicious, with a crispy crust and smoky flavor.

Turkey Club

Makes: 4 servings   *Serving Size: 1 club*   *Prep Time: 5 minutes*

- **4** tsp light mayonnaise
- **4** whole-wheat sandwich thins
- **8** ounces thinly sliced reduced-sodium deli turkey breast
- **4** slices turkey bacon, cooked
- **4** romaine lettuce leaves, torn into pieces
- **1** tomato, sliced into 8 thin slices

1 Spread 1 tsp mayonnaise on 1 half of a sandwich thin. Top with 2 ounces turkey breast, 1 slice turkey bacon, 1 lettuce leaf, and 2 slices tomato. Place other sandwich thin half on top of sandwich.

2 Repeat process for remaining three sandwiches.

Exchanges/Choices
1 1/2 Starch   2 Lean Meat

Calories 205
 Calories from Fat 55
Total Fat . . . . .6.0 g
 Saturated Fat . . . . .1.0 g
 Trans Fat . . . . .0.0 g
Cholesterol. . . . . 30 mg
Sodium . . . . 660 mg
Potassium. . . . . 430 mg
Total Carbohydrate . . . . . . 24 g
 Dietary Fiber . . . . 6 g
 Sugars . . . . 3 g
Protein . . . . 19 g
Phosphorus . . . . 265 mg

Dietitian's Tip

If your meal plan calls for more meat, you can add some extra lean deli ham to this sandwich.

Apple and Raisin Stuffed Pork Chops LC

Makes: 4 servings   *Serving Size: 1 pork chop*   *Prep Time: 20 minutes*

4	4-ounce center-cut pork chops
1	tsp canola oil
1/4	cup finely diced red onion
1/2	cup peeled, finely diced apple
2	Tbsp raisins
1/2	tsp minced garlic
1 1/2	Tbsp brandy or apple cider vinegar
1/4	cup fat-free, low-sodium chicken broth
1/4	tsp each nutmeg, cinnamon, sage, salt (optional), and ground black pepper

1 Prepare an indoor or outdoor grill. Prepare pork chops by slicing a 2-inch pocket in the side of each chop and set aside.

2 In a large sauté pan, heat oil over medium-high heat. Add onions and cook until they are caramelized (brown in color but not burned, about 7 minutes). Add apples and raisins and cook until the apples become soft.

3 Add garlic and cook for 30 seconds. Add brandy (or vinegar), chicken broth, and spices; cook until all of the moisture is reduced. Set aside to cool slightly.

4 Use a small spoon and gently stuff pork chops with apple mixture. Use only one or two spoonfuls of stuffing and do not overstuff chops.

5 Grill chops over medium-high heat for about 5–8 minutes per side or until done.

Exchanges/Choices
1/2 Carbohydrate   3 Lean Meat

Calories	155
Calories from Fat	55
Total Fat	6.0 g
Saturated Fat	1.8 g
Trans Fat	0.0 g
Cholesterol	45 mg
Sodium	65 mg
Potassium	285 mg
Total Carbohydrate	7 g
Dietary Fiber	1 g
Sugars	5 g
Protein	17 g
Phosphorus	115 mg

Chef's Tip

Take care not to overstuff the pork chops in this recipe. If you do, the stuffing will burst out during cooking and create quite a mess!

Grilled Tomatoes GF LC

Makes: 4 servings   *Serving Size: 1 tomato*   *Prep Time: 5 minutes*

4	medium tomatoes, sliced into 1/2-inch-thick slices
1	Tbsp olive oil
1/2	tsp salt (optional)
1/4	tsp ground black pepper
1/4	tsp cayenne pepper

1 Prepare an indoor or outdoor grill. Brush each side of each tomato slice lightly with olive oil.

2 Sprinkle salt (optional), pepper, and cayenne pepper on one side of each slice.

3 Grill tomatoes over medium heat for 2 minutes on each side.

Exchanges/Choices
1 Vegetable   1 Fat

Calories	55
Calories from Fat	30
Total Fat	3.5 g
Saturated Fat	0.5 g
Trans Fat	0.0 g
Cholesterol	0 mg
Sodium	5 mg
Potassium	295 mg
Total Carbohydrate	5 g
Dietary Fiber	2 g
Sugars	3 g
Protein	1 g
Phosphorus	30 mg

Chef's Tip

Here's a great way to use those extra tomatoes from the garden. Grilling vegetables adds a unique flavor.

JULY

WEEK 2

DAY 1
Tangy Tarragon
   Turkey Burgers   228
Red Potato Salad   229

DAY 2
Beef and Broccoli   230

DAY 3
Taco Salad with
   Black Beans   231

DAY 4
Tuna Salad with
   Pasta   232

DAY 5
Orange-Glazed
   Pork Loin
   Medallions   233
Mediterranean
   Couscous   234

GROCERY LIST

Fresh Produce
Broccoli—2 heads
Celery—2 stalks
Dill—1 bunch
Garlic—2 cloves
Lettuce, romaine—2 heads
Onion, red—1
Onion, yellow or white—1
Orange—1
Potatoes, red, new—3 pounds
Tomatoes, large—3

Meat, Poultry, & Fish
Beef sirloin, boneless—
   1 pound
Pork tenderloin—1 pound
Turkey bacon—8 slices
Turkey, ground, 93% lean—
   1 3/4 pound

Grains, Bread, & Pasta
Hamburger buns,
   whole-wheat—4
Pasta, elbow macaroni,
   whole-wheat—8 ounces

Dairy & Cheese
Cheese, sharp cheddar,
   75% reduced-fat,
   shredded—3/4 cup
Eggs
Sour cream, fat-free—1/2 cup
Yogurt, Greek, plain,
   fat-free—1/2 cup

Canned Goods & Sauces
Beans, black, canned—1 cup
Broth, beef, fat-free, low-
   sodium, 14.5-ounce can—1
Hot pepper sauce
Soy sauce, lite
Tuna, packed in water,
   12-ounce can—1

Staples, Seasonings, & Baking Needs
Black pepper, ground
Cornstarch
Mayonnaise, light
Mustard, Dijon
Nonstick cooking spray
Oil, canola
Oil, sesame
Sage
Salt
Sugar
Sugar substitute
Tarragon
Vinegar, rice wine

Miscellaneous
Chilies, red, whole, dried—2
Orange juice—1 3/4 cups
Salsa
Tortilla chips, baked

Tangy Tarragon Turkey Burgers

Makes: 4 servings *Serving Size: 1 burger* *Prep Time: 15 minutes*

3/4	pound 93% lean ground turkey
2	Tbsp dried tarragon
1/4	cup orange juice
1	tsp orange zest
1/4	tsp salt (optional)
1/4	tsp ground black pepper
1	garlic clove, minced
1/2	Tbsp hot pepper sauce
4	whole-wheat hamburger buns
8	medium tomato slices
4	lettuce leaves

1 Prepare an indoor or outdoor grill. Combine first 8 ingredients in a bowl. Divide turkey into 4 equal portions, shaping each into a 1/2-inch-thick patty.

2 Place patties on grill rack; grill 7 minutes on each side or until done. (Or coat a large nonstick skillet with cooking spray and cook patties over medium heat for 3–4 minutes per side, or until juices run clear.)

3 Serve burgers on buns with 2 tomato slices and 1 lettuce leaf.

Exchanges/Choices

1 1/2 Starch	1 Vegetable
2 Lean Meat	1/2 Fat

Calories	265
Calories from Fat	80
Total Fat	9.0 g
Saturated Fat	2.2 g
Trans Fat	0.1 g
Cholesterol	65 mg
Sodium	280 mg
Potassium	485 mg
Total Carbohydrate	26 g
Dietary Fiber	4 g
Sugars	6 g
Protein	21 g
Phosphorus	275 mg

Dietitian's Tip

Turkey burgers are traditionally lower in fat compared to beef burgers. However, this does not compromise any flavor in this recipe—the combination of orange, tarragon, and turkey makes for a mouthwatering burger.

Red Potato Salad GF

Makes: 10 servings *Serving Size: 1 cup* *Prep Time: 30 minutes*

3 pounds red new potatoes, quartered

1 cup finely diced red onion

1/2 cup finely diced celery

8 slices turkey bacon, cooked and cut into 1-inch strips

5 hard-boiled egg whites, sliced

1/2 cup light mayonnaise

1/2 cup fat-free sour cream

1/2 tsp salt (optional)

1/4 tsp ground black pepper

2 Tbsp fresh dill

1 Place potatoes in a large saucepan; cover with water. Bring to a boil; cook 12 minutes or longer until tender. Drain; cool.

2 In a large bowl, mix together remaining ingredients. Add potatoes and toss gently.

Exchanges/Choices
2 Starch 1/2 Carbohydrate
1/2 Fat

Calories	220
Calories from Fat	45
Total Fat	5.0 g
Saturated Fat	1.0 g
Trans Fat	0.0 g
Cholesterol	10 mg
Sodium	295 mg
Potassium	695 mg
Total Carbohydrate	37 g
Dietary Fiber	3 g
Sugars	4 g
Protein	8 g
Phosphorus	190 mg

Dietitian's Tip

Here's a twist on traditional potato salad, with a lot less fat but a unique, great taste.

Beef and Broccoli LC

Makes: 6 servings   *Serving Size: 1/6 recipe*   *Prep Time: 15 minutes*

2	tsp lite soy sauce
1/4	tsp sugar
1/4	tsp salt (optional)
1	pound boneless beef sirloin, cut across the grain into 1/4-inch-thick slices
1	Tbsp cornstarch
1	Tbsp lite soy sauce
1	Tbsp rice wine vinegar
1/4	cup fat-free, low-sodium beef broth or water
1	packet sugar substitute
1	tsp sesame oil
2	tsp canola oil nonstick cooking spray
1	garlic clove, minced

2	dried whole red chilies or 1/2 tsp crushed red pepper flakes
4	cups broccoli florets
1/4	cup water

1 In a small bowl, whisk together soy sauce, sugar, and salt (optional). Add beef and marinate for 20 minutes in the refrigerator.

2 Meanwhile, dissolve cornstarch in soy sauce and vinegar in a small bowl. Whisk in broth, sugar substitute, and sesame oil and set aside.

3 Heat canola oil and a generous amount of cooking spray in a large nonstick skillet or wok over high heat. Stir-fry beef for 2 minutes and remove from pan. Coat pan again with cooking spray and add garlic and whole chilies or red pepper flakes. Stir-fry for 30 seconds, then add broccoli and stir-fry 2 more minutes.

4 Add water and steam broccoli, covered, for 1 1/2–2 minutes, or until it is tender-crisp. Stir sauce and add it to pan along with beef and bring to a boil.

5 Reduce heat and simmer for 2 minutes, or until sauce is thickened and beef is heated through. Remove whole chilies before serving.

Exchanges/Choices

1 Vegetable   2 Lean Meat

Calories	135
Calories from Fat	45
Total Fat	5.0 g
Saturated Fat	1.3 g
Trans Fat	0.1 g
Cholesterol	30 mg
Sodium	215 mg
Potassium	360 mg
Total Carbohydrate	5 g
Dietary Fiber	1 g
Sugars	2 g
Protein	17 g
Phosphorus	155 mg

Dietitian's Tip

In traditional recipes, fat provides a lot of the flavor. If you add bold flavors instead, such as the garlic and red chilies in this recipe, you can enjoy great taste without extra calories.

Taco Salad with Black Beans GF

Makes: 7 servings   *Serving Size: about 1 3/4 cups*   *Prep Time: 20 minutes*

1	pound 93% lean ground turkey
1 1/2	cups salsa
5	cups chopped romaine lettuce
1	cup canned black beans, rinsed and drained
3/4	cup shredded 75% reduced-fat, sharp cheddar cheese
2	large tomatoes, chopped
1 1/2	cups crumbled baked tortilla chips

1 In a large nonstick skillet, brown ground turkey over high heat. Add salsa and bring to a boil. Set aside.

2 In a large salad bowl, add lettuce. Place cooked turkey on top of lettuce in center. Top with black beans, cheese, tomatoes, and tortilla chips.

Exchanges/Choices

1 Starch	1 Vegetable
2 Lean Meat	1/2 Fat

Calories 225
  Calories from Fat 65
Total Fat . . . . .7.0 g
  Saturated Fat . . . . .2.2 g
  Trans Fat . . . . .0.1 g
Cholesterol. . . . . 55 mg
Sodium . . . . 560 mg
Potassium. . . . . 640 mg
Total Carbohydrate . . . . . . 21 g
  Dietary Fiber . . . . 5 g
  Sugars . . . . 4 g
Protein . . . . 22 g
Phosphorus . . . . 285 mg

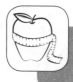

Chef's Tip

This recipe is just as tasty if it is made with diced chicken breast.

Tuna Salad with Pasta

Makes: 7 servings   *Serving Size: about 1 cup*   *Prep Time: 15 minutes*

8	ounces whole-wheat elbow macaroni, uncooked
1/2	cup chopped onion
1	cup chopped celery
1/2	cup fat-free plain Greek yogurt
1/4	cup light mayonnaise
1	12-ounce can tuna packed in water, drained
1/4	tsp salt (optional)
1/4	tsp ground black pepper

1 Cook pasta according to package directions, omitting salt. Drain and rinse under cold water.

2 In a salad bowl, add all ingredients and toss well. Refrigerate before serving.

Exchanges/Choices

2 Starch   1 Lean Meat

Calories	190
Calories from Fat	25
Total Fat	3.0 g
Saturated Fat	0.5 g
Trans Fat	0.0 g
Cholesterol	20 mg
Sodium	230 mg
Potassium	270 mg
Total Carbohydrate	27 g
Dietary Fiber	3 g
Sugars	3 g
Protein	15 g
Phosphorus	190 mg

Dietitian's Tip

If you want to reduce carbs even further, you can eliminate the pasta and serve the tuna salad in a lettuce wrap.

Orange-Glazed Pork Loin Medallions GF LC

Makes: 4 servings   *Serving Size: 4 ounces*   *Prep Time: 15 minutes*

Glaze

1 1/2	cups orange juice
2	Tbsp Dijon mustard
4	Tbsp rice wine vinegar
1/2	tsp dried sage

Pork

1	pound pork tenderloin, sliced into 1/2-inch-thick medallions
1/4	tsp salt (optional)
1/4	tsp ground black pepper nonstick cooking spray

1 In a small bowl, whisk together glaze ingredients.

2 Season tenderloin well with salt (optional) and pepper. Coat a medium sauté pan with cooking spray. Sear pork medallions over high heat on both sides for about 2 minutes. Remove meat from pan.

3 Add glaze mixture to pan and let it reduce by half or until it becomes thicker (a glaze consistency). Add meat back to pan for 30 seconds, cooking the meat in glaze on both sides.

Exchanges/Choices

1 Fruit	3 Lean Meat

Calories	170
Calories from Fat	30
Total Fat	3.5 g
Saturated Fat	1.0 g
Trans Fat	0.0 g
Cholesterol	60 mg
Sodium	225 mg
Potassium	555 mg
Total Carbohydrate	12 g
Dietary Fiber	0 g
Sugars	9 g
Protein	23 g
Phosphorus	220 mg

Chef's Tip

It is best to sear meat in a sauté pan that is not nonstick. That way the meat will turn a deep golden brown.

Mediterranean Couscous

Makes: 8 servings   *Serving Size: 1/2 cup*   *Prep Time: 5 minutes*

1	10-ounce box whole-wheat couscous
1/4	cup golden raisins
2	Tbsp pine nuts
1/4	tsp salt (optional)
1/4	tsp ground black pepper

1 Cook couscous according to package directions, omitting oil or butter. Fluff the cooked couscous with a fork.

2 Gently fold in raisins, pine nuts, salt (optional), and pepper. Serve warm.

Exchanges/Choices
2 Starch

Calories 160
Calories from Fat 15
Total Fat . . . . .1.5 g
Saturated Fat . . . . .0.2 g
Trans Fat . . . . .0.0 g
Cholesterol. . . . . 0 mg
Sodium . . . . 0 mg
Potassium. . . . . 105 mg
Total Carbohydrate . . . . . . 31 g
Dietary Fiber . . . . 3 g
Sugars . . . . 3 g
Protein . . . . 5 g
Phosphorus . . . . 80 mg

Chef's Tip

This quick and easy side dish can be a great accompaniment to many meals.

JULY

WEEK 3

GROCERY LIST

Fresh Produce
Basil—1 bunch
Bell peppers, green—3
Bell peppers, red—3
Bell peppers, yellow or
  orange—2
Garlic—1 head
Greens, field, mixed—4 cups
Lemon—1
Mushrooms, button—2 pints
Onions, red, large—2
Onion, yellow or white—1
Oregano—1 bunch
Pears, medium—2
Tarragon—1 bunch
Tomatoes—2
Zucchini, medium—1

Meat, Poultry, & Fish
Beef, flank steaks, 4 ounces
  each—4
Chicken breasts, boneless,
  skinless—1 pound
Orange roughy fillets,
  4 ounces each—4

Grains, Bread, & Pasta
Lasagna, whole-wheat—
  16 noodles
Pasta, orzo, whole-wheat—
  2 cups cooked
Pasta, penne, whole-
  wheat—16 ounces

Dairy & Cheese
Cheese, goat—1/4 cup
  crumbled
Cheese, Parmesan—1 small
  block
Cheese, ricotta, fat-free—
  1 cup
Eggs
Half-and-half, fat-free—
  1 pint
Margarine, trans-fat-free

Canned Goods & Sauces
Broth, chicken, fat-free,
  low-sodium, 14.5-ounce
  can—1
Pasta sauce, marinara, low-
  sodium, 16-ounce jar—1

Staples, Seasonings, & Baking Needs
Black pepper, ground
Cornstarch
Garlic salt
Honey
Nonstick cooking spray
Oil, olive
Parsley
Salt
Splenda Brown Sugar Blend
Vinegar, balsamic

Miscellaneous
Bamboo skewers—8
Pecans—1/4 cup
Salad dressing, Italian,
  fat-free—1/2 cup
Wine, white

Grilled Flank Steak with Onion Rings GF LC

Makes: 4 servings   *Serving Size: 1 steak*   *Prep Time: 5 minutes*

4 4-ounce flank steaks
1/2 tsp salt (optional)
1/4 tsp ground black pepper
2 large red onions, cut into 1/2-inch-thick rings
1 Tbsp olive oil

1 Prepare an indoor or outdoor grill. Season both sides of steaks with salt (optional) and pepper. Set aside.

2 In a large bowl, toss onion rings with oil to coat.

3 Place steaks and onions on grill over medium-high heat. Grill steaks for 5 minutes on each side. Grill onions for 6–7 minutes on each side.

Exchanges/Choices
2 Vegetable   3 Lean Meat
1 Fat

Calories 225
  Calories from Fat 80
Total Fat . . . . .9.0 g
  Saturated Fat . . . . .3.0 g
  Trans Fat . . . . .0.0 g
Cholesterol. . . . . 40 mg
Sodium . . . . 50 mg
Potassium. . . . . 445 mg
Total Carbohydrate . . . . . . 12 g
  Dietary Fiber . . . . 2 g
  Sugars . . . . 5 g
Protein . . . . 23 g
Phosphorus . . . . 205 mg

Chef's Tip

Be sure to slice flank steak against the grain for maximum tenderness.

Orzo Salad

Makes: 4 servings   *Serving Size: 1/2 cup*   *Prep Time: 5 minutes*

2	cups cooked whole-wheat orzo pasta
1/4	cup fat-free, low-sodium chicken broth
1	Tbsp chopped fresh basil
1	Tbsp chopped fresh oregano
1	Tbsp chopped fresh tarragon
1/4	tsp salt (optional)
1/4	tsp ground black pepper

1 Toss all ingredients in a large bowl.

2 Refrigerate and serve cold.

Exchanges/Choices
1 Starch

Calories 90
  Calories from Fat 0
Total Fat . . . . 0.0 g
  Saturated Fat . . . . 0.1 g
  Trans Fat . . . . 0.0 g
Cholesterol . . . . 0 mg
Sodium . . . . 35 mg
Potassium . . . . 55 mg
Total Carbohydrate . . . . . . 19 g
  Dietary Fiber . . . . 2 g
  Sugars . . . . 1 g
Protein . . . . 4 g
Phosphorus . . . . 65 mg

Dietitian's Tip

Fresh herbs are a great way to add flavor to foods without adding extra fat or sodium. You may want to test your green thumb by growing your own small herb garden—it's easier than you may think!

Three-Pepper Pasta Salad with Goat Cheese

Makes: 10 servings   *Serving Size: 1 cup*   *Prep Time: 15 minutes*

Dressing

1/2	cup balsamic vinegar
2	Tbsp olive oil
1/2	tsp garlic salt (optional)
1/4	tsp ground black pepper
2	Tbsp honey

Salad

16	ounces whole-wheat penne pasta, uncooked
2	medium green bell peppers, finely diced
2	medium yellow or orange bell peppers, finely diced
2	medium red bell peppers, finely diced
1/4	cup crumbled goat cheese
2	Tbsp chopped fresh basil

1 In a small bowl, whisk together dressing ingredients.

2 Cook pasta according to package directions, omitting salt. Drain and rinse under cold water.

3 In a large salad bowl, toss cooled pasta with remaining salad ingredients. Drizzle dressing over pasta and toss to coat.

Exchanges/Choices

2 1/2 Starch   1 Vegetable
1/2 Fat

Calories	255
Calories from Fat	45
Total Fat	5.0 g
Saturated Fat	1.4 g
Trans Fat	0.0 g
Cholesterol	5 mg
Sodium	25 mg
Potassium	235 mg
Total Carbohydrate	46 g
Dietary Fiber	6 g
Sugars	10 g
Protein	8 g
Phosphorus	130 mg

Dietitian's Tip

Goat cheese is a fat source in this recipe, but you only need to use a small amount for a lot of flavor. If you don't like goat cheese, try substituting feta or Parmesan.

Orange Roughy with Citrus Cream Sauce

Makes: 4 servings   *Serving Size: 1 fillet*   *Prep Time: 10 minutes*

nonstick cooking spray
4   4-ounce orange roughy fillets
1/4   tsp salt (optional)
1/4   tsp ground black pepper
1   pint fat-free half-and-half
2   Tbsp cornstarch
1   tsp olive oil
2   garlic cloves, minced
1/4   cup white wine
1/4   cup lemon juice (juice of 1 lemon)
1   Tbsp lemon zest
1/4   cup crumbled goat cheese

1 Preheat oven to 350°F. Coat a shallow baking dish with cooking spray. Season both sides of each orange roughy fillet with salt (optional) and pepper.

2 Place fillets in baking dish and bake for 15 minutes or until fish flakes with a fork.

3 Meanwhile, in a medium bowl, whisk together half-and-half and cornstarch to make a slurry. Set aside.

4 Heat oil and cooking spray in a medium nonstick skillet over medium-high heat. Sauté garlic for 30 seconds. Add wine, lemon juice, and lemon zest and let it reduce by half. Add slurry and bring to a boil. Reduce heat and simmer for 3 minutes.

5 Pour 1/4 cup sauce over each fillet and top with 1 Tbsp goat cheese.

Exchanges/Choices
1 Carbohydrate   3 Lean Meat

Calories 215
    Calories from Fat 45
Total Fat . . . . .5.0 g
    Saturated Fat . . . . .2.2 g
    Trans Fat . . . . .0.0 g
Cholesterol. . . . . 75 mg
Sodium . . . . 235 mg
Potassium. . . . . 470 mg
Total Carbohydrate . . . . . . 17 g
    Dietary Fiber . . . . 0 g
    Sugars . . . . 7 g
Protein . . . . 23 g
Phosphorus . . . . 330 mg

Dietitian's Tip

This fish is great served with a green vegetable, such as asparagus, broccoli, or Brussels sprouts.

Veggie Lasagna Roulades

Makes: 8 servings   *Serving Size: 2 roulades*   *Prep Time: 40 minutes*

16	whole-wheat lasagna noodles
1	cup fat-free ricotta cheese
1/4	cup freshly grated Parmesan cheese
1	Tbsp dried parsley
1	egg
	nonstick cooking spray
1	cup mushrooms, finely diced
1	medium zucchini, finely diced
2	tomatoes, seeded and finely diced
3	garlic cloves, minced
1/4	tsp salt (optional)
1/4	tsp ground black pepper
16	ounces low-sodium marinara pasta sauce

1 Preheat oven to 350°F. Cook lasagna noodles according to package directions, omitting salt. Drain. Lay out noodles on wax paper.

2 In a medium bowl, mix ricotta, Parmesan cheese, parsley, and egg. Set aside.

3 Coat a large nonstick skillet with cooking spray. Sauté mushrooms, zucchini, tomato, and garlic over high heat for 5–7 minutes. Remove from heat and let cool.

4 Fold vegetables into cheese mixture. Add salt (optional) and pepper. Heap 2 Tbsp cheese mixture at the end of each noodle.

5 Starting at the cheese mixture end, roll noodle to the other end. Secure with a toothpick. Repeat for remaining noodles.

6 Coat baking dish with cooking spray. Place roulades side by side in the dish. Pour sauce over roulades and bake for 20 minutes.

Exchanges/Choices

2 Starch   1 Vegetable
1 Lean Meat

Calories	245
Calories from Fat	35
Total Fat	4.0 g
Saturated Fat	0.9 g
Trans Fat	0.0 g
Cholesterol	35 mg
Sodium	220 mg
Potassium	510 mg
Total Carbohydrate	39 g
Dietary Fiber	6 g
Sugars	6 g
Protein	14 g
Phosphorus	240 mg

Chef's Tip

This recipe is a fun twist on regular lasagna.

Chicken Kabobs GF LC

Makes: 4 servings　　　　*Serving Size: 2 skewers*　　　　*Prep Time: 20 minutes*

1　pint button mushrooms

1　large onion, sliced into 1-inch chunks

1　red bell pepper, sliced into 1-inch chunks

1　green bell pepper, sliced into 1-inch chunks

1　pound boneless, skinless chicken breasts, cut into 1-inch cubes

8　bamboo skewers, soaked in warm water

1/2　cup fat-free Italian dressing

1 Prepare an indoor or outdoor grill.

2 Assemble kabobs by alternating mushrooms, onions, peppers, and chicken cubes on each skewer (making 8 skewers).

3 Brush all sides of kabobs with Italian dressing. Grill over medium heat for 10 minutes, turning occasionally.

Exchanges/Choices

2 Vegetable　　　3 Lean Meat

Calories 190
　Calories from Fat 30
Total Fat . . . . .3.5 g
　Saturated Fat . . . . .1.0 g
　Trans Fat . . . . .0.0 g
Cholesterol. . . . . 65 mg
Sodium . . . . 415 mg
Potassium. . . . . 570 mg
Total Carbohydrate . . . . . . 13 g
　Dietary Fiber . . . . 3 g
　Sugars . . . . 8 g
Protein . . . . 27 g
Phosphorus . . . . 275 mg

Dietitian's Tip

Kabobs are a great way to work vegetables and protein into your meal plan. Serve over brown rice or quinoa for a well-balanced meal.

Pear Pecan Salad GF LC

Makes: 8 servings   *Serving Size: 1/2 cup*   *Prep Time: 20 minutes*

2	tsp trans-fat-free margarine
1	tsp Splenda Brown Sugar Blend
1/4	cup chopped pecans
2	medium pears, diced
4	cups mixed field greens
2	Tbsp balsamic vinegar
2	tsp olive oil
1	tsp honey

1 Preheat oven to 350°F. Combine margarine and brown sugar in a small bowl and microwave for 30 seconds to melt margarine. Add pecans and toss to coat.

2 Spread pecan mixture in a small baking dish and bake for 15 minutes. Remove from oven and set aside to cool.

3 In a large salad bowl, toss together pears and greens.

4 In a small bowl, whisk together remaining ingredients. Drizzle dressing over salad and toss to coat. Serve with 1/2 Tbsp pecan mixture sprinkled on top of each serving.

Exchanges/Choices
1/2 Fruit   1 Fat

Calories 80
　Calories from Fat 40
Total Fat . . . . .4.5 g
　Saturated Fat . . . . .0.6 g
　Trans Fat . . . . .0.0 g
Cholesterol. . . . . 0 mg
Sodium . . . . 15 mg
Potassium. . . . . 135 mg
Total Carbohydrate . . . . . . 10 g
　Dietary Fiber . . . . 2 g
　Sugars . . . . 6 g
Protein . . . . 1 g
Phosphorus . . . . 25 mg

Chef's Tip

Nuts can be a great addition to any salad, offering different texture and flavor—transforming any recipe into a truly unique dish.

JULY
WEEK 4

GROCERY LIST

Fresh Produce
Asparagus—1 1/4 pounds
Bell peppers, green—2
Bell peppers, red—2
Cabbage—1 head
Carrots—2
Lettuce, romaine—2 heads
Onions, red—2
Onion, yellow or white,
    large—1
Scallions—4
Squash, yellow, medium—2
Tomatoes—3
Zucchini, medium—2

Meat, Poultry, & Fish
Beef, ground, 95% lean—
    3/4 pound
Chicken breasts, boneless,
    skinless, 4 ounces each—8
Pork cutlets, boneless, lean,
    4 ounces each—4
Salmon fillets, 4 ounces
    each—4

Grains, Bread, & Pasta
Bran flakes—1 cup
Bread crumbs, whole-
    wheat—1/4 cup
Hamburger buns, whole-
    wheat—5
Tortillas, whole-wheat,
    low-carb, 10-inch—4

Dairy & Cheese
Cheese, Parmesan—1 large
    block
Cream cheese, fat-free—
    4 ounces
Cream cheese, reduced-fat,
    tub—8 ounces
Eggs
Sour cream, fat-free—1/2 cup

Canned Goods & Sauces
Barbeque sauce—1 bottle
Pineapple, crushed, packed
    in juice—1 cup

Staples, Seasonings,
& Baking Needs
Black pepper, ground
Flour, all-purpose
Garlic powder
Nonstick cooking spray
Oil, canola
Oil, sesame
Onion powder
Sesame seeds
Splenda Sugar Blend
Sugar substitute
Thyme
Vanilla extract
Vinegar, balsamic
Vinegar, rice wine

Miscellaneous
Almonds, sliced—3 Tbsp
Aluminum foil
Baking cups, paper—15
Cookies, vanilla wafers,
    reduced-fat—12
Onion soup mix, 1-ounce
    package—1
Pecans, chopped—1/2 cup
Pie filling, cherry, light,
    21-ounce can—1
Ramen-style noodles,
    3-ounce package—1
Salad dressing, Caesar,
    reduced-fat—1/4 cup
Salad dressing, Italian,
    fat-free—1/2 cup
Salad dressing, Ranch,
    reduced-fat—1/4 cup

Salmon Packet with Asparagus GF LC

Makes: 4 servings　　　　　*Serving Size: 1 packet*　　　　　*Prep Time: 10 minutes*

4	12 × 19-inch sheets aluminum foil
	nonstick cooking spray
1 1/4	pound fresh asparagus, ends trimmed
4	4-ounce salmon fillets
4	tsp dried thyme
6	Tbsp freshly grated Parmesan cheese
1/4	cup balsamic vinegar

1 Prepare an indoor or outdoor grill. Spray aluminum foil with cooking spray.

2 Place 1/4 pound asparagus on each sheet of foil. Place salmon fillet on top of asparagus. Sprinkle 1 tsp thyme, 1 1/2 Tbsp Parmesan cheese, and 1 Tbsp balsamic vinegar over salmon.

3 Bring up sides of foil. Double-fold top and ends to seal packet (leave a little room in the packet for air circulation). Repeat for remaining 3 packets.

4 Place packets in covered outdoor grill over medium-high heat and cook for 12–14 minutes until salmon flakes with a fork.

Exchanges/Choices
1 Vegetable　　　　4 Lean Meat
1 Fat

Calories 245
　Calories from Fat 100
Total Fat . . . . .11.0 g
　Saturated Fat . . . . .2.4 g
　Trans Fat . . . . .0.0 g
Cholesterol. . . . . 85 mg
Sodium . . . . 135 mg
Potassium. . . . . 530 mg
Total Carbohydrate . . . . 6 g
　Dietary Fiber . . . . 2 g
　Sugars . . . . 3 g
Protein . . . . 28 g
Phosphorus . . . . 325 mg

Chef's Tip

These packets can also be baked in the oven. Place packets on a baking sheet and bake at 450°F for 18–20 minutes. Cooking vegetables and fish this way can't get any easier!

Chicken Caesar Wrap

Makes: 4 servings   *Serving Size: 1 wrap*   *Prep Time: 20 minutes*

4	4-ounce boneless, skinless chicken breasts
1/4	tsp ground black pepper
4	cups chopped romaine lettuce
1	tomato, seeded and finely diced
1/4	cup freshly grated Parmesan cheese
1/4	cup reduced-fat Caesar dressing
4	10-inch whole-wheat, low-carb tortillas

1 Prepare an indoor or outdoor grill. Season chicken breasts with pepper. Grill chicken for 4–6 minutes per side.

2 Remove chicken from grill and chop into 1-inch pieces.

3 In a large bowl, toss together lettuce, tomato, Parmesan cheese, and chicken. Drizzle with Caesar dressing and toss to coat.

4 Place 1 1/2 cups chicken mixture into 1 tortilla and wrap.

5 Repeat procedure for 3 remaining wraps.

Exchanges/Choices

1 Starch   4 Lean Meat

Calories 275
  Calories from Fat 90
Total Fat . . . . 10.0 g
  Saturated Fat . . . . 2.2 g
  Trans Fat . . . . 0.0 g
Cholesterol. . . . . 70 mg
Sodium . . . . 590 mg
Potassium. . . . . 445 mg
Total Carbohydrate . . . . . . 23 g
  Dietary Fiber . . . . 13 g
  Sugars . . . . 3 g
Protein . . . . 35 g
Phosphorus . . . . 365 mg

Dietitian's Tip

You can use whole-wheat tortillas for these wraps to increase dietary fiber.

Pecan Chicken Salad

Makes: 5 servings   *Serving Size: 1 cup salad and 3–4 chicken strips*   *Prep Time: 15 minutes*

	nonstick cooking spray
1	cup bran flake crumbs
1/2	cup chopped pecans
1/2	tsp garlic powder
1/2	tsp onion powder
1	egg
2	egg whites
2	Tbsp all-purpose flour
4	4-ounce boneless, skinless chicken breasts
6	cups chopped romaine lettuce
1	cup shredded carrots
1/2	cup finely diced red onion
1/4	cup reduced-fat Ranch dressing

1 Preheat oven to 350°F. Coat a shallow baking pan with cooking spray.

2 In a medium bowl, combine bran flake crumbs, pecans, garlic powder, and onion powder.

3 In a separate bowl, lightly beat egg and egg whites.

4 Place flour in a separate bowl.

5 Dip each side of chicken breast in flour, then egg mixture, then bran flake and pecan mixture.

6 Place chicken breasts in baking pan. Spray chicken lightly with cooking spray and bake 30–35 minutes, until juices run clear.

7 In a large salad bowl, toss together lettuce, carrots, onion, and dressing. Remove chicken from pan and slice into 1-inch-thick strips.

8 Place a heaping cup of salad mixture on a plate and arrange 3–4 chicken strips on top. Repeat for remaining 4 salads.

Exchanges/Choices

1 Starch	1 Vegetable
3 Lean Meat	1 1/2 Fat

Calories 305
  Calories from Fat 125
Total Fat . . . . 14.0 g
  Saturated Fat . . . . 2.0 g
  Trans Fat . . . . 0.0 g
Cholesterol . . . . 90 mg
Sodium . . . . 350 mg
Potassium . . . . 565 mg
Total Carbohydrate . . . . . . 22 g
  Dietary Fiber . . . . 5 g
  Sugars . . . . 6 g
Protein . . . . 25 g
Phosphorus . . . . 305 mg

Dietitian's Tip

To reduce the fat content of this recipe, use fat-free Ranch dressing.

BBQ Pork Cutlets

Makes: 4 servings   *Serving Size: 1 cutlet*   *Prep Time: 5 minutes*

4	4-ounce lean boneless pork cutlets
1/2	cup bottled barbecue sauce
1	cup canned, crushed pineapple with juice
1/4	tsp ground black pepper nonstick cooking spray

1 Preheat oven to 350°F.

2 Place one cutlet between two sheets of plastic wrap and, using a meat tenderizer or rolling pin, pound the cutlet to 1/4-inch thickness. Repeat for remaining 3 cutlets. Set aside.

3 In a medium bowl, combine barbecue sauce, pineapple, and pepper.

4 Coat a large, shallow baking dish with cooking spray. Line the bottom of the dish with the pork cutlets and cover with barbecue sauce mixture.

5 Bake for 20 minutes or until pork is done.

Exchanges/Choices
1 Carbohydrate   3 Lean Meat
1/2 Fat

Calories	245
Calories from Fat	70
Total Fat	8.0 g
Saturated Fat	2.9 g
Trans Fat	0.0 g
Cholesterol	70 mg
Sodium	385 mg
Potassium	440 mg
Total Carbohydrate	19 g
Dietary Fiber	1 g
Sugars	14 g
Protein	22 g
Phosphorus	200 mg

Chef's Tip

Ask your butcher to prepare fresh cutlets for you. He can even pound them out for you, saving prep time.

Marinated Grilled Veggies GF LC

Makes: 8 servings　　　　*Serving Size: 1/8 recipe*　　　　*Prep Time: 30 minutes*

2 green bell peppers, seeded and sliced into quarters

2 red bell peppers, seeded and sliced into quarters

2 medium zucchini, sliced into 1/4-inch-thick slices lengthwise

2 medium yellow squash, sliced into 1/4-inch-thick slices lengthwise

1 large onion, sliced into 1/4-inch-thick rings

1/2 cup fat-free Italian dressing

1 Prepare an indoor or outdoor grill.

2 Toss together all ingredients in a large bowl and marinate in the refrigerator for 20 minutes.

3 Place vegetables on grill over medium heat. Grill for 4 minutes on all sides.

Exchanges/Choices
2 Vegetable

Calories 50
　Calories from Fat 5
Total Fat . . . . 0.5 g
　Saturated Fat . . . . 0.1 g
　Trans Fat . . . . 0.0 g
Cholesterol . . . . 0 mg
Sodium . . . . 185 mg
Potassium . . . . 455 mg
Total Carbohydrate . . . . . . 11 g
　Dietary Fiber . . . . 3 g
　Sugars . . . . 7 g
Protein . . . . 2 g
Phosphorus . . . . 80 mg

Dietitian's Tip

Don't be afraid to grill these or your other favorite vegetables . . . they are delicious!

Onion Burger

Makes: 5 servings *Serving Size: 1 burger* *Prep Time: 5 minutes*

3/4 pound 95% lean ground beef
1/2 1-ounce package onion soup mix
1 egg
1/4 cup whole-wheat bread crumbs
5 whole-wheat hamburger buns
10 medium tomato slices
10 lettuce leaves
5 thin slices red onion

1 Prepare an indoor or outdoor grill.

2 Combine beef, soup mix, egg, and bread crumbs in a medium bowl and mix well to incorporate. Divide mixture into 5 equal portions and shape into 1/2-inch-thick patties.

3 Place burgers on grill over medium-high heat and grill 7 minutes on each side or until well done (meat should not be pink on the inside).

4 Serve each burger on a whole-wheat bun with 2 slices tomato, 2 lettuce leaves, and 1 onion slice.

Exchanges/Choices
1 1/2 Starch 1 Vegetable
2 Lean Meat

Calories 260
  Calories from Fat 65
Total Fat . . . . .7.0 g
  Saturated Fat . . . . 2.3 g
  Trans Fat . . . . .0.1 g
Cholesterol. . . . . 80 mg
Sodium . . . . 545 mg
Potassium. . . . . 520 mg
Total Carbohydrate . . . . . . 30 g
  Dietary Fiber . . . . 5 g
  Sugars . . . . 7 g
Protein . . . . 20 g
Phosphorus . . . . 275 mg

Dietian's Tip

Summer wouldn't be complete without a great grilled burger! Try ground turkey in this recipe instead of beef.

Asian Coleslaw LC

Makes: 7 servings   *Serving Size: 1 cup*   *Prep Time: 10 minutes*

4   cups shredded cabbage
1   cup shredded carrots
4   scallions, sliced
1   3-ounce package ramen-style noodles, uncooked and crushed
2   Tbsp sesame seeds
3   Tbsp sliced almonds, toasted
1   flavor packet from ramen-style noodles
1   packet sugar substitute
3   Tbsp rice wine vinegar
1   Tbsp canola oil
1   tsp sesame oil

1 In a large bowl, toss cabbage, carrots, scallions, and crushed noodles together.

2 In a large nonstick skillet, sauté the sesame seeds and almonds over low-medium heat for 2 minutes or until toasted; set aside.

3 In a small bowl, whisk together remaining ingredients. Pour dressing over the salad and toss to coat. Sprinkle sesame seeds and almonds over top of salad.

Exchanges/Choices
1/2 Starch   1 Vegetable
1 1/2 Fat

Calories 130
  Calories from Fat 70
Total Fat . . . . .8.0 g
  Saturated Fat . . . . .1.2 g
  Trans Fat . . . . .0.0 g
Cholesterol. . . . . 0 mg
Sodium . . . . 155 mg
Potassium. . . . . 190 mg
Total Carbohydrate. . . . . . 14 g
  Dietary Fiber . . . . 2 g
  Sugars . . . . 3 g
Protein . . . . 3 g
Phosphorus . . . . 60 mg

Chef's Tip

Buy packaged shredded cabbage at the store to save time.

Cherry Tarts

Makes: 15 servings   *Serving Size: 1 tart*   *Prep Time: 10 minutes*

8   ounces reduced-fat tub cream cheese
4   ounces fat-free cream cheese
1/2   cup fat-free sour cream
1   egg
2   egg whites
1/2   cup Splenda Sugar Blend
1   Tbsp vanilla extract
15   paper baking cups
15   reduced-fat vanilla wafers
1   21-ounce can light cherry pie topping

1 Preheat oven to 350°F. Combine cream cheeses, sour cream, egg, egg whites, Splenda, and vanilla extract. Beat until smooth.

2 Line muffin pan with paper baking cups and place 1 vanilla wafer in the bottom of each cup.

3 Fill each muffin cup with about 1/4 cup cream cheese mixture.

4 Place muffin pan in oven and bake 40–45 minutes or until lightly golden brown.

5 Let cool and top each tart with 1 Tbsp cherry pie filling.

Exchanges/Choices
1 1/2 Carbohydrate   1/2 Fat

Calories 130
  Calories from Fat 30
Total Fat . . . . .3.5 g
  Saturated Fat . . . . .1.9 g
  Trans Fat . . . . .0.0 g
Cholesterol . . . . 25 mg
Sodium . . . . 160 mg
Potassium . . . . 115 mg
Total Carbohydrate . . . . . . 20 g
  Dietary Fiber . . . . 0 g
  Sugars . . . . 16 g
Protein . . . . 3 g
Phosphorus . . . . 85 mg

Dietitian's Tip

You can easily make this recipe gluten-free by substituting a gluten-free cookie for the vanilla wafer. Just make sure to verify all the other ingredients you are using are gluten-free.

AUGUST

Embrace Ethnicity

This month, try foods from around the world without packing on vacation pounds. Don't be intimated by these diverse ethnic recipes. By experimenting with different foods, you're adding more variety to your diet, which is a key component to good nutrition. You'll also keep from getting bored this month and see that healthy eating can be very interesting. Take a look at the Moroccan Pork, Hungarian Goulash, Mediterranean Chicken, and Kung Pao Chicken . . . just to name a few.

Tiramisu (page 288)

This version of the traditional Italian dessert is lighter, but you can expect the same bold, rich flavors.

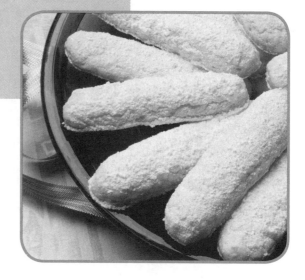

GF gluten-free recipe, but always check ingredients for gluten.

LC these recipes contain 15 grams of carbohydrate or less per serving.

NEW new recipe for the second edition.

AUGUST RECIPES

AUGUST

WEEK 1

DAY 1
Chicken Marsala   256

DAY 2
Pork Chop Suey   257
Fried Rice   258

DAY 3
Crab Tostadas   259

DAY 4
Curried Eggplant
    Couscous   260

DAY 5
Spicy Szechwan
    Beef   261
Spring Rolls   262

GROCERY LIST

Fresh Produce
Avocado—1
Broccoli—2 heads
Cabbage, Napa—1 head
Carrots—3
Celery—2 stalks
Cilantro—1 bunch
Cucumbers, medium—2
Eggplant—1
Garlic—1 clove
Mushrooms—1 pint
Scallions—1 large bunch
Sugar snap peas—3 cups

Meat, Poultry, & Fish
Beef tenderloin—1 pound
Chicken breasts, boneless,
    skinless, 4 ounces each—4
Crabmeat, imitation—
    1/2 pound
Pork chops, boneless—
    1 pound

Grains, Bread, & Pasta
Couscous, whole-wheat,
    10-ounce box—1
Rice, brown—1 bag
Tortillas, corn, 6-inch—5

Dairy & Cheese
Egg substitute—1 cup
Sour cream, fat-free—2 Tbsp

Canned Goods & Sauces
Bamboo shoots, 8-ounce
    cans—2
Bean sprouts, 15-ounce
    can—1

Broth, chicken, fat-free,
    low-sodium, 14.5-ounce
    cans—5
Hot pepper sauce
Preserves, apricot,
    sugar-free—1 jar
Soy sauce, lite
Water chestnuts, 8-ounce
    can—1

Frozen Foods
Peas, 10-ounce package—1

**Staples, Seasonings,
& Baking Needs**
Black pepper, ground
Cornstarch
Curry powder
Flour, all-purpose
Lemon juice
Nonstick cooking spray
Oil, canola
Oil, olive
Oil, sesame
Salt
Vinegar, rice wine

Miscellaneous
Chilies, red, whole, dried—3
Raisins, golden—1/4 cup
Rice paper wrappers,
    6-inch—10
Salsa
Wine, Marsala

Chicken Marsala LC

Makes: 4 servings   *Serving Size: 1 chicken breast*   *Prep Time: 5 minutes*

nonstick cooking spray

4   4-ounce boneless, skinless chicken breasts
4   cups sliced mushrooms
1   garlic clove, minced
1   Tbsp all-purpose flour
1/2 cup Marsala wine
1   14.5-ounce can fat-free, low-sodium chicken broth
1/4 tsp salt (optional)
1/4 tsp ground black pepper

1 Coat a large nonstick skillet with cooking spray. Over medium-high heat, sauté chicken breasts for 6 minutes on each side. Remove from pan and set aside.

2 Spray pan again with cooking spray and reduce heat to medium. Add mushrooms and garlic and sauté until all the liquid is evaporated. Add flour, stirring well to coat the mushrooms. Cook for 1 more minute. Add wine, stirring well to incorporate the flour. Add broth and turn heat to high. Let simmer for 5 minutes. Add salt (optional) and pepper.

3 Serve sauce over chicken breasts.

Exchanges/Choices
1/2 Carbohydrate   3 Lean Meat

Calories 185
Calories from Fat 25
Total Fat . . . . .3.0 g
Saturated Fat . . . . .0.8 g
Trans Fat . . . . .0.0 g
Cholesterol. . . . . 65 mg
Sodium . . . . 315 mg
Potassium. . . . . 520 mg
Total Carbohydrate . . . . 7 g
Dietary Fiber . . . . 1 g
Sugars . . . . 3 g
Protein . . . . 28 g
Phosphorus . . . . 255 mg

Chef's Tip

Serve over whole-grain egg noodles, and save time by buying pre-sliced mushrooms.

Pork Chop Suey LC

Makes: 4 servings　　　　*Serving Size: 1 cup*　　　　*Prep Time: 10 minutes*

nonstick cooking spray
1　pound boneless pork chops, cut into 1-inch strips
2　celery stalks, thinly sliced
1　cup canned bean sprouts, rinsed and drained
1　cup canned water chestnuts, rinsed, drained, and sliced
1　14.5-ounce can fat-free, low-sodium chicken broth
1　Tbsp cornstarch
1 1/2　Tbsp lite soy sauce

1 Coat a large nonstick skillet or wok with cooking spray and stir-fry pork over high heat for 4 minutes. Remove pork from pan.

2 Spray pan again with cooking spray and reduce heat to medium. Stir-fry the celery, bean sprouts, and water chestnuts for about 5 minutes. Add pork back to pan.

3 In a small bowl, whisk together chicken broth and cornstarch. Pour over pork and vegetables in the pan and bring to a boil. Add soy sauce, reduce heat, and simmer for 3 minutes.

Exchanges/Choices
1 Vegetable　　3 Lean Meat
1/2 Fat

Calories	205
Calories from Fat	65
Total Fat	7.0 g
Saturated Fat	2.6 g
Trans Fat	0.0 g
Cholesterol	60 mg
Sodium	545 mg
Potassium	530 mg
Total Carbohydrate	9 g
Dietary Fiber	2 g
Sugars	2 g
Protein	24 g
Phosphorus	220 mg

Chef's Tip

You can use chicken breasts instead of pork in this recipe.

Fried Rice

Makes: 8 servings   *Serving Size: 1/2 cup*   *Prep Time: 10 minutes*

4 cups cooked brown rice, chilled
2 Tbsp fat-free, low-sodium chicken broth
2 Tbsp rice wine vinegar
1 Tbsp lite soy sauce
1/2 tsp salt (optional)
1 tsp sesame oil
1/4 tsp ground black pepper
nonstick cooking spray
1 Tbsp canola oil
1 cup egg substitute
1 bunch scallions, finely chopped (about 1 cup)
1 10-ounce package frozen peas, thawed

1 Spread rice in a shallow baking pan and separate grains with a fork.

2 In a small bowl, whisk together broth, vinegar, soy sauce, salt (optional), sesame oil, and black pepper. Set aside.

3 Coat a large nonstick skillet or wok with cooking spray and heat canola oil over moderately high heat until hot. Stir-fry egg substitute until scrambled, about 30 seconds. Add scallions and stir-fry 1 minute.

4 Add peas and stir-fry until heated through. Add rice and stir-fry, stirring frequently, 2–3 minutes, or until heated through.

5 Stir liquid and add to fried rice, tossing to coat evenly.

Exchanges/Choices

2 Starch	1/2 Fat

Calories 175
  Calories from Fat 30
Total Fat . . . . .3.5 g
  Saturated Fat . . . . .0.4 g
  Trans Fat . . . . 0.0 g
Cholesterol. . . . . 0 mg
Sodium . . . . 165 mg
Potassium. . . . . 160 mg
Total Carbohydrate . . . . . . 29 g
  Dietary Fiber . . . . 4 g
  Sugars . . . . 3 g
Protein . . . . 8 g
Phosphorus . . . . 115 mg

Dietitian's Tip

This version of a classic favorite contains a lot less fat but is just as delicious.

Crab Tostadas

Makes: 5 servings   *Serving Size: 1 tostada*   *Prep Time: 5 minutes*

5	6-inch corn tortillas
1	avocado, mashed
1/2	pound shredded imitation crabmeat
1	Tbsp lemon juice
1	Tbsp sliced scallions
1	tsp chopped cilantro
2	Tbsp fat-free sour cream
3	Tbsp salsa

1 Preheat oven to 400°F. Place corn tortillas on a baking sheet and bake for 5 minutes or until crisp.

2 In a medium bowl, combine remaining ingredients and mix well.

3 Spoon crab mixture on tortillas.

Exchanges/Choices

1 Starch   1/2 Carbohydrate
1 Lean Meat

Calories	150
Calories from Fat	45
Total Fat	5.0 g
Saturated Fat	0.9 g
Trans Fat	0.0 g
Cholesterol	10 mg
Sodium	460 mg
Potassium	275 mg
Total Carbohydrate	22 g
Dietary Fiber	4 g
Sugars	4 g
Protein	6 g
Phosphorus	230 mg

Chef's Tip

Avocados are easy to ripen. Put them in a paper bag with an apple for 2–3 days at room temperature. When they turn dark purple or black and are soft to the touch, they're ready to eat! Garnish these tasty tostadas with shredded lettuce, chopped tomatoes, and a touch of hot salsa for an extra kick.

Curried Eggplant Couscous

Makes: 10 servings   *Serving Size: 1/2 cup*   *Prep Time: 5 minutes*

2 cups fat-free, low-sodium chicken broth, divided
1 cup uncooked whole-wheat couscous
1/2 tsp salt (optional)
1/4 tsp ground black pepper
2 Tbsp all-purpose flour
1 Tbsp curry powder
1 eggplant, cubed (about 4 cups)
2 tsp olive oil
1 cup shredded carrots
1/4 cup golden raisins

1 In a medium saucepan, bring 1 1/4 cups chicken broth to a boil; reserve remaining 3/4 cup. Add 1 cup uncooked couscous. Cover and remove from heat. Let stand for 5 minutes and fluff with fork.

2 In a large mixing bowl, combine salt (optional), pepper, flour, and curry powder. Add eggplant and toss to coat.

3 Add oil to a large nonstick skillet over medium-high heat. Add eggplant and stir-fry for 5 minutes. Add remaining 3/4 cup chicken broth and stir well to incorporate the flour. Add carrots and raisins and cook 1 more minute. Stir in couscous and mix well.

Exchanges/Choices
1 Starch   1 Vegetable

Calories 110
  Calories from Fat 10
Total Fat . . . . .1.0 g
  Saturated Fat . . . . .0.2 g
  Trans Fat . . . . .0.0 g
Cholesterol. . . . . 0 mg
Sodium . . . . 110 mg
Potassium. . . . . 180 mg
Total Carbohydrate . . . . . . 22 g
  Dietary Fiber . . . . 3 g
  Sugars . . . . 4 g
Protein . . . . 4 g
Phosphorus . . . . 55 mg

Chef's Tip

This recipe is a perfect example of marrying different flavors—spicy curry, sweet raisins, and creamy eggplant—into a real palate-pleaser.

Spicy Szechwan Beef

Makes: 6 servings　　　　　*Serving Size: 1/6 recipe*　　　　　*Prep Time: 10 minutes*

nonstick cooking spray
1　tsp sesame oil
1　pound beef tenderloin, sliced into 1-inch strips
1/4　cup cashews
3　cups sugar snap peas
4　cups broccoli florets (about 2 heads)
1　cup canned bamboo shoots, rinsed and drained

2　scallions, thinly sliced
1　14.5-ounce can fat-free, reduced-sodium chicken broth
3　Tbsp lite soy sauce
2　tsp hot pepper sauce
1　Tbsp cornstarch
3　dried whole red chilies

1 Coat a large nonstick skillet with cooking spray and heat oil over medium-high heat. Add beef and stir-fry for 3 minutes. Remove beef from pan.

2 Spray pan again with cooking spray; add cashews and stir-fry for 1 minute. Add sugar snap peas, broccoli, bamboo shoots, and scallions and stir-fry for 5 minutes over medium heat. Add beef back to pan.

3 In a small bowl, whisk together broth, soy sauce, hot pepper sauce, and cornstarch. Pour over meat and vegetables in pan. Add chilies. Bring to a boil, reduce heat, and simmer for 2 minutes.

4 Remove chilies before serving.

Exchanges/Choices
2 Vegetable　　2 Lean Meat
1/2 Fat

Calories 190
　Calories from Fat 70
Total Fat . . . . .8.0 g
　Saturated Fat . . . . .2.2 g
　Trans Fat . . . . .0.0 g
Cholesterol. . . . . 40 mg
Sodium . . . . 540 mg
Potassium. . . . . 520 mg
Total Carbohydrate . . . . . . 11 g
　Dietary Fiber . . . . 3 g
　Sugars . . . . 4 g
Protein . . . . 19 g
Phosphorus . . . . 220 mg

Dietitian's Tip

Cashews are a good source of monounsaturated fat and vitamin E . . . plus they add great flavor and crunchiness to any dish.

Spring Rolls

Makes: 5 servings *Serving Size: 2 rolls* *Prep Time: 20 minutes*

Spring Rolls

1/2 cup canned bamboo shoots, rinsed, drained, and shredded
2   medium carrots, cut into thin sticks
2   medium cucumbers, seeded and cut into thin sticks
3   cups Napa cabbage, finely shredded
10 6-inch rice paper wrappers

Dipping Sauce

1/2 cup sugar-free apricot preserves
1   Tbsp lite soy sauce
1/2 tsp hot pepper sauce
1/4 tsp sesame oil

1 In a large bowl, toss bamboo shoots, carrots, cucumber, and cabbage. Divide into 10 equal portions.

2 Soak one rice paper skin in warm water until softened, about 30 seconds. Lay rice paper on a clean, flat surface. Place one portion of the vegetable mixture in the center of the rice paper. Fold the left and right sides into the middle until almost touching. Roll paper from the bottom to form the roll. Repeat for remaining rice papers. Set aside.

3 Combine sauce ingredients in a small saucepan over high heat. Bring to a boil, stirring constantly. Boil for 2 minutes. Serve warm with cold spring rolls for dipping.

Exchanges/Choices

1/2 Starch   1/2 Carbohydrate
1 Vegetable

Calories	90
Calories from Fat	5
Total Fat	0.5 g
Saturated Fat	0.1 g
Trans Fat	0.0 g
Cholesterol	0 mg
Sodium	175 mg
Potassium	340 mg
Total Carbohydrate	24 g
Dietary Fiber	2 g
Sugars	4 g
Protein	2 g
Phosphorus	60 mg

Dietitian's Tip

You can make this recipe gluten-free by eliminating the soy sauce or by using gluten-free soy sauce. Just make sure all the other ingredients are gluten-free.

AUGUST

WEEK 2

DAY 1
Apple Chicken
  Salad   264

DAY 2
Tasty "Fried"
  Chicken   265
Spicy Greens   266

DAY 3
Greek Lemon Rice
  Soup   267

DAY 4
Kung Pao Chicken   268

DAY 5
Souvlaki   269
Moussaka   270

GROCERY LIST

Fresh Produce
Apples, medium—2
Bell pepper, red, medium—1
Carrots—2
Celery—1 head
Cucumber—1
Eggplant, large—1
Garlic—1 head
Greens, collard, turnip,
  mustard, or kale—
  3 pounds
Greens, field, mixed
  (mesclun)—6 cups
Lemon—1
Mushrooms, Portobello,
  large—2
Onions, yellow or white—2
Tomatoes, cherry—1 cup

Meat, Poultry, & Fish
Chicken breasts, boneless,
  skinless—2 pounds
Pork chops, boneless—
  1 1/4 pounds

Grains, Bread, & Pasta
Pita pockets, whole-wheat—5
Rice, brown—1 bag

Dairy & Cheese
Cheese, Parmesan—1 block
Eggs
Yogurt, plain, fat-free—
  8 ounces

Canned Goods & Sauces
Broth, chicken, fat-free,
  low-sodium, 14.5-ounce
  cans—6
Hot pepper sauce
Soy sauce, lite
Tomatoes, crushed, 15-ounce
  can—1
Water chestnuts, 8-ounce
  can—1

Staples, Seasonings, & Baking Needs
Black pepper, ground
Cayenne pepper
Cinnamon
Cornstarch
Flour, all-purpose
Garlic salt
Lemon juice
Liquid smoke
Mustard, Dijon
Nonstick cooking spray
Oil, olive
Oil, sesame
Onion powder
Oregano
Salt
Splenda Brown Sugar Blend
Thyme
Vinegar, rice wine
Vinegar, white balsamic

Miscellaneous
Bamboo skewers
Cereal, cornflakes—1 box
Peanuts, chopped—1/4 cup
Walnuts, chopped—1/2 cup

Apple Chicken Salad [NEW]

Makes: 4 servings   *Serving Size: 1 1/2 cups salad*   *Prep Time: 15 minutes*

Dressing

1/4	cup white balsamic vinegar
1	Tbsp olive oil
1	Tbsp Splenda Brown Sugar Blend
1/4	tsp salt (optional)
1/4	tsp ground black pepper
1	tsp Dijon mustard
1	tsp minced garlic

Salad

6	cups mesclun (mixed field greens) salad mix
10	ounces cooked boneless, skinless chicken breast, sliced
2	medium apples, cored and sliced
1/2	cup chopped walnuts
1	cup cherry tomatoes, halved

1 In a small bowl, whisk dressing ingredients together. Set aside.

2 In a large salad bowl, toss salad ingredient together. Drizzle salad with dressing and toss gently to coat.

Exchanges/Choices

1/2 Fruit	1/2 Carbohydrate
1 Vegetable	3 Lean Meat
2 Fat	

Calories	335
Calories from Fat	145
Total Fat	16.0 g
Saturated Fat	2.2 g
Trans Fat	0.0 g
Cholesterol	60 mg
Sodium	105 mg
Potassium	605 mg
Total Carbohydrate	24 g
Dietary Fiber	5 g
Sugars	15 g
Protein	26 g
Phosphorus	255 mg

Chef's Tip

Sweeter apples like pink lady or honeycrisp work best in this salad, but any apple will do.

Tasty "Fried" Chicken

Makes: 4 servings   *Serving Size: 1 chicken breast*   *Prep Time: 15 minutes*

nonstick cooking spray
1 1/2   cups cornflake crumbs
1/2   tsp dried thyme
1/2   tsp garlic salt
1/2   tsp onion powder
1   egg
2   egg whites
1   tsp hot pepper sauce (optional)
2   Tbsp all-purpose flour
4   4-ounce boneless, skinless chicken breasts

1 Preheat oven to 350°F. Coat a shallow baking pan with cooking spray.

2 In a medium bowl, combine cornflake crumbs, thyme, garlic salt, and onion powder.

3 In a separate bowl, lightly beat egg and egg whites. Add hot pepper sauce and mix well.

4 Place flour in a separate bowl.

5 Dip each side of the chicken breast in flour, then egg mixture, then cornflake mixture.

6 Place chicken breasts in baking pan. Spray chicken lightly with cooking spray and bake 30–35 minutes, until juices run clear.

Exchanges/Choices
1 1/2 Starch   3 Lean Meat

Calories 250
  Calories from Fat 35
Total Fat . . . . 4.0 g
  Saturated Fat . . . . 1.2 g
  Trans Fat . . . . 0.0 g
Cholesterol. . . . . 110 mg
Sodium . . . . 440 mg
Potassium. . . . . 270 mg
Total Carbohydrate . . . . . . 22 g
  Dietary Fiber . . . . 1 g
  Sugars . . . . 2 g
Protein . . . . 29 g
Phosphorus . . . . 220 mg

Chef's Tip

You will be amazed at how great this baked chicken tastes. The cornflakes retain their crunchiness, providing a fried-like texture and excellent flavor.

Spicy Greens LC

Makes: 4 servings   *Serving Size: 1 cup*   *Prep Time: 20 minutes*

2	pounds mixed greens of choice (collard, turnip, mustard, or kale)
1	14.5-ounce can fat-free, low-sodium chicken broth
1	medium onion, chopped
2	garlic cloves, minced
1/4	tsp cayenne pepper
1/2	tsp ground black pepper
1	tsp liquid smoke

1 Wash greens thoroughly. Discard tough stems and cut greens into pieces.

2 Place greens in a large soup pot. Add chicken broth, onion, and garlic. Simmer, covered, for 30–45 minutes or until tender. Season with cayenne pepper, black pepper, and liquid smoke.

Exchanges/Choices
3 Vegetable

Calories	70
Calories from Fat	5
Total Fat	0.5 g
Saturated Fat	0.1 g
Trans Fat	0.0 g
Cholesterol	0 mg
Sodium	290 mg
Potassium	425 mg
Total Carbohydrate	13 g
Dietary Fiber	5 g
Sugars	3 g
Protein	5 g
Phosphorus	75 mg

Dietitian's Tip

Greens are a good source of folic acid. Folic acid may help protect against heart disease and helps lower the risk of birth defects, such as spina bifida.

Greek Lemon Rice Soup

Makes: 10 servings   *Serving Size: 1 cup*   *Prep Time: 5 minutes*

4	14.5-ounce cans fat-free, low-sodium chicken broth
1	cup rice, uncooked
1/4	cup lemon juice (juice of 1 lemon)
2	eggs
2	Tbsp cold water
2	Tbsp cornstarch
1/2	tsp salt (optional)
1/2	tsp ground black pepper

1 Bring chicken broth to a boil in a large soup pot. Add rice and reduce to a simmer for 20 minutes.

2 In a large bowl, whisk together lemon juice, eggs, water, and cornstarch.

3 Pour one ladle of the hot broth into the egg mixture, whisking constantly to temper the eggs. Repeat with two more ladles of soup.

4 Reduce heat to low. Add tempered egg mixture to soup, stirring constantly until fully incorporated. Remove from heat. Add salt (optional) and pepper.

Exchanges/Choices
1 Starch

Calories	100
Calories from Fat	10
Total Fat	1.0 g
Saturated Fat	0.3 g
Trans Fat	0.0 g
Cholesterol	35 mg
Sodium	425 mg
Potassium	170 mg
Total Carbohydrate	18 g
Dietary Fiber	0 g
Sugars	1 g
Protein	4 g
Phosphorus	65 mg

Chef's Tip

You can add cooked chicken (cut into small cubes) to this soup for a little protein and flavor boost.

Kung Pao Chicken

Makes: 4 servings   *Serving Size: 1 cup chicken and 1/2 cup rice*   *Prep Time: 10 minutes*

2   Tbsp cornstarch
1/2 cup fat-free, low-sodium chicken broth
2   Tbsp rice wine vinegar
2   Tbsp lite soy sauce
1/2 tsp hot pepper sauce
1   tsp Splenda Brown Sugar Blend
2   tsp sesame oil, divided
1   garlic clove, minced
     nonstick cooking spray

1   pound boneless, skinless chicken breasts, cubed
1   medium red bell pepper, finely diced
1/2 cup finely diced carrots
1   8-ounce can water chestnuts, rinsed, drained, and chopped
1/4 cup chopped peanuts
2   cups brown rice, cooked

1 In a small bowl, combine cornstarch and chicken broth and whisk until cornstarch dissolves. Add vinegar, soy sauce, hot pepper sauce, Splenda Brown Sugar Blend, 1 tsp sesame oil, and garlic; stir well and set aside.

2 In a large nonstick skillet or wok, heat cooking spray and 1 tsp sesame oil over medium-high heat. Add chicken breast and cook for 4 minutes. Remove from pan and set aside.

3 Add peppers, carrots, water chestnuts, and peanuts to pan. Stir-fry for 4 minutes. Add chicken broth mixture to skillet and bring to a boil. Add chicken back to pan and simmer for 3 minutes.

4 Serve over brown rice.

Chef's Tip

No need to order out for Chinese food. Make your own low-fat version—you won't even taste the difference!

Exchanges/Choices

2 Starch   1 Vegetable
3 Lean Meat   1 Fat

Calories	385
Calories from Fat	100
Total Fat	11.0 g
Saturated Fat	2.0 g
Trans Fat	0.0 g
Cholesterol	65 mg
Sodium	510 mg
Potassium	545 mg
Total Carbohydrate	39 g
Dietary Fiber	5 g
Sugars	5 g
Protein	31 g
Phosphorus	335 mg

Souvlaki

Makes: 5 servings   *Serving Size: 1 stuffed pita*   *Prep Time: 20 minutes*

5   whole-wheat pita pockets
1 1/4   pounds boneless pork chops, cut into 1-inch cubes
1/2   cup lemon juice
2   garlic cloves, sliced
1   Tbsp dried oregano
1   cucumber, peeled, seeded, and shredded (about 1 1/2 cups)
8   ounces fat-free plain yogurt
1   small garlic clove, minced
1/4   tsp salt (optional)
1/4   tsp ground black pepper bamboo skewers, soaked in warm water

1 Prepare an indoor or outdoor grill.

2 Slice one side of each pita to open pocket, but do not cut all the way through. Set aside.

3 In a medium bowl, combine pork cubes, lemon juice, garlic, and oregano. Marinate in refrigerator for 15 minutes.

4 In a medium bowl, mix cucumber, yogurt, garlic, salt (optional), and pepper. Set aside.

5 Skewer 6–7 pork cubes on each bamboo skewer and grill over medium-high heat for 3 minutes on each side.

6 Toast pita bread and fill each pita with 1/2 cup pork and 1/2 cup sauce.

Exchanges/Choices
2 Starch   1/2 Carbohydrate
3 Lean Meat

Calories 340
  Calories from Fat 80
Total Fat . . . . .9.0 g
  Saturated Fat . . . . .2.9 g
  Trans Fat . . . . .0.0 g
Cholesterol. . . . . 60 mg
Sodium . . . . 380 mg
Potassium. . . . . 595 mg
Total Carbohydrate . . . . . . 37 g
  Dietary Fiber . . . . 5 g
  Sugars . . . . 5 g
Protein . . . . 29 g
Phosphorus . . . . 360 mg

Chef's Tip

These traditional Greek shish kabobs make an excellent light summer meal. They're great at a picnic.

Moussaka GF

Makes: 8 servings   *Serving Size: 1/8 recipe*   *Prep Time: 15 minutes*

1 large eggplant, unpeeled, cut into 1/4-inch-thick rounds
1 Tbsp olive oil
  nonstick cooking spray
1 large onion, thinly sliced
1 cup finely chopped carrots
1 cup finely chopped celery
1 garlic clove, minced
2 large portobello mushrooms, cut into 1/2-inch pieces
1 tsp dried oregano
1/2 tsp ground cinnamon
1 15-ounce can crushed tomatoes
1/2 tsp salt (optional)
1/4 tsp ground black pepper
1/4 cup freshly grated Parmesan cheese

Exchanges/Choices
3 Vegetable   1/2 Fat

Calories 100	
Calories from Fat 20	
Total Fat . . . . 2.5 g	
Saturated Fat . . . . 0.7 g	
Trans Fat . . . . 0.0 g	
Cholesterol . . . . 0 mg	
Sodium . . . . 130 mg	
Potassium . . . . 510 mg	
Total Carbohydrate . . . . . . 17 g	
Dietary Fiber . . . . 4 g	
Sugars . . . . 8 g	
Protein . . . . 4 g	
Phosphorus . . . . 95 mg	

1 Preheat oven to 425°F. Brush both sides of eggplant rounds with olive oil. Arrange in a single layer on a baking sheet. Bake 10 minutes. Turn eggplant and continue baking until tender, about 15 minutes.

2 While eggplant is roasting, coat a large nonstick skillet with cooking spray. Over medium-high heat, add onion, carrots, and celery. Sauté until onion is clear, about 7 minutes.

3 Stir in garlic and mushrooms. Sauté until liquid evaporates, about 10 minutes. Add oregano, cinnamon, and tomatoes. Cook until mixture is thick, about 10 minutes. Add salt (optional) and pepper.

4 Reduce oven temperature to 350°F. Coat a shallow baking dish with cooking spray. Arrange half of eggplant rounds in single layer in dish. Spoon half of tomato mixture evenly over eggplant. Sprinkle with 2 Tbsp Parmesan cheese. Repeat layering with remaining eggplant, tomato mixture, and 2 Tbsp cheese, ending with cheese.

5 Bake until heated through and cheese is golden brown on top, about 20 minutes.

Chef's Tip

Traditional moussaka calls for a béchamel, or white cream sauce. We skipped that high-fat addition with an end result that's just as tasty.

AUGUST

WEEK 3

DAY 1
Spaghetti with Turkey
Meatballs   272

DAY 2
Mushroom
Chicken   273
Italian Green
Beans   274

DAY 3
Vegetable Paella   275

DAY 4
Cajun Shrimp   276

DAY 5
Mediterranean
Chicken   277
Cucumber Tomato
Salad   278

GROCERY LIST

Fresh Produce
Bell peppers, green—2
Bell peppers, red—2
Cucumbers, large—2
Garlic—2 heads
Mushrooms, sliced—1 quart
Onions, yellow or white—4
Parsley, Italian (flat leaf)—
   1/4 cup
Tomatoes, medium—2
Zucchini—1

Meat, Poultry, & Fish
Chicken breasts, boneless,
   skinless—2 3/4 pounds
Shrimp, peeled and
   deveined—12 ounces
Turkey, ground, 93% lean—
   1 1/2 pounds

Grains, Bread, & Pasta
Bread crumbs, Italian-
   style—1/3 cup
Linguine, whole-wheat—12
   ounces
Rice, brown—1 bag

Dairy & Cheese
Cheese, Asiago—1 small
   block
Cheese, Parmesan, freshly
   shredded—1/3 cup
Margarine, trans-fat-free

Canned Goods & Sauces
Beans, cannellini, 15-ounce
   can—1
Broth, chicken, fat-free,
   low-sodium, 14.5-ounce
   cans—5
Marinara pasta sauce,
   reduced-sodium,
   24.5-ounce jars—2
Tomatoes, diced, no-salt-
   added, 15-ounce cans—3

Frozen Foods
Green beans, Italian, cut—
   1-pound bag

Staples, Seasonings,
& Baking Needs
Basil
Black pepper, ground
Cayenne pepper
Nonstick cooking spray
Oil, olive
Onion powder
Oregano
Paprika
Salt
Vinegar, balsamic
Vinegar, red wine

Miscellaneous
Wine, white

Spaghetti with Turkey Meatballs

Makes: 8 servings   *Serving Size: 1 cup meatball sauce*   *Prep Time: 15 minutes*
(about 2–3 meatballs)

1	tsp olive oil
4	garlic cloves, minced
2	24.5-ounce reduced-sodium jars marinara pasta sauce
1 1/2	pounds 93% lean ground turkey
1	egg
1/3	cup freshly shredded Parmesan cheese
1/4	cup chopped fresh Italian (flat leaf) parsley
1/3	cup Italian-style bread crumbs
1 1/2	tsp dried minced onion
1/4	tsp ground black pepper
12	ounces whole-wheat linguine, uncooked

1 In a large saucepan, heat oil and garlic over medium heat and sauté for 30 seconds. Add pasta sauce.

2 In a medium bowl, combine all remaining ingredients except linguine and mix well. Form meat into small balls (makes about 30 meatballs).

3 Add meatballs to sauce. Bring to a boil; reduce heat and simmer for about 1 hour; stirring occasionally.

4 Cook pasta according to package directions, omitting salt. Drain.

5 Serve meatball sauce over linguine.

Exchanges/Choices

3 Starch   3 Lean Meat
1 1/2 Fat

Calories	450
Calories from Fat	145
Total Fat	16.0 g
Saturated Fat	3.3 g
Trans Fat	0.1 g
Cholesterol	85 mg
Sodium	600 mg
Potassium	880 mg
Total Carbohydrate	48 g
Dietary Fiber	8 g
Sugars	9 g
Protein	29 g
Phosphorus	360 mg

Dietitian's Tip

If you want to reduce carbs, serve the meatballs and sauce over cooked spaghetti squash instead.

Mushroom Chicken LC NEW

Makes: 8 servings   *Serving Size: 4 ounces chicken and mushrooms*   *Prep Time: 15 minutes*

2 pounds boneless, skinless chicken breasts
1 tsp salt (optional)
1/2 tsp ground black pepper
1 Tbsp olive oil
1 Tbsp trans-fat-free margarine
4 cups sliced mushrooms
1 garlic clove, minced
1 cup fat-free, low-sodium chicken broth
2 Tbsp balsamic vinegar
1/2 cup Asiago cheese, shredded

1 Preheat oven to 350°F.

2 Season the chicken with salt (optional) and pepper.

3 Heat olive oil in an oven-safe skillet over medium-high heat. Add chicken and sear on 2 minutes on each side.

4 Remove chicken from pan. Add margarine and mushrooms and sauté for about 5 minutes. Add garlic and sauté for 30 seconds.

5 Add chicken broth and balsamic vinegar and simmer until the liquid is reduced by half.

6 Add chicken back to pan. Place pan in oven and bake for 15 minutes. Top chicken with cheese and bake 5 more minutes.

Exchanges/Choices
4 Lean Meat

Calories 180
  Calories from Fat 65
Total Fat . . . . .7.0 g
  Saturated Fat . . . . .2.1 g
  Trans Fat . . . . .0.0 g
Cholesterol. . . . . 70 mg
Sodium . . . . 170 mg
Potassium. . . . . 335 mg
Total Carbohydrate. . . . . . . 2 g
  Dietary Fiber . . . . 0 g
  Sugars . . . . 1 g
Protein . . . . 26 g
Phosphorus . . . . 235 mg

Chef's Tip

You can use this same cooking method for other meats like pork tenderloin or chops, but leave off the cheese and top with chopped fresh basil instead.

Italian Green Beans GF LC

Makes: 6 servings *Serving Size: 1/2 cup* *Prep Time: 5 minutes*

1	pound frozen Italian cut green beans or fresh green beans, sliced
1	Tbsp olive oil
1	small onion, diced
2	garlic cloves, minced
1	15-ounce can no-salt-added diced tomatoes
1/4	tsp dried basil
1/4	tsp dried oregano

1 Steam green beans until tender-crisp. Set aside.

2 Heat olive oil in a medium nonstick skillet over medium-high heat. Sauté onions until clear. Add garlic; sauté 30 seconds. Add tomatoes, basil, and oregano and simmer for 15–20 minutes.

3 Pour tomato mixture over steamed green beans and mix well.

Exchanges/Choices
2 Vegetable   1/2 Fat

Calories 80
  Calories from Fat 20
Total Fat . . . . .2.5 g
  Saturated Fat . . . . .0.4 g
  Trans Fat . . . . .0.0 g
Cholesterol. . . . . 0 mg
Sodium . . . . 215 mg
Potassium. . . . . 365 mg
Total Carbohydrate . . . . . . 14 g
  Dietary Fiber . . . . 5 g
  Sugars . . . . 4 g
Protein . . . . 3 g
Phosphorus . . . . 60 mg

Chef's Tip

Italian green beans are wider and thicker than regular green beans. They're usually found in the frozen food aisle of your market.

Vegetable Paella

Makes: 6 servings   *Serving Size: 1 cup*   *Prep Time: 15 minutes*

1	Tbsp olive oil
1	red bell pepper, diced
1	onion, diced
2	large garlic cloves, minced
1/4	cup white wine
1 1/2	cups uncooked brown rice
2	14.5-ounce cans fat-free, low-sodium chicken broth
1	15-ounce can no-salt-added diced tomatoes, drained
1 1/2	tsp paprika
1/2	tsp salt (optional)
1/4	tsp ground black pepper
1	15-ounce can cannellini beans, rinsed and drained

1 Add oil to a large nonstick skillet over medium-high heat. Sauté bell pepper and onion for 3–4 minutes. Add garlic and sauté for 30 seconds.

2 Add wine and cook until liquid is reduced by half, about 3 minutes.

3 Stir in rice, broth, tomatoes, paprika, salt (optional), and pepper. Bring to a boil. Reduce heat and simmer for 35 minutes.

4 Stir in beans and simmer for 3 more minutes.

Exchanges/Choices
3 Starch   1 Vegetable
1/2 Fat

Calories	305
Calories from Fat	35
Total Fat	4.0 g
Saturated Fat	0.7 g
Trans Fat	0.0 g
Cholesterol	0 mg
Sodium	415 mg
Potassium	625 mg
Total Carbohydrate	53 g
Dietary Fiber	6 g
Sugars	5 g
Protein	10 g
Phosphorus	265 mg

Chef's Tip

Feel free to add shrimp to this dish if you would like an additional protein source.

Cajun Shrimp LC

Makes: 5 servings   *Serving Size: 1/5 recipe*   *Prep Time: 10 minutes*

2 tsp olive oil, divided
1 green bell pepper, thinly sliced
1 red bell pepper, thinly sliced
1 small onion, thinly sliced
1 garlic clove, minced
12 ounces peeled and deveined raw shrimp
1 14.5-ounce can fat-free, low-sodium chicken broth
1 tsp paprika
1 tsp onion powder
1/4 tsp cayenne pepper
1/2 tsp ground black pepper

1 Add 1 tsp olive oil to a large nonstick skillet over medium-high heat. Add peppers and onion and stir-fry for 5 minutes. Remove from pan and set aside.

2 Add remaining 1 tsp olive oil to pan and reduce heat to medium. Add garlic and shrimp and sauté for 1–2 minutes or until shrimp is done. Add peppers back to pan.

3 Pour chicken broth, paprika, onion powder, cayenne pepper, and black pepper in pan and bring to a simmer for 1 minute.

Exchanges/Choices
1 Vegetable   2 Lean Meat

Calories	115
Calories from Fat	25
Total Fat	3.0 g
Saturated Fat	0.6 g
Trans Fat	0.0 g
Cholesterol	110 mg
Sodium	610 mg
Potassium	365 mg
Total Carbohydrate	6 g
Dietary Fiber	2 g
Sugars	3 g
Protein	16 g
Phosphorus	185 mg

Chef's Tip

Shrimp could be served over quinoa or quinoa pasta, if desired.

Mediterranean Chicken

Makes: 5 servings   *Serving Size: about 1 1/3 cups*   *Prep Time: 13 minutes*

1   cup brown rice, uncooked
    nonstick cooking spray
3/4 pound boneless, skinless chicken
    breasts, cubed
1/4 tsp ground black pepper
1   Tbsp olive oil
3   garlic cloves, minced
1   cup diced zucchini
1   green bell pepper, diced
1/2 cup diced onion
1   15-ounce can no-salt-added diced
    tomatoes with juice
1   cup fat-free, low-sodium chicken
    broth
1   Tbsp dried oregano
1/2 tsp salt (optional)

1 Cook rice according to package directions, omitting salt.

2 Coat a large nonstick skillet or wok with cooking spray. Season chicken with black pepper and sauté over medium-high heat for 3–4 minutes. Remove chicken from pan.

3 Add olive oil and garlic to skillet and sauté 30 seconds. Add zucchini, green pepper, and onion and sauté 3–4 minutes. Add chicken back to pan along with diced tomatoes, chicken broth, oregano, and salt (optional).

4 Bring to a boil; reduce heat and simmer 6–7 minutes. Add cooked rice to pan and mix well.

Exchanges/Choices
2 Starch   1 Vegetable
2 Lean Meat

Calories	275
Calories from Fat	55
Total Fat	6.0 g
Saturated Fat	1.1 g
Trans Fat	0.0 g
Cholesterol	40 mg
Sodium	175 mg
Potassium	550 mg
Total Carbohydrate	37 g
Dietary Fiber	4 g
Sugars	4 g
Protein	19 g
Phosphorus	275 mg

Chef's Tip

This dish is as tasty as it is beautiful. Garnish it with a few sprigs of fresh oregano for an extra flair.

Cucumber Tomato Salad GF LC

Makes: 5 servings   *Serving Size: 1/5 recipe*   *Prep Time: 10 minutes*

2 large cucumbers, peeled, seeded, and diced
2 medium tomatoes, seeded and diced
1 Tbsp olive oil
2 Tbsp red wine vinegar
1/2 tsp salt (optional)
dash ground black pepper

1 In a medium bowl, toss cucumbers and tomatoes.

2 Drizzle oil and vinegar over vegetables and toss to coat. Season with salt (optional) and pepper.

Exchanges/Choices
1 Vegetable   1/2 Fat

Calories 45
  Calories from Fat 25
Total Fat . . . . 3.0 g
  Saturated Fat . . . . 0.4 g
  Trans Fat . . . . 0.0 g
Cholesterol . . . . 0 mg
Sodium . . . . 0 mg
Potassium . . . . 225 mg
Total Carbohydrate . . . . 4 g
  Dietary Fiber . . . . 1 g
  Sugars . . . . 2 g
Protein . . . . 1 g
Phosphorus . . . . 30 mg

Chef's Tip

For added flavor, sprinkle some feta cheese on top of this salad.

AUGUST
WEEK 4

DAY 1
Greek Lemon Chicken
and Quinoa   280

DAY 2
Hungarian
Goulash   281

DAY 3
Cuban Black Beans and
Pork   282

DAY 4
Stuffed Turkey Meatloaf
Balls   283
Ratatouille   285

DAY 5
Moroccan Pork
with Caramelized
Radicchio   286
Stuffed Tomatoes   287

**DESSERT OF
THE MONTH**
Tiramisu   288

GROCERY LIST

Fresh Produce
Bell peppers, green—2
Bell pepper, red—1
Cilantro—1 bunch
Eggplant—1
Garlic—1 head
Mushrooms, cremini
    (baby bella)—8 ounces
Onions, yellow or white—3
Oregano—1 bunch
Potatoes, Idaho, medium—2
Radicchio—1 head
Tomatoes, beefsteak, large
    (9–10 ounces each)—4
Zucchini—3

Meat, Poultry, & Fish
Beef, sirloin steak—1 pound
Chicken breasts, boneless,
    skinless, 4 ounces each—4
Pork chops, boneless, 4 ounces
    each—4
Pork tenderloin—1 pound
Turkey, ground, 93% lean—
    1 pound

Grains, Bread, & Pasta
Oats, rolled, old-fashioned—
    1/2 cup
Quinoa—1 box
Ronzoni Healthy Harvest Whole
    Grain egg noodles—6 ounces

Dairy & Cheese
Cheese, goat, crumbled—1/4 cup
Cheese, Parmesan—1 small block
Cream cheese, fat-free—5 ounces
Cream cheese, light—7 ounces
Eggs
Sour cream, fat-free—1/2 cup

Canned Goods & Sauces
Beans, black, 16-ounce cans—2
Broth, chicken, fat-free, low-
    sodium, 14.5-ounce cans—2
Broth, vegetable, fat-free, low-
    sodium, 14.5-ounce can—1
Tomatoes, crushed, 15-ounce
    can—1
Worcestershire sauce

Frozen Foods
Corn—1 small bag
Whipped topping, fat-free—
    8 ounces

Staples, Seasonings,
& Baking Needs
Black pepper, ground
Cayenne pepper
Cinnamon
Cumin
Flour, all-purpose
Ketchup
Lemon juice
Lime juice
Mustard, dry
Nonstick cooking spray
Oil, canola
Oil, olive
Oregano
Paprika
Red pepper flakes
Salt
Sugar
Sugar, powdered
Vinegar, balsamic
Vinegar, apple cider

Miscellaneous
Cocoa, unsweetened—3 Tbsp
Coffee, instant granules—2 Tbsp
Cookies, ladyfingers—24
Pudding mix, instant, vanilla,
    1-ounce package—1

Greek Lemon Chicken and Quinoa GF

Makes: 4 servings   *Serving Size: 1 chicken breast and 1/2 cup quinoa*   *Prep Time: 35 minutes*

3	Tbsp fresh lemon juice
2	tsp olive oil
3	garlic cloves, minced
1	tsp chopped fresh oregano (or 1/4 tsp dried oregano)
4	4-ounce boneless, skinless chicken breasts nonstick cooking spray
1/4	tsp salt (optional)
1/4	tsp ground black pepper
2	cups cooked quinoa

1 In a medium bowl, whisk together lemon juice, olive oil, garlic, and oregano. Add chicken breasts to marinade and turn to coat. Marinate chicken in refrigerator for 30 minutes.

2 Coat a large nonstick skillet with cooking spray. Remove chicken from marinade and season well with salt (optional) and pepper. Reserve marinade. Cook chicken over high heat for about 5–7 minutes on each side. Add reserved marinade to pan and bring to a boil for 1 minute.

3 Serve chicken breasts over quinoa.

Exchanges/Choices

1 1/2 Starch   3 Lean Meat
1/2 Fat

Calories	285
Calories from Fat	80
Total Fat	9.0 g
Saturated Fat	1.7 g
Trans Fat	0.0 g
Cholesterol	65 mg
Sodium	65 mg
Potassium	375 mg
Total Carbohydrate	21 g
Dietary Fiber	3 g
Sugars	2 g
Protein	28 g
Phosphorus	320 mg

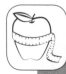

Dietitian's Tip

Quinoa contains more high-quality protein than any other grain, and it's gluten-free. Steamed broccoli and carrots would make a great side dish for this entrée.

Hungarian Goulash

Makes: 8 servings   *Serving Size: 1 cup*   *Prep Time: 15 minutes*

6 ounces Ronzoni Healthy Harvest Whole Grain egg noodles, uncooked
nonstick cooking spray
1 pound sirloin steak, sliced into thin 1-inch pieces
1 medium onion, thinly sliced
2 medium Idaho potatoes, peeled and diced
2 Tbsp ketchup
1/2 tsp Worcestershire sauce
2 Tbsp all-purpose flour
2 14.5-ounce cans fat-free, low-sodium chicken broth
2 garlic cloves, minced
1 tsp dry mustard
1 Tbsp paprika
1/2 tsp salt (optional)
1/4 tsp ground black pepper
1/2 cup fat-free sour cream

1 Cook whole-grain egg noodles according to package directions, omitting salt. Drain.

2 Coat a large nonstick skillet with cooking spray over high heat. Add sirloin and sauté for 3–4 minutes. Remove from pan and set aside.

3 Add onion to pan and sauté for 5–6 minutes or until onions begin to brown. Add potatoes and continue to sauté.

4 In a medium bowl, whisk together remaining ingredients except sour cream. Pour mixture over potatoes and onions and bring to a boil. Reduce heat and simmer for 20 minutes or until potatoes are soft.

5 Add steak back to pan and stir in sour cream.

Exchanges/Choices
2 Starch   1 Lean Meat

Calories	210
Calories from Fat	25
Total Fat	3.0 g
Saturated Fat	1.0 g
Trans Fat	0.1 g
Cholesterol	25 mg
Sodium	350 mg
Potassium	475 mg
Total Carbohydrate	30 g
Dietary Fiber	4 g
Sugars	3 g
Protein	17 g
Phosphorus	200 mg

Chef's Tip

This version tastes just like your grandmother's! You can substitute fat-free sour cream for regular in any recipe and still achieve wonderful creaminess and flavor.

Cuban Black Beans and Pork

Makes: 5 servings   *Serving Size: 1/2 cup beans*   *Prep Time: 5 minutes*

2	tsp canola oil
1	pound pork tenderloin, cut into 1-inch chunks
1	large onion, chopped
1	green bell pepper, cut into 1/2-inch strips
4	large garlic cloves, minced
1	tsp cumin
1/2	Tbsp dried oregano
2	16-ounce cans black beans, rinsed and drained
1	cup canned fat-free, reduced-sodium vegetable broth
1	Tbsp apple cider vinegar
1/2	tsp crushed red pepper flakes (optional)

1 In a large saucepan, heat oil over medium heat. Add pork and sauté for 4 minutes. Add onion, green pepper, garlic, cumin, and oregano and sauté additional 5 minutes.

2 Add black beans, vegetable broth, vinegar, and red pepper flakes to pan and simmer for 15 minutes.

Exchanges/Choices

1 1/2 Starch   1 Vegetable
3 Lean Meat

Calories	280
Calories from Fat	45
Total Fat	5.0 g
Saturated Fat	1.1 g
Trans Fat	0.0 g
Cholesterol	50 mg
Sodium	270 mg
Potassium	815 mg
Total Carbohydrate	31 g
Dietary Fiber	10 g
Sugars	5 g
Protein	28 g
Phosphorus	330 mg

Dietitian's Tip

This dish is a great combination of lean protein (pork tenderloin) and healthy carbs (beans)!

Stuffed Turkey Meatloaf Balls

Makes: 8 meatloaf balls　　　*Serving Size: 2 meatloaf balls*　　　*Prep Time: 20 minutes*

Filling

	nonstick cooking spray
1	Tbsp olive oil
8	ounces cremini (baby bella) mushrooms, chopped
1/2	medium onion, chopped
2	garlic cloves, chopped
1	tsp dried oregano
1/4	tsp ground black pepper
1/4	cup freshly grated Parmesan cheese

Meatloaf

1	pound 93% lean ground turkey
1/2	cup old-fashioned rolled oats
2	egg whites
2	garlic cloves, minced
1/2	medium onion, minced
1	medium zucchini, shredded
1/2	tsp salt (optional)
1/4	tsp ground black pepper

Glaze

1/2	cup ketchup
1/4	cup balsamic vinegar

1 Preheat oven to 375°F. Coat a large baking sheet with cooking spray.

2 Heat olive oil in a medium sauté pan over medium-high heat. Add the filling ingredients except the Parmesan cheese and sauté until mushrooms and onions are tender and have expelled all of their liquid. Remove from heat, stir in the Parmesan cheese and set aside to cool.

3 In a mixing bowl, combine the meatloaf ingredients until incorporated.

(continued on next page)

Exchanges/Choices

1/2 Starch	1/2 Carbohydrate
2 Vegetable	4 Lean Meat
1 Fat	

Calories	350
Calories from Fat	135
Total Fat	15.0 g
Saturated Fat	3.5 g
Trans Fat	0.1 g
Cholesterol	90 mg
Sodium	490 mg
Potassium	905 mg
Total Carbohydrate	26 g
Dietary Fiber	3 g
Sugars	13 g
Protein	30 g
Phosphorus	390 mg

Stuffed Turkey Meatloaf Balls (Continued)

4 Once the filling is cool, pulse the filling in a food processor until minced but still slightly chunky. Do not purée into a paste.

5 Divide meatloaf mixture into 8 equal portions. Flatten one portion onto your hand to form a patty. Place a heaping 1 Tbsp of mushroom mixture into center of the patty and close your hand to form a ball around the mushroom mixture. Repeat for remaining meatloaf balls. Place onto the sprayed baking sheet and bake for 35 minutes.

6 In a small bowl, whisk together ketchup and balsamic vinegar. After the meatloaf balls have baked for 35 minutes, brush each meatloaf ball generously with half the glaze. Return to the oven for 5 minutes, then brush the remaining glaze on the meatloaf balls and bake for 5 more minutes.

Chef's Tip

These meatloaf balls aren't your grandmother's meatloaf. They are a fun party food and kids love them, too. Adding the oatmeal increases the fiber content and they are flavorful and satisfying. Serve with a green salad and creamy polenta for a fancy Italian meal.

▲ American Diabetes Association.
My Food Advisor

This is an original recipe from the American Diabetes Association's online nutrition resource, **Recipes for Healthy Living**—your one-stop shop for diabetes-friendly recipes, meal plans, and other nutrition tips. Sign up today for the FREE *Recipes for Healthy Living* newsletter and to get access to the website by visiting **www.diabetes.org/recipes**.

Ratatouille GF LC

Makes: 6 servings   *Serving Size: 1 cup*   *Prep Time: 15 minutes*

1	Tbsp olive oil
2	garlic cloves, minced
1	medium eggplant, cubed
2	small zucchini, sliced
1	green bell pepper, chopped
1	cup canned crushed tomatoes
1/2	tsp salt (optional)
1/4	tsp ground black pepper

1 Heat oil in a large nonstick skillet over medium-high heat. Add garlic and sauté 30 seconds.

2 Add remaining ingredients and cook 10–15 minutes, stirring occasionally, until vegetables are tender.

Exchanges/Choices
2 Vegetable   1/2 Fat

Calories 70
  Calories from Fat 20
Total Fat . . . . .2.5 g
  Saturated Fat . . . . .0.4 g
  Trans Fat . . . . .0.0 g
Cholesterol. . . . . 0 mg
Sodium . . . . 60 mg
Potassium. . . . . 480 mg
Total Carbohydrate . . . . . . 11 g
  Dietary Fiber . . . . 5 g
  Sugars . . . . 5 g
Protein . . . . 2 g
Phosphorus . . . . 55 mg

Chef's Tip

This classic side dish is just as good when served the next day.

Moroccan Pork with Caramelized Radicchio GF LC

Makes: 4 servings   *Serving Size: 1 pork chop*   *Prep Time: 10 minutes*

1   tsp cumin
1   tsp paprika
1/4 tsp cayenne pepper
1/4 tsp ground cinnamon
1/4 tsp dry mustard
4   4-ounce boneless pork chops
2   tsp olive oil
    nonstick cooking spray
1   head radicchio, chopped
1   tsp sugar
1/2 tsp salt (optional)
1/4 tsp ground black pepper

1 In a small bowl, combine the first 5 ingredients and mix well. Dredge one side of each pork chop in spice mixture.

2 Add oil and a generous amount of cooking spray to a large nonstick skillet over high heat. Place chops spice side down in the skillet. Cook for 6 minutes on each side. Remove from pan and set aside.

3 Spray skillet generously again and add radicchio to pan. Sauté radicchio for 2 minutes. Add sugar, salt (optional), and pepper. Sauté 5–6 more minutes or until radicchio begins to caramelize. Serve radicchio on top of each pork chop.

Exchanges/Choices
3 Lean Meat   1 Fat

Calories 190
  Calories from Fat 90
Total Fat . . . . 10.0 g
  Saturated Fat . . . . 2.9 g
  Trans Fat . . . . 0.0 g
Cholesterol . . . . 60 mg
Sodium . . . . 55 mg
Potassium . . . . 445 mg
Total Carbohydrate . . . . 4 g
  Dietary Fiber . . . . 1 g
  Sugars . . . . 1 g
Protein . . . . 22 g
Phosphorus . . . . 195 mg

Dietitian's Tip

Most people just use radicchio in salads. You won't believe how good it tastes caramelized in this recipe. Try cooking other leafy salad greens—they add fantastic texture and flavor to other dishes!

Stuffed Tomatoes GF LC

Makes: 8 servings   *Serving Size: 1/2 tomato*   *Prep Time: 15 minutes*

2   cups frozen corn, thawed
1   large red bell pepper, diced
4   large beefsteak tomatoes (each about 9–10 ounces)
1   Tbsp olive oil
2   Tbsp fresh lime juice
1   garlic clove, minced
2   Tbsp chopped fresh cilantro
1/2 tsp salt (optional)
1/4 tsp ground black pepper
1/4 cup crumbled goat cheese

1 Toss corn and bell pepper in a medium bowl and set aside.

2 Cut tomatoes horizontally in half. Using a small spoon, scoop center of tomatoes into small bowl, leaving a shell. Discard tomato seeds and juices and chop tomato meat; add to corn mixture.

3 In a small bowl, whisk together oil, lime juice, garlic, cilantro, salt (optional), and pepper. Drizzle over corn mixture. Spoon corn salad into tomato shells.

4 Sprinkle each tomato with 1 Tbsp goat cheese and serve cold.

Exchanges/Choices
1/2 Starch   1 Vegetable
1/2 Fat

Calories	95
Calories from Fat	35
Total Fat	4.0 g
Saturated Fat	1.4 g
Trans Fat	0.0 g
Cholesterol	5 mg
Sodium	25 mg
Potassium	405 mg
Total Carbohydrate	14 g
Dietary Fiber	3 g
Sugars	5 g
Protein	4 g
Phosphorus	90 mg

Dietitian's Tip

Tomatoes offer great nutritional value. Not only are they a good source of vitamins A and C, but they also contain a pigment called lycopene, which may slow the development of some cancers.

Tiramisu

Makes: 16 servings　　　*Serving Size: 1/2 cup*　　　*Prep Time: 35 minutes*

1	cup cold water
1	1-ounce package sugar-free vanilla instant pudding mix
1/2	cup powdered sugar
7	ounces light cream cheese
5	ounces fat-free cream cheese
8	ounces fat-free whipped topping
1	cup hot water
2	Tbsp instant coffee granules
24	ladyfingers
3	Tbsp unsweetened cocoa, divided

1 In a medium bowl, combine cold water, vanilla pudding mix, and powdered sugar and stir with whisk. Chill 20 minutes.

2 Add cream cheeses to pudding mixture and beat with a mixer at medium speed until well blended. Fold in whipped topping.

3 In a small bowl or mug, mix hot water and coffee granules.

4 Split ladyfingers in half lengthwise. Arrange 16 ladyfinger halves flat side down in a trifle or large glass bowl. Drizzle ladyfingers with coffee. Spread 1/3 of the pudding mixture over the ladyfingers and sprinkle with 1 Tbsp cocoa. Repeat layers, ending with cocoa.

5 Cover and chill 4 hours or longer.

Exchanges/Choices

1 Carbohydrate	1 Fat

Calories 115
　Calories from Fat 30
Total Fat . . . . .3.5 g
　Saturated Fat . . . . .1.9 g
　Trans Fat . . . . .0.0 g
Cholesterol. . . . . 30 mg
Sodium . . . . 205 mg
Potassium. . . . . 95 mg
Total Carbohydrate . . . . . . 16 g
　Dietary Fiber . . . . 0 g
　Sugars . . . . 13 g
Protein . . . . 3 g
Phosphorus . . . . 140 mg

Dietitian's Tip

You can still enjoy dessert if you have diabetes . . . just enjoy it in moderation! This one is beautiful when served in a trifle bowl.

SEPTEMBER

Super Salad Meals

Treat yourself to a quick and hearty salad like you've never had before. This month features one salad per week that's not your typical lettuce and tomato. Salads can be a quick way to work a variety of food groups into a meal, and they're also are a great way to increase your vegetable intake. This month's salads are created into a complete meal by adding a variety of different tastes and textures, such as with the Mandarin Orange Chicken Salad and the Southwest Salad.

Zucchini and Green Pepper Frittata (page 318)
Spinach Salad with Warm Bacon Dressing (page 319)
This frittata and delicious salad will delight and amaze your taste buds. Together, these dishes may look impressive, but they're so easy to make!

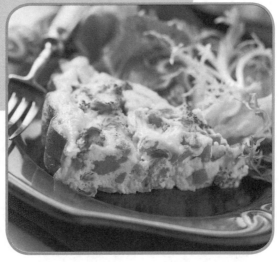

 gluten-free recipe, but always check ingredients for gluten.

 these recipes contain 15 grams of carbohydrate or less per serving.

 new recipe for the second edition.

SEPTEMBER RECIPES

SEPTEMBER

WEEK 1

DAY 1
Chicken Caesar
  Salad   292

DAY 2
Shrimp Fajitas   293
Broccoli
  Amandine   294

DAY 3
Beef Tips with
  Mushroom
  Gravy   295
Roasted Brussels
  Sprouts   296

DAY 4
Black-Eyed Pea
  Soup   297

DAY 5
Chicken Couscous
  Salad   298

GROCERY LIST

Fresh Produce
Bell pepper, green—1
Bell pepper, red—1
Broccoli florets, 12-ounce
  bag—1
Carrot—1
Garlic—2 cloves
Greens, field, mixed—4 cups
Lemons—3
Lettuce, romaine, 10-ounce
  bag—1
Mushrooms, sliced—1 pint
Onions, yellow or white—2

Meat, Poultry, & Fish
Beef tenderloin tips—
  1 pound
Chicken breasts, boneless,
  skinless—2 pounds
Shrimp—1 pound
Turkey bacon—8 slices

Grains, Bread, & Pasta
Couscous, whole-wheat—
  1 box
Tortillas, corn, 6 inches—8

Dairy & Cheese
Cheese, Parmesan—1 block
Milk, fat-free—1/4 cup
Sour cream, fat-free—1/4 cup

Canned Goods & Sauces
Black-eyed peas, 15.5-ounce
  cans—2
Broth, beef, fat-free, low-
  sodium, 14.5-ounce
  can—1
Broth, chicken, fat-free,
  low-sodium, 14.5-ounce
  cans—3

Frozen Foods
Brussels sprouts—1 pound
Spinach—1 small package

Staples, Seasonings, & Baking Needs
Black pepper, ground
Cayenne pepper
Chili powder
Cornstarch
Cumin
Honey
Mayonnaise, light
Mustard, dry
Nonstick cooking spray
Oil, canola
Oil, olive
Red pepper flakes
Salt

Miscellaneous
Almonds, slivered—3 Tbsp
Walnuts, chopped—1/4 cup

Chicken Caesar Salad GF LC

Makes: 6 servings   *Serving Size: 1/6 recipe*   *Prep Time: 10 minutes*

Dressing

2	Tbsp light mayonnaise
1/4	cup fat-free sour cream
1/4	cup fat-free milk
2	Tbsp lemon juice
1/2	tsp dry mustard
3	Tbsp freshly grated Parmesan cheese
1/4	tsp salt (optional)
	dash ground black pepper

Salad

1	pound boneless, skinless chicken breasts
1	10-ounce bag romaine lettuce
2	Tbsp freshly grated Parmesan cheese

1 Prepare an indoor or outdoor grill. In a medium bowl, whisk together dressing ingredients. Reserve 1/2 cup of dressing.

2 Add chicken breasts to remaining dressing and marinate in the refrigerator for 15 minutes.

3 Remove chicken breasts from marinade and grill over medium-high heat for 5–6 minutes on each side or until done. Slice grilled chicken into strips.

4 In a large bowl, toss together salad ingredients. Drizzle with reserved dressing and toss well to coat.

5 Divide salad among 6 plates and top with sliced chicken.

Exchanges/Choices
1/2 Carbohydrate   2 Lean Meat

Calories	135
Calories from Fat	40
Total Fat	4.5 g
Saturated Fat	1.4 g
Trans Fat	0.0 g
Cholesterol	50 mg
Sodium	160 mg
Potassium	290 mg
Total Carbohydrate	5 g
Dietary Fiber	1 g
Sugars	2 g
Protein	19 g
Phosphorus	180 mg

Dietitian's Tip

Caesar salad dressing is typically very high in fat, but we've solved that problem by using light mayo, fat-free sour cream, and fat-free milk.

Shrimp Fajitas GF

Makes: 4 servings   *Serving Size: 2 fajitas*   *Prep Time: 10 minutes*

nonstick cooking spray
2   tsp canola oil
1   medium red bell pepper, cut into 1/4-inch strips
1   medium green bell pepper, cut into 1/4-inch strips
1   medium onion, cut into 1/4-inch strips
10 ounces peeled and deveined uncooked shrimp
2   Tbsp water
1   tsp chili powder
1/2 tsp cumin
1/4 tsp cayenne pepper
1/4 tsp ground black pepper
8   6-inch corn tortillas, warmed

1 Coat a large nonstick skillet with cooking spray and add oil; heat over medium-high heat. Sauté peppers for 10 minutes. Add remaining ingredients except tortillas and cook for another 5 minutes or until shrimp is done.

2 Fill each tortilla with 1/8 of shrimp and pepper mixture.

Exchanges/Choices
1 1/2 Starch   1 Vegetable
2 Lean Meat

Calories 235
   Calories from Fat 40
Total Fat . . . . 4.5 g
   Saturated Fat . . . . 0.6 g
   Trans Fat . . . . 0.0 g
Cholesterol . . . . 115 mg
Sodium . . . . 615 mg
Potassium . . . . 430 mg
Total Carbohydrate . . . . . . 30 g
   Dietary Fiber . . . . 5 g
   Sugars . . . . 4 g
Protein . . . . 19 g
Phosphorus . . . . 335 mg

Chef's Tip

Bell peppers come in a variety of colors—try orange and yellow peppers in this dish for a colorful and tasty meal.

Broccoli Amandine GF LC NEW

Makes: 6 servings   *Serving Size: 1/2 cup*   *Prep Time: 5 minutes*

	nonstick cooking spray
1	12-ounce bag broccoli florets
1 1/2	Tbsp olive oil
2	garlic cloves, minced
3	Tbsp slivered almonds
1/8	tsp ground black pepper
1	Tbsp lemon juice
1	Tbsp freshly grated Parmesan cheese

1 Preheat oven to 425°F. Spray a baking sheet with cooking spray.

2 In a small bowl, mix together broccoli, olive oil, garlic, almonds, and black pepper. Pour mixture onto baking sheet.

3 Bake for 10–12 minutes, until broccoli tips are slightly brown.

4 Pour broccoli into a bowl and mix in lemon juice and Parmesan cheese.

Exchanges/Choices
1 Vegetable   1 Fat

Calories	75
Calories from Fat	55
Total Fat	6.0 g
Saturated Fat	0.8 g
Trans Fat	0.0 g
Cholesterol	0 mg
Sodium	30 mg
Potassium	225 mg
Total Carbohydrate	5 g
Dietary Fiber	2 g
Sugars	1 g
Protein	3 g
Phosphorus	65 mg

Dietitian's Tip

You've probably had green beans amandine, now you have to try broccoli amandine. Almonds and nuts contain heart-healthy monounsaturated and polyunsaturated fats. The American Heart Association recommends eating at least 4 servings per week of nuts, legumes, or seeds.

△. American Diabetes Association.
MyFood**Advisor**

This is an original recipe from the American Diabetes Association's online nutrition resource, **Recipes for Healthy Living**—your one-stop shop for diabetes-friendly recipes, meal plans, and other nutrition tips. Sign up today for the FREE *Recipes for Healthy Living* newsletter and to get access to the website by visiting **www.diabetes.org/recipes**.

Beef Tips with Mushroom Gravy LC

Makes: 4 servings   *Serving Size: 1/4 recipe*   *Prep Time: 10 minutes*

nonstick cooking spray
1   pound beef tenderloin tips
1   pint sliced mushrooms
1   cup fat-free, low-sodium beef broth
1   Tbsp cornstarch
1/2   tsp salt (optional)
1/4   tsp ground black pepper

1 Coat a large nonstick skillet with cooking spray over high heat. Add beef tips to skillet and sauté for 5–6 minutes or until browned well. Remove beef from pan and set aside. Cover beef.

2 Add mushrooms to pan and sauté for 4–5 minutes.

3 In a small bowl, whisk together broth and cornstarch. Pour over mushrooms and bring to a boil, scraping brown bits up from the bottom of the pan. Reduce heat and simmer for 2 minutes.

4 Stir in salt (optional) and pepper. Return beef tips and any juice and stir into gravy.

Exchanges/Choices
3 Lean Meat

Calories	160
Calories from Fat	55
Total Fat	6.0 g
Saturated Fat	2.2 g
Trans Fat	0.0 g
Cholesterol	60 mg
Sodium	155 mg
Potassium	410 mg
Total Carbohydrate	3 g
Dietary Fiber	0 g
Sugars	1 g
Protein	23 g
Phosphorus	205 mg

Chef's Tip

Serve this home-style favorite next to Roasted Brussels Sprouts (page 296).

American Diabetes Association.
MyFood**Advisor**

This is an original recipe from the American Diabetes Association's online nutrition resource, **Recipes for Healthy Living**—your one-stop shop for diabetes-friendly recipes, meal plans, and other nutrition tips. Sign up today for the FREE *Recipes for Healthy Living* newsletter and to get access to the website by visiting **www.diabetes.org/recipes**.

Roasted Brussels Sprouts GF LC NEW

Makes: 5 servings   *Serving Size: 6 Brussels sprouts*   *Prep Time: 5 minutes*

nonstick cooking spray
1 pound frozen Brussels sprouts, thawed
2 Tbsp olive oil
1/2 tsp ground black pepper
3 slices turkey bacon, cut into 1-inch pieces

1 Preheat oven to 400°F. Spray a baking sheet with cooking spray.

2 Place Brussels sprouts in a bowl and add oil; toss to coat.

3 Add pepper and bacon and mix well.

4 Place Brussels sprouts on a baking sheet and bake for 35–40 minutes or until they are crisp on the outside.

Exchanges/Choices
1 Vegetable   1 1/2 Fat

Calories 95
  Calories from Fat 55
Total Fat . . . . 6.0 g
  Saturated Fat . . . . 0.9 g
  Trans Fat . . . . 0.0 g
Cholesterol . . . . 5 mg
Sodium . . . . 85 mg
Potassium . . . . 290 mg
Total Carbohydrate . . . . 7 g
  Dietary Fiber . . . . 4 g
  Sugars . . . . 2 g
Protein . . . . 5 g
Phosphorus . . . . 90 mg

Dietitian's Tip

Brussels sprouts are low in calories and carbohydrate, which means they are good for blood glucose. Roasting is a great way to enhance their flavor.

Black-Eyed Pea Soup

Makes: 8 servings   *Serving Size: 1 cup*   *Prep Time: 10 minutes*

2	tsp olive oil
5	slices turkey bacon, chopped
1	small onion, finely diced
1	cup shredded carrots
1/4	cup frozen chopped spinach, thawed and drained
2	15.5-ounce cans black-eyed peas, rinsed and drained
3	14.5-ounce cans fat-free, low-sodium chicken broth
1/2	tsp salt (optional)
1/4	tsp ground black pepper
1/4	tsp crushed red pepper flakes

1 Add oil to a large soup pot over high heat. Add bacon and sauté for 3 minutes or until bacon is crispy. Add onion and sauté 4 minutes or until clear. Add carrots and spinach. Sauté 3–4 minutes.

2 Add remaining ingredients and bring to a boil. Reduce heat and simmer for 20 minutes.

Exchanges/Choices

1 Starch   1 Lean Meat

Calories	140
Calories from Fat	25
Total Fat	3.0 g
Saturated Fat	0.8 g
Trans Fat	0.0 g
Cholesterol	5 mg
Sodium	305 mg
Potassium	425 mg
Total Carbohydrate	19 g
Dietary Fiber	6 g
Sugars	4 g
Protein	9 g
Phosphorus	170 mg

Dietitian's Tip

Soups can be a great way to incorporate more legumes and beans into your diet. Beans and legumes, such as lentils, pinto beans, red beans, and navy beans, are low in fat and a great source of fiber.

Chicken Couscous Salad

Makes: 6 servings   *Serving Size: 1/6 recipe*   *Prep Time: 15 minutes*

Dressing
1/4	cup lemon juice
2	Tbsp honey
2	Tbsp olive oil
1/4	tsp salt (optional)
	dash ground black pepper

Salad
4	cups cooked and cooled whole-wheat couscous
2	cups cooked, chopped chicken breast meat
1/4	cup chopped walnuts, toasted
4	cups mixed field greens

1 In a medium bowl, whisk together dressing ingredients and set aside.

2 In another medium bowl, toss couscous, chicken, and walnuts. Drizzle dressing over couscous and toss to coat.

3 Arrange field greens on a plate and mound 1 cup of couscous salad in center. Repeat for remaining 5 plates.

Exchanges/Choices
1 1/2 Starch   1/2 Carbohydrate
2 Lean Meat   1 Fat

Calories	290
Calories from Fat	90
Total Fat	10.0 g
Saturated Fat	1.4 g
Trans Fat	0.0 g
Cholesterol	40 mg
Sodium	50 mg
Potassium	300 mg
Total Carbohydrate	34 g
Dietary Fiber	5 g
Sugars	6 g
Protein	20 g
Phosphorus	160 mg

Chef's Tip

This recipe shows you how to mix different textures and flavors for a unique and outstanding meal.

SEPTEMBER
WEEK 2

DAY 1
Asian Beef Noodle
    Salad   300

DAY 2
Chicken Fingers   301
Savory Grits   302

DAY 3
Salad Niçoise   303

DAY 4
Grilled Veal
    Chops   304
Braised Red
    Cabbage   305

DAY 5
Taco Pizza   306

GROCERY LIST

Fresh Produce
Apples, Granny Smith,
    small—2
Cabbage, red—1 head
Carrots, medium—2
Cucumbers medium—2
Green beans—4 cups
Lettuce, romaine—1 head
Lime—1
Mint—1 bunch
Potatoes, red, new—
    1/2 pound
Salad greens, mixed—8 cups
Scallions—1 bunch
Tomatoes—2
Tomatoes, grape—24

Meat, Poultry, & Fish
Beef, ground, 95% lean—
    1/2 pound
Beef, top sirloin steak—
    1 pound
Chicken breasts, boneless,
    skinless—1 pound
Veal chops, boneless,
    4 ounces each—4

Grains, Bread, & Pasta
Cereal, brown rice—1 small
    box
Grits—1 small box
Pasta, angel hair, whole-
    wheat—8 ounces
Pizza crust, whole-wheat,
    12-inch prepackaged—1

Dairy & Cheese
Cheese, cheddar, reduced-fat,
    shredded—3 ounces
Cheese, Mexican-
    style, reduced-fat,
    shredded—2/3 cup
Eggs

Canned Goods & Sauces
Broth, chicken, fat-free,
    low-sodium, 14.5-ounce
    can—1
Hot pepper sauce
Soy sauce, lite
Tuna, packed in water,
    6-ounce cans—2

Staples, Seasonings, & Baking Needs
Allspice
Black pepper, ground
Cayenne pepper
Chili powder
Cumin
Flour, all-purpose
Honey
Mustard, Dijon
Nonstick cooking spray
Oil, olive
Oil, sesame
Onion salt
Salt
Vinegar, apple cider
Vinegar, red wine
Vinegar, rice wine

Miscellaneous
Peanut butter
Peanuts, unsalted, roasted—
    3 Tbsp
Salad dressing, Italian,
    light—2 Tbsp
Salsa
Sesame seeds

Asian Beef Noodle Salad

Makes: 6 servings   *Serving Size: 1/6 recipe*   *Prep Time: 15 minutes*

Dressing
- **2** Tbsp smooth peanut butter
- **3** Tbsp fresh lime juice
- **1/4** tsp cayenne pepper
- **1/2** cup chopped fresh mint

Salad
- **8** ounces whole-wheat angel hair pasta, uncooked
- **2** Tbsp lite soy sauce
- **2** Tbsp rice wine vinegar
- **1** pound top sirloin steak, cut into 3-inch strips
- **2** tsp sesame oil
   nonstick cooking spray
- **2** medium cucumbers, peeled, seeded, and sliced into thin sticks
- **2** medium carrots, shredded
- **4** scallions, cut diagonally
- **3** Tbsp roasted unsalted peanuts, coarsely chopped
- **2** Tbsp sesame seeds, toasted

1 In a medium bowl, whisk together dressing ingredients. Set aside.

2 Cook pasta according to package directions, omitting salt; drain and rinse under cold water to cool.

3 In a medium bowl, whisk together soy sauce and rice wine vinegar. Add beef and toss to coat.

4 Add the sesame oil and a generous amount of cooking spray to a large sauté pan or wok over high heat. Stir-fry beef in batches; set aside to cool slightly.

5 In a large salad bowl, toss remaining ingredients, except sesame seeds, with cooled pasta. Drizzle the dressing over the salad and toss to coat.

6 Arrange 6 portions of the salad on salad plates and top with a portion of beef. Garnish with toasted sesame seeds.

Chef's Tip

This recipes makes for a great lunch dish. It's easy and impressive!

Exchanges/Choices

2 Starch	1 Vegetable
3 Lean Meat	1 Fat

Calories	345
Calories from Fat	110
Total Fat	12.0 g
Saturated Fat	2.5 g
Trans Fat	0.1 g
Cholesterol	30 mg
Sodium	265 mg
Potassium	545 mg
Total Carbohydrate	35 g
Dietary Fiber	7 g
Sugars	4 g
Protein	25 g
Phosphorus	300 mg

Chicken Fingers

Makes: 5 servings   *Serving Size: 3 chicken strips*   *Prep Time: 15 minutes*

nonstick cooking spray
1/2   cup all-purpose flour
1/2   tsp salt (optional)
1/4   tsp ground black pepper
1   egg
2   egg whites
1/2   tsp hot pepper sauce
2   cups crispy brown rice cereal, crushed
1   pound boneless, skinless chicken breasts, cut into strips (about 15 strips)

1 Preheat oven to 350°F. Coat a large baking dish with cooking spray.

2 Combine flour, salt (optional), and pepper and spread out on a plate. In a medium bowl, whisk together egg, egg whites, and hot pepper sauce. Spread crushed cereal out on a plate.

3 Dredge each strip in flour, dip in egg mixture, then roll in cereal, coating completely.

4 Line strips in the bottom of the baking dish and spray generously with cooking spray. Bake for 25 minutes.

Exchanges/Choices
1 1/2 Starch   3 Lean Meat

Calories 215
 Calories from Fat 30
Total Fat . . . . .3.5 g
 Saturated Fat . . . . .1.0 g
 Trans Fat . . . . .0.0 g
Cholesterol. . . . . 85 mg
Sodium . . . . 85 mg
Potassium. . . . . 240 mg
Total Carbohydrate . . . . . . 21 g
 Dietary Fiber . . . . 1 g
 Sugars . . . . 2 g
Protein . . . . 24 g
Phosphorus . . . . 210 mg

Chef's Tip

Use warmed barbecue sauce or low-fat Ranch dressing as dipping sauces for these crispy chicken fingers.

Savory Grits LC

Makes: 7 servings   *Serving Size: 1/2 cup*   *Prep Time: 10 minutes*

3 1/2	cups water
3/4	cup grits
1/2	tsp salt (optional)
3	ounces reduced-fat shredded cheddar cheese
1/4	cup chopped scallions

1 In a medium saucepan, bring water to a boil. Stir in grits and salt (optional), stirring vigorously. Reduce heat and simmer covered for 15–20 minutes, stirring occasionally.

2 Stir in cheese and scallions until cheese melts.

Exchanges/Choices

1 Starch   1/2 Fat

Calories	90
Calories from Fat	25
Total Fat	3.0 g
Saturated Fat	1.5 g
Trans Fat	0.0 g
Cholesterol	5 mg
Sodium	105 mg
Potassium	40 mg
Total Carbohydrate	13 g
Dietary Fiber	1 g
Sugars	0 g
Protein	4 g
Phosphorus	85 mg

Dietitian's Tip

This tasty recipe is a healthy version of the old Southern favorite.

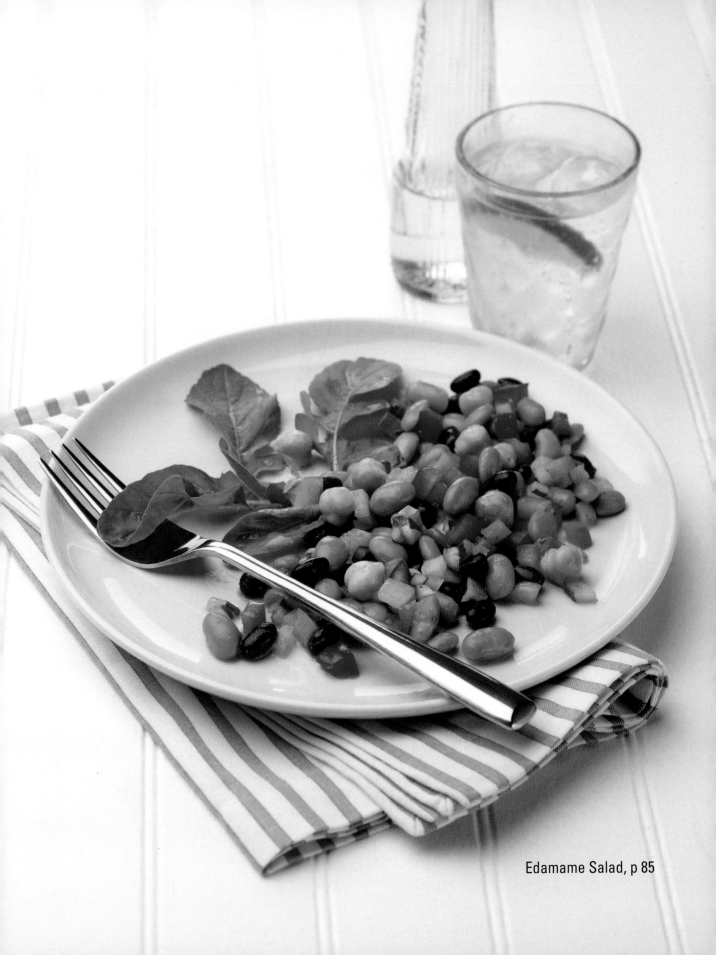

Edamame Salad, p 85

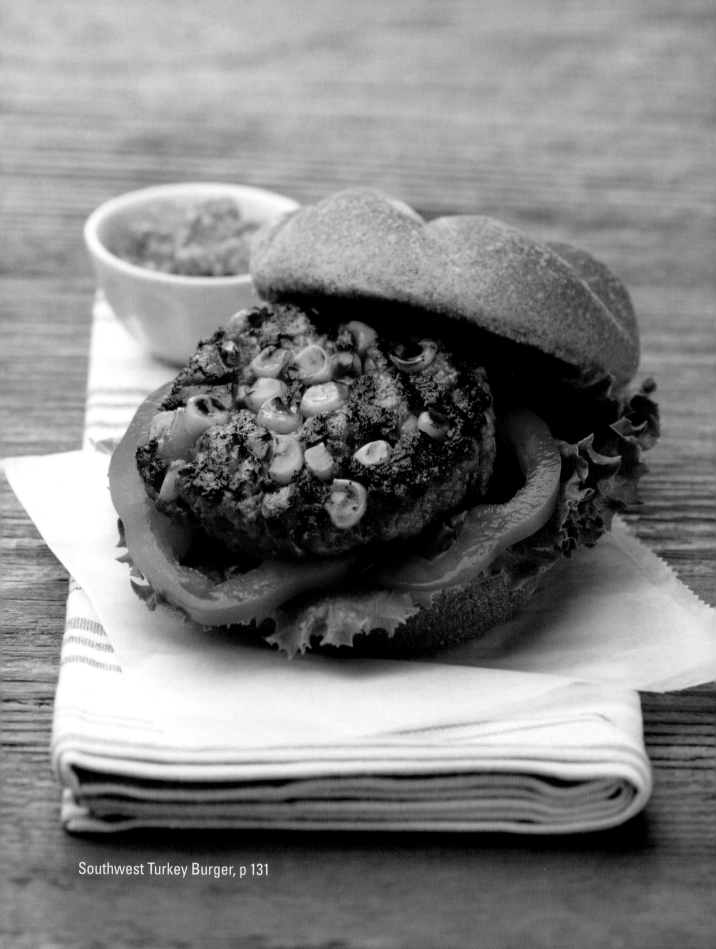

Southwest Turkey Burger, p 131

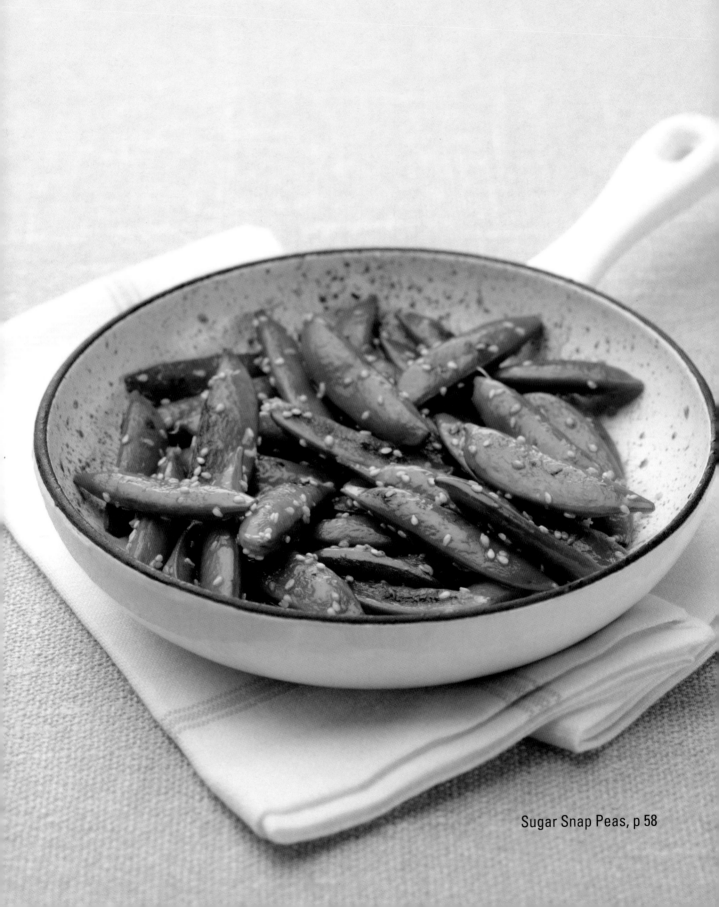

Sugar Snap Peas, p 58

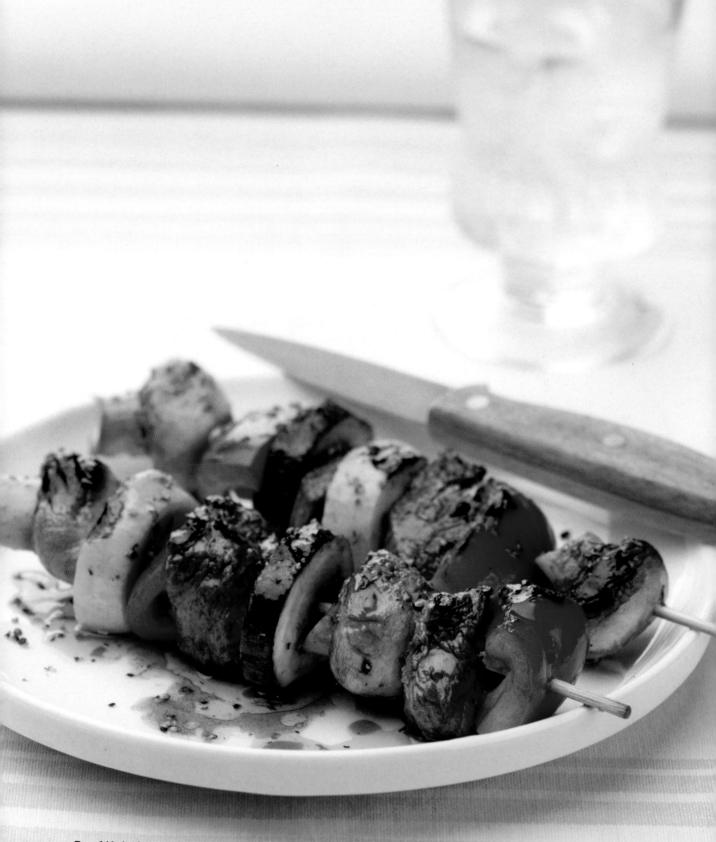
Beef Kabobs, p 197

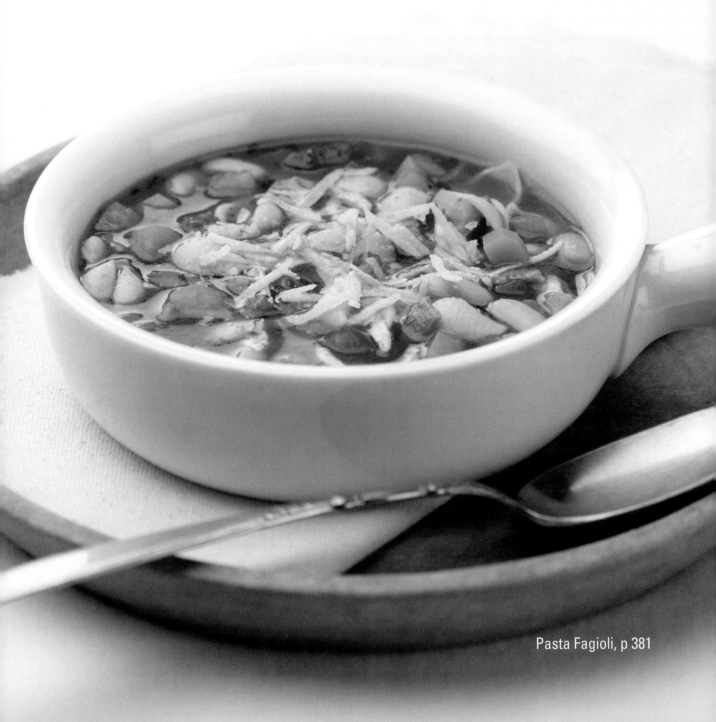

Pasta Fagioli, p 381

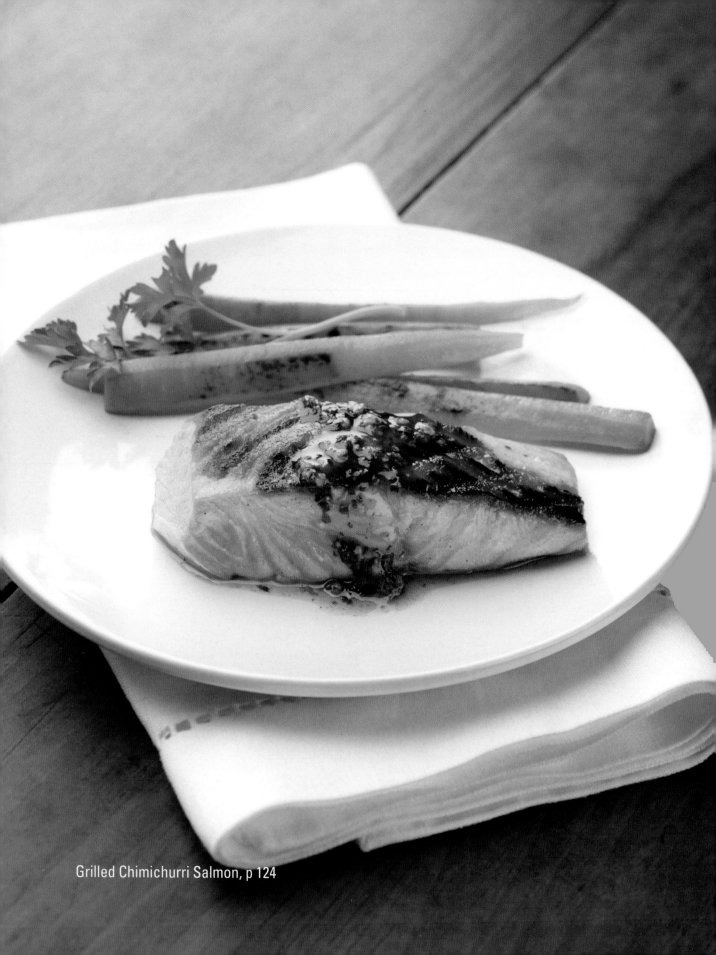

Grilled Chimichurri Salmon, p 124

Salad Niçoise GF

Makes: 4 servings *Serving Size: 1/4 recipe* *Prep Time: 20 minutes*

Dressing

1/4	cup red wine vinegar
2	Tbsp Dijon mustard
2	Tbsp olive oil

Salad

4	cups chopped romaine lettuce
2	6-ounce cans tuna packed in water, drained
4	cups green beans, steamed to tender-crisp and cooled
1/2	pound red new potatoes, boiled and quartered
4	hard-boiled egg whites, quartered
2	cups diced tomatoes

1 In a small bowl, whisk together dressing ingredients; set aside.

2 Place 1 cup romaine lettuce on a plate and top with 1/4 of the tuna, 1 cup green beans, 4 potato quarters, 4 egg white slices, and 1/4 of the tomatoes.

3 Drizzle 1/4 of the dressing over salad. Repeat procedure for remaining 3 salads.

Exchanges/Choices

1 Starch	2 Vegetable
2 Lean Meat	1 Fat

Calories	265
Calories from Fat	70
Total Fat	8.0 g
Saturated Fat	1.2 g
Trans Fat	0.0 g
Cholesterol	30 mg
Sodium	495 mg
Potassium	950 mg
Total Carbohydrate	27 g
Dietary Fiber	7 g
Sugars	6 g
Protein	23 g
Phosphorus	250 mg

Chef's Tip

This French classic is easy and delicious.

Grilled Veal Chops GF LC

Makes: 4 servings   *Serving Size: 1 veal chop*   *Prep Time: 5 minutes*

4   4-ounce boneless veal chops
2   Tbsp light Italian dressing
1/2 tsp salt (optional)
1/4 tsp ground black pepper

1 Prepare an indoor or outdoor grill. Trim any visible fat from chops. Brush each side with dressing. Season well with salt (optional) and pepper.

2 Grill for 4–6 minutes on each side over medium heat.

Exchanges/Choices
4 Lean Meat

Calories 175
 Calories from Fat 65
Total Fat . . . . 7.0 g
 Saturated Fat . . . . 1.9 g
 Trans Fat . . . . 0.0 g
Cholesterol. . . . . 90 mg
Sodium . . . . 150 mg
Potassium. . . . . 225 mg
Total Carbohydrate . . . . . . 1 g
 Dietary Fiber . . . . 0 g
 Sugars . . . . 1 g
Protein . . . . 25 g
Phosphorus . . . . 175 mg

Chef's Tip

You can use pork instead of veal in this recipe.

Braised Red Cabbage

Makes: 4 servings   *Serving Size: 1/2 cup*   *Prep Time: 10 minutes*

1	14.5-ounce can fat-free, low-sodium chicken broth
1/2	cup apple cider vinegar
2	Tbsp red wine vinegar
1	Tbsp honey
1/2	tsp allspice
1/4	tsp salt (optional)
4	cups shredded red cabbage
2	small Granny Smith apples, grated

1 In a large saucepan, bring broth, vinegars, honey, allspice, and salt (optional) to a boil.

2 Add cabbage and apples. Reduce heat and simmer uncovered for 30 minutes.

Exchanges/Choices
1/2 Fruit   1 Vegetable

Calories 75
  Calories from Fat 0
Total Fat . . . . .0.0 g
  Saturated Fat . . . . .0.0 g
  Trans Fat . . . . .0.0 g
Cholesterol. . . . . 0 mg
Sodium . . . . 275 mg
Potassium. . . . . 325 mg
Total Carbohydrate . . . . . . 17 g
  Dietary Fiber . . . . 2 g
  Sugars . . . . 12 g
Protein . . . . 2 g
Phosphorus . . . . 45 mg

Chef's Tip

Use the large holes on your cheese grater to grate the apples.

Taco Pizza

Makes: 8 servings   *Serving Size: 1 slice*   *Prep Time: 15 minutes*

Pizza

1/2	pound 95% lean ground beef
1/3	cup water
1/2	tsp cumin
1/2	Tbsp chili powder
1/8	tsp cayenne pepper
1/2	tsp onion salt (optional)
1	12-inch prepackaged whole-wheat pizza crust
1 1/2	cups salsa
2/3	cup reduced-fat shredded Mexican-style cheese

Salad

8	cups mixed salad greens
24	grape tomatoes

1 Preheat oven to 450°F.

2 Brown beef in a large nonstick skillet over medium-high heat until thoroughly cooked and no longer pink. Drain fat. Add water, cumin, chili powder, cayenne pepper, and onion salt (optional). Simmer 2–4 minutes.

3 Place pizza crust on baking sheet. Spread salsa over pizza crust.

4 Spoon taco meat over pizza crust and distribute evenly. Top with cheese. Bake 10 minutes or until pizza crust is crisp and cheese is melted.

5 Serve each slice of pizza with a side salad: 1 cup salad greens and 3 grape tomatoes.

Exchanges/Choices

1 Starch   1 Vegetable
1 Med-Fat Meat

Calories	180
Calories from Fat	55
Total Fat	6.0 g
Saturated Fat	2.5 g
Trans Fat	0.0 g
Cholesterol	25 mg
Sodium	560 mg
Potassium	500 mg
Total Carbohydrate	22 g
Dietary Fiber	5 g
Sugars	4 g
Protein	13 g
Phosphorus	210 mg

Chef's Tip

If you prefer, you can top this pizza with the side salad after baking.

SEPTEMBER

WEEK 3

DAY 1
Mandarin Orange
Chicken Salad   308

DAY 2
Baked Perch   309
Cauliflower "Potato"
Salad   310

DAY 3
Southwest Salad   311

DAY 4
Philly Cheesesteak
Wraps   312
Broccoli
Casserole   313

DAY 5
Thai-Spiced Roasted
Chicken   314

GROCERY LIST

Fresh Produce
Bell pepper, yellow or
orange—1
Broccoli—2 heads
Cauliflower—1 head
Celery—2 stalks
Garlic—3 cloves
Lettuce—1 head
Lettuce, romaine, 10-ounce
bags—2
Mushrooms, button—1 pint
Onions, yellow or white—2
Scallions—2
Tomatoes—1

Meat, Poultry, & Fish
Beef, flank steak—10 ounces
Chicken, whole, roaster—
5 1/2 pounds
Chicken breasts, boneless,
skinless—3/4 pound
Perch fillets, 4 ounces
each—4
Turkey, ground, 93% lean—
3/4 pound

Grains, Bread, & Pasta
Tortillas, whole-wheat, low-
carb, 10-inch—4

Dairy & Cheese
Cheese, cheddar,
50% reduced-fat,
shredded—1/2 cup
Cheese, sharp cheddar, 75%
reduced-fat, shredded—
1 cup
Cream cheese, fat-free—
2 Tbsp
Milk, fat-free—1/2 cup
Yogurt, Greek, plain, fat-
free—1/2 cup

Canned Goods & Sauces
Beans, black, 16-ounce
can—1
Broth, beef, fat-free, low-
sodium, 14.5-ounce
can—1
Chickpeas (garbanzo beans),
15-ounce can—1
Oranges, mandarin,
11-ounce cans—2
Soup, cream of celery,
condensed, reduced-fat,
10.75-ounce can—1
Soy sauce, lite
Sweet pickle relish—1 jar
Tomatoes, crushed, 15-ounce
can—1

Staples, Seasonings, & Baking Needs
Basil
Black pepper, ground
Cayenne pepper
Chili powder
Cumin
Curry powder
Mustard, yellow
Nonstick cooking spray
Oil, canola
Oil, olive
Oil, sesame
Oregano
Salt
Splenda Sugar Blend

Miscellaneous
Orange juice—1/2 cup
Salad dressing, Italian, fat-
free—1/2 cup

Mandarin Orange Chicken Salad

Makes: 4 servings   *Serving Size: 1/4 recipe*   *Prep Time: 35 minutes*

Salad

1/2	cup orange juice
1	tsp canola oil
1	Tbsp lite soy sauce
1	garlic clove, sliced
3/4	pound boneless, skinless chicken breasts
	nonstick cooking spray
1	10-ounce bag romaine lettuce
2	11-ounce cans mandarin oranges packed in juice, drained (reserve 1/4 cup juice)

Dressing

1/2	cup fat-free Italian dressing
1/4	cup reserved mandarin orange juice

1 Preheat boiler. Combine orange juice, canola oil, soy sauce, and garlic in a large mixing bowl. Place chicken in bowl and marinate in the refrigerator for 15 minutes.

2 Coat broiler with cooking spray and place chicken on broiler rack. Broil 3 inches away from heat until lightly brown (about 4 minutes on each side).

3 Cut cooked chicken into cubes. In a large salad bowl, toss lettuce, chicken, and mandarin oranges.

4 In a small bowl, whisk together dressing ingredients. Drizzle dressing over salad and toss well to coat.

Exchanges/Choices

1 Fruit   3 Lean Meat

Calories	180
Calories from Fat	30
Total Fat	3.5 g
Saturated Fat	0.8 g
Trans Fat	0.0 g
Cholesterol	50 mg
Sodium	495 mg
Potassium	535 mg
Total Carbohydrate	17 g
Dietary Fiber	3 g
Sugars	13 g
Protein	20 g
Phosphorus	205 mg

Chef's Tip

Instead of broiling the chicken, you can also grill it on an indoor or outdoor grill.

Baked Perch GF LC

Makes: 4 servings   *Serving Size: 1 fillet*   *Prep Time: 10 minutes*

nonstick cooking spray

4	4-ounce perch fillets
1	15-ounce can crushed tomatoes
2	garlic cloves, minced
2	tsp chili powder
1/2	tsp cumin
1	tsp dried oregano
1/2	tsp salt (optional)

1 Preheat oven to 350°F.

2 Coat a shallow baking dish with cooking spray. Arrange perch fillets in bottom of dish.

3 In a small bowl, mix remaining ingredients and pour over fish fillets. Bake for 15–20 minutes or until fish flakes easily.

Exchanges/Choices
2 Vegetable   3 Lean Meat

Calories 155
  Calories from Fat 20
Total Fat . . . . 2.5 g
  Saturated Fat . . . . 0.4 g
  Trans Fat . . . . 0.0 g
Cholesterol . . . . 50 mg
Sodium . . . . 240 mg
Potassium . . . . 670 mg
Total Carbohydrate . . . . . . 9 g
  Dietary Fiber . . . . 3 g
  Sugars . . . . 5 g
Protein . . . . 24 g
Phosphorus . . . . 295 mg

Dietitian's Tip

Fish is always a great protein choice. Just remember that baked or broiled fish is much healthier than fried.

Cauliflower "Potato" Salad GF LC 🌟

Makes: 5 servings   *Serving Size: heaping 1/2 cup*   *Prep Time: 20 minutes*

1	head cauliflower with stem, chopped into 1-inch pieces
1	cup water
1/2	cup fat-free plain Greek yogurt
1	Tbsp olive oil
1	tsp Splenda Sugar Blend
1	tsp yellow mustard
2	Tbsp sweet pickle relish
1/4	tsp salt (optional)
1/8	tsp ground black pepper
2	scallions (white and green parts), minced
2	celery stalks, small dice

1 Over medium-high heat, add the cauliflower and water to a large pot with a lid. Steam cauliflower for about 12 minutes, until very tender. Drain, cool, and dry the cauliflower.

2 In a medium bowl, whisk together the yogurt, olive oil, Splenda, mustard, relish, salt (optional), and black pepper.

3 Once the cauliflower has cooled, using a fork, roughly mash the cauliflower so all of the pieces are about the same size. Do not mash until creamy; just break up the cauliflower into uniform pieces.

4 Add the cauliflower, scallions, and celery to the dressing and stir to incorporate.

Exchanges/Choices
2 Vegetable   1/2 Fat

Calories	80
Calories from Fat	25
Total Fat	3.0 g
Saturated Fat	0.5 g
Trans Fat	0.0 g
Cholesterol	0 mg
Sodium	125 mg
Potassium	490 mg
Total Carbohydrate	10 g
Dietary Fiber	3 g
Sugars	6 g
Protein	5 g
Phosphorus	100 mg

Chef's Tip

This recipe is best made the night before and allowed to marinate in the refrigerator overnight, but it can be served right away as well.

🔺 American Diabetes Association.
My Food Advisor

This is an original recipe from the American Diabetes Association's online nutrition resource, **Recipes for Healthy Living**—your one-stop shop for diabetes-friendly recipes, meal plans, and other nutrition tips. Sign up today for the FREE *Recipes for Healthy Living* newsletter and to get access to the website by visiting **www.diabetes.org/recipes**.

Southwest Salad GF

Makes: 6 servings   *Serving Size: 1/6 recipe*   *Prep Time: 15 minutes*

1   small onion, diced
3/4   pound 93% lean ground turkey
2   tsp chili powder
1/2   tsp cumin
1/4   tsp cayenne pepper
1   15.5-ounce can black beans, rinsed and drained
1   15-ounce can chickpeas (garbanzo beans), rinsed and drained
1   large tomato, seeded and diced
4   cups chopped romaine lettuce
1/3   cup reduced-fat shredded cheddar cheese

1 Add onion and ground turkey to a large nonstick skillet over medium-high heat. Cook about 8–10 minutes or until turkey is cooked through (no longer pink).

2 Add chili powder, cumin, and cayenne pepper and cook 2 more minutes. Gently stir in beans, garbanzo beans, and tomato. Cook 2 more minutes. Set aside to cool slightly.

3 Toss meat mixture with lettuce in a large bowl. Sprinkle with cheese.

Exchanges/Choices
1 1/2 Starch   1 Vegetable
2 Lean Meat   1/2 Fat

Calories 250
   Calories from Fat 70
Total Fat . . . . 8.0 g
   Saturated Fat . . . . 2.2 g
   Trans Fat . . . . 0.1 g
Cholesterol . . . . 45 mg
Sodium . . . . 230 mg
Potassium . . . . 595 mg
Total Carbohydrate . . . . . . 26 g
   Dietary Fiber . . . . 8 g
   Sugars . . . . 5 g
Protein . . . . 21 g
Phosphorus . . . . 295 mg

Chef's Tip

Chickpeas are also known as garbanzo beans.

Philly Cheesesteak Wrap NEW

Makes: 4 servings   *Serving Size: 1 wrap*   *Prep Time: 15 minutes*

1 tsp olive oil
nonstick cooking spray
1 small onion, small dice
1 cup button mushrooms, stemmed and small dice
1 yellow or orange bell pepper, stemmed, seeded, and small dice
10 ounces flank steak, chopped fine
2 Tbsp fat-free cream cheese
1/2 cup 75% reduced-fat shredded sharp cheddar cheese
1/4 cup fat-free, low-sodium beef broth
1/2 tsp salt (optional)

1/4 tsp ground black pepper
4 10-inch whole-wheat, low-carb tortillas
2 cups shredded lettuce

1 Add olive oil and a generous amount of cooking spray to a large sauté pan over medium high heat. Add onion, mushrooms and bell pepper to the pan and sauté until vegetables are beginning to soften, about 5 minutes.

2 Turn the heat up to high and add flank steak to the pan with the vegetables and continue to sauté until meat is just beginning to brown, 5–7 minutes.

3 Add cream cheese, cheddar cheese, beef broth, salt (optional), and black pepper. Continue to cook, stirring constantly, until cheese is melted and a sauce forms.

4 Warm the whole-wheat wraps in the microwave for 20 seconds. Divide the meat mixture evenly among the wraps, add 1/2 cup shredded lettuce, and fold the sides in first, then roll to wrap.

Exchanges/Choices
1 Starch   1 Vegetable
3 Lean Meat

Calories	255
Calories from Fat	90
Total Fat	10.0 g
Saturated Fat	2.7 g
Trans Fat	0.0 g
Cholesterol	30 mg
Sodium	515 mg
Potassium	495 mg
Total Carbohydrate	25 g
Dietary Fiber	13 g
Sugars	4 g
Protein	29 g
Phosphorus	395 mg

Dietian's Tip

If you are following a gluten-free diet, you can purchase gluten-free tortillas and broth.

.American Diabetes Association.
MyFoodAdvisor

This is an original recipe from the American Diabetes Association's online nutrition resource, **Recipes for Healthy Living**—your one-stop shop for diabetes-friendly recipes, meal plans, and other nutrition tips. Sign up today for the FREE *Recipes for Healthy Living* newsletter and to get access to the website by visiting **www.diabetes.org/recipes**.

Broccoli Casserole LC

Makes: 8 servings *Serving Size: 1/2 cup* *Prep Time: 10 minutes*

4	cups broccoli florets, steamed
1	10.75-ounce can reduced-fat condensed cream of celery soup
1/2	cup fat-free milk
1/2	cup 50% reduced-fat shredded cheddar cheese
1/8	tsp ground black pepper

1 Preheat oven to 350°F.

2 In a large bowl, combine all ingredients. Pour into a medium casserole dish and bake for 30 minutes.

Exchanges/Choices
1/2 Carbohydrate   1/2 Fat

Calories 55
 Calories from Fat 20
Total Fat . . . . .2.5 g
 Saturated Fat . . . . .1.4 g
 Trans Fat . . . . .0.0 g
Cholesterol. . . . . 5 mg
Sodium . . . . 330 mg
Potassium. . . . . 185 mg
Total Carbohydrate . . . . 6 g
 Dietary Fiber . . . . 1 g
 Sugars . . . . 2 g
Protein . . . . 4 g
Phosphorus . . . . 85 mg

Dietitian's Tip

Broccoli is a cruciferous vegetable, like cauliflower and Brussels sprouts, and may help protect you against some cancers. Broccoli also has plenty of vitamins A and C, folic acid, and lots of fiber!

Thai-Spiced Roasted Chicken GF LC

Makes: 8 servings   *Serving Size: 3 ounces chicken and*   *Prep Time: 15 minutes*
                                         4 potato wedges

1   5 1/2-pound whole roaster
    chicken
1   tsp salt (optional), divided
1   tsp ground black pepper, divided
1   Tbsp sesame oil
1   Tbsp curry powder
1   Tbsp dried basil
    nonstick cooking spray

1 Preheat oven to 450°F. Remove and discard giblet and neck from chicken cavity. Trim excess fat around neck and cavity opening. Rinse chicken with cold water and pat dry.

2 Season inside of cavity with 1/2 tsp salt (optional) and 1/2 tsp pepper. Starting at the neck, loosen skin around breast using your finger. Rub entire chicken (including breast meat under the skin) with sesame oil.

3 In a small bowl, mix curry and basil together. Rub half of mixture onto the breasts under the skin and rub the entire chicken with remaining mixture.

4 Place chicken breast side up into a roasting pan coated with cooking spray. Season with remaining salt (optional) and pepper.

5 Bake for 30 minutes. After 30 minutes, reduce heat to 350°F and bake for an additional 45 minutes. Remove skin before serving.

Exchanges/Choices
4 Lean Meat   1/2 Fat

Calories 210
  Calories from Fat 80
Total Fat . . . . 9.0 g
  Saturated Fat . . . . 2.3 g
  Trans Fat . . . . 0.0 g
Cholesterol . . . . 90 mg
Sodium . . . . 85 mg
Potassium . . . . 265 mg
Total Carbohydrate . . . . 1 g
  Dietary Fiber . . . . 0 g
  Sugars . . . . 0 g
Protein . . . . 29 g
Phosphorus . . . . 200 mg

Chef's Tip

To make this chicken Italian-style, substitute olive oil for sesame oil and dried oregano for the curry powder.

SEPTEMBER

WEEK 4

GROCERY LIST

Fresh Produce
Basil—1 bunch
Bell peppers, green,
    medium—2
Bell peppers, red, medium—2
Blueberries—1 pint
Broccoli—1 head
Carrots—7
Lemons—3
Mushrooms, sliced—1/2 pint
Onion, yellow or white—1
Parsley, Italian (flat leaf)—
    1 bunch
Salad greens, field, mixed—
    9 cups
Spinach, 10-ounce bag—1
Strawberries—1 pound
Tarragon—1 bunch
Tomatoes, plum (Roma),
    ripe—4
Zucchini, medium—2

Meat, Poultry, & Fish
Beef, top sirloin steak,
    boneless—1 pound
Chicken breasts, boneless,
    skinless—3/4 pound
Crabmeat, imitation—
    3/4 pound
Pork tenderloin, ground—
    1 pound
Turkey bacon—6 slices

Grains, Bread, & Pasta
Oats, old-fashioned—1 cup
Pasta, penne, whole-
    wheat—8 ounces
Pasta, shells, quinoa,
    medium—8 ounces
Rice, brown—1 bag

Dairy & Cheese
Cheese, mozzarella, fresh—
    5 ounces
Cheese, Parmesan—1 small
    block
Eggs
Margarine, trans-fat-free
Milk, fat-free—1/4 cup

Canned Goods & Sauces
Broth, beef, fat-free, low-
    sodium, 14.5-ounce
    can—1
Broth, chicken, fat-free,
    low-sodium, 14.5-ounce
    can—1
Soy sauce, lite

Staples, Seasonings, &
Baking Needs
Black pepper, ground
Black peppercorns
Cinnamon
Cornstarch
Flour, all-purpose
Garlic powder
Honey
Mayonnaise, light
Mustard, Dijon
Nonstick cooking spray
Oil, olive
Salt
Splenda Brown Sugar Blend
Splenda Sugar Blend
Sugar substitute
Vinegar, apple cider
Vinegar, balsamic

Miscellaneous
Pecans, chopped—1/2 cup

Crab Pasta Salad

Makes: 6 servings *Serving Size: 1/6 recipe* *Prep Time: 15 minutes*

Dressing
1/4	cup light mayonnaise
1	Tbsp lemon juice
2	Tbsp chopped fresh tarragon
	dash ground black pepper

Salad
8	ounces medium quinoa pasta shells, uncooked
3/4	pound chopped imitation crabmeat
1	medium red bell pepper, diced
1	medium green bell pepper, diced
1	large carrot, diced

1 In a small bowl, whisk together dressing ingredients; set aside.

2 Cook pasta according to package directions, omitting salt; drain and rinse under cold water until cooled.

3 In a large bowl, toss together cooled pasta with remaining salad ingredients. Drizzle dressing over salad and toss well to coat.

Exchanges/Choices
2 Starch	1/2 Carbohydrate
1 Vegetable	1/2 Fat

Calories	235
Calories from Fat	30
Total Fat	3.5 g
Saturated Fat	0.5 g
Trans Fat	0.0 g
Cholesterol	15 mg
Sodium	570 mg
Potassium	415 mg
Total Carbohydrate	44 g
Dietary Fiber	4 g
Sugars	7 g
Protein	8 g
Phosphorus	355 mg

Chef's Tip

Imitation crabmeat is also known as surimi. It has an excellent flavor and is much lower in cost than crab or lobster meat. Look for it in the fresh or frozen seafood section of your market.

Pork Stir-Fry

Makes: 4 servings   *Serving Size: 1/4 recipe*   *Prep Time: 15 minutes*

1   pound ground pork tenderloin
    nonstick cooking spray
2   cups broccoli florets
1   medium red bell pepper, thinly
    sliced
1/2 pint sliced mushrooms
1/2 cup fat-free, low-sodium chicken
    broth
2   tsp cornstarch
2   Tbsp lite soy sauce
1/2 tsp garlic powder
2   cups cooked brown rice

1 Cook pork in a large nonstick skillet or wok over medium-high heat for 5–7 minutes or until no longer pink. Drain any excess fat and remove from pan.

2 Coat the pan with cooking spray. Add broccoli, bell pepper, and mushrooms and sauté for 5–6 minutes. Add pork back to pan.

3 In a small bowl, whisk broth, cornstarch, soy sauce, and garlic powder. Pour over mixture and bring to a boil. Reduce heat and simmer 2–3 minutes. Serve over brown rice.

Exchanges/Choices
1 1/2 Starch   1 Vegetable
3 Lean Meat

Calories 285
  Calories from Fat 55
Total Fat . . . . 6.0 g
  Saturated Fat . . . . 1.7 g
  Trans Fat . . . . 0.0 g
Cholesterol . . . . 65 mg
Sodium . . . . 430 mg
Potassium . . . . 680 mg
Total Carbohydrate . . . . . . 30 g
  Dietary Fiber . . . . 3 g
  Sugars . . . . 3 g
Protein . . . . 29 g
Phosphorus . . . . 360 mg

Dietitian's Tip

Tired of chicken stir-fry? Try this dish for a nice change.

Zucchini and Green Pepper Frittata GF LC NEW

Makes: 8 servings   *Serving Size: 1 slice*   *Prep Time: 10 minutes*

3	eggs
6	egg whites
1/4	cup fat-free milk
2	Tbsp fresh basil, minced, divided
1/2	tsp salt (optional)
1/4	tsp ground black pepper
1	Tbsp olive oil
2	cups shredded zucchini (1 large or 2 medium zucchini)
1	medium onion, thinly sliced
1	green bell pepper, small dice
1/4	cup freshly grated Parmesan cheese

1 Preheat oven to 400°F.

2 In a medium bowl, whisk together eggs, egg whites, milk, 1 Tbsp basil, salt (optional), and pepper.

3 Add olive oil to a medium oven-safe nonstick sauté pan over medium-high heat. Add zucchini, onion, and bell pepper. Sauté until soft, about 7–9 minutes. Reduce heat to low.

4 Pour egg mixture over the zucchini and onions. Drag a flat plastic spatula through the egg and vegetable mixture several times to form large, wet curds, scraping the bottom and sides of the pan at the same time. Shake the pan to even out the mixture and press the top of it lightly with the spatula to flatten it out.

5 Sprinkle the top of frittata evenly with Parmesan cheese and put in the oven to bake for 10 minutes.

6 After baking for 10 minutes, put the frittata under the broiler for 3–4 minutes or until cheese is golden brown.

7 Slide the frittata out of the pan onto a serving platter or a cutting board. Slice into 8 pie slices. Garnish with remaining fresh basil.

Chef's Tip

This is a great summer brunch or dinner dish using vegetables out of the garden. Don't be afraid to add other fresh vegetables to this frittata, like tomatoes, summer squash, or mushrooms. Serve it with a fresh salad made with field greens and a light balsamic vinaigrette.

Exchanges/Choices

1 Vegetable   1 Lean Meat
1/2 Fat

Calories	80
Calories from Fat	35
Total Fat	4.0 g
Saturated Fat	1.2 g
Trans Fat	0.0 g
Cholesterol	65 mg
Sodium	110 mg
Potassium	245 mg
Total Carbohydrate	5 g
Dietary Fiber	1 g
Sugars	3 g
Protein	7 g
Phosphorus	85 mg

Spinach Salad with Warm Bacon Dressing GF LC

Makes: 8 servings   *Serving Size: 1/2 cup*   *Prep Time: 5 minutes*

nonstick cooking spray
- **6** slices turkey bacon, diced
- **1/2** cup apple cider vinegar
- **1** Tbsp olive oil
- **2** Tbsp honey
- **1/4** tsp salt (optional)
- **1** 10-ounce bag fresh spinach leaves, torn

1 Coat a small sauté pan with cooking spray and heat over medium-high heat. Add bacon and sauté 3 minutes or until bacon is crispy. Add remaining ingredients except spinach and bring to a boil. Boil for 5–7 minutes or until slightly thickened.

2 Place spinach in a large bowl. Drizzle hot dressing over spinach and toss to coat.

September is National Cholesterol Education Month. High fat intake can cause too much cholesterol to build up in your bloodstream! Watch your fat intake.

Exchanges/Choices
1/2 Carbohydrate   1/2 Fat

Calories	65
Calories from Fat	30
Total Fat	3.5 g
Saturated Fat	0.8 g
Trans Fat	0.0 g
Cholesterol	5 mg
Sodium	165 mg
Potassium	235 mg
Total Carbohydrate	6 g
Dietary Fiber	1 g
Sugars	5 g
Protein	3 g
Phosphorus	45 mg

Chef's Tip

Turkey bacon is an excellent, healthier substitute for real bacon. Use it in any recipe—you won't be able to tell the difference!

Chicken Pasta Salad with Fresh Mozzarella

Makes: 9 servings　　*Serving Size: 1 cup pasta salad and 1 cup mixed greens*　　*Prep Time: 15 minutes*

Dressing
- **5**　Tbsp balsamic vinegar
- **2**　Tbsp olive oil
- **1/2**　tsp Dijon mustard

Salad
- **8**　ounces whole-wheat penne pasta, uncooked
- **3/4**　pound boneless, skinless chicken breasts, cooked and cubed
- **4**　ripe plum (Roma) tomatoes, diced
- **1/4**　cup chopped flat-leaf parsley
- **5**　ounces fresh mozzarella cheese, cubed
- **9**　cups shredded mixed field greens

1 In a small bowl, whisk together dressing ingredients; set aside.

2 Cook pasta according to package directions, omitting salt. Drain pasta and run under cold water until pasta is cooled. In a large bowl, toss cooled pasta with remaining salad ingredients, except field greens. Place each serving of the pasta salad over 1 cup mixed greens.

3 Drizzle dressing on top and toss well to coat.

Exchanges/Choices

1 1/2 Starch　　2 Lean Meat
1/2 Fat

Calories	220
Calories from Fat	65
Total Fat	7.0 g
Saturated Fat	2.4 g
Trans Fat	0.0 g
Cholesterol	30 mg
Sodium	125 mg
Potassium	270 mg
Total Carbohydrate	24 g
Dietary Fiber	4 g
Sugars	3 g
Protein	15 g
Phosphorus	180 mg

Chef's Tip

This is a refreshing and beautiful dish that is easy to prepare.

Steak au Poivre LC

Makes: 4 servings   *Serving Size: 1/4 recipe*   *Prep Time: 5 minutes*

1	pound boneless top sirloin steak
1/2	tsp salt (optional)
1/2	tsp ground black pepper nonstick cooking spray
1	tsp black peppercorns, crushed
1/2	cup fat-free, low-sodium beef broth

1 Trim any visible fat from sirloin. Season both sides with salt (optional) and pepper.

2 Coat a medium oven-safe skillet with cooking spray over high heat. Sear both sides of steak for 3–4 minutes or until brown. Place skillet in oven and bake for 10 minutes. Remove from oven.

3 Remove steak from pan and set aside. Cover steak. Place skillet back on stove over high heat. Add remaining ingredients to skillet and bring to a boil for 5–7 minutes or until sauce is reduced by one-fourth. Pour sauce over steak.

Exchanges/Choices
3 Lean Meat

Calories	140
Calories from Fat	40
Total Fat	4.5 g
Saturated Fat	1.6 g
Trans Fat	0.1 g
Cholesterol	40 mg
Sodium	110 mg
Potassium	320 mg
Total Carbohydrate	1 g
Dietary Fiber	0 g
Sugars	0 g
Protein	23 g
Phosphorus	185 mg

Chef's Tip

Find whole black peppercorns in the spice aisle of your market.

Carrot Salad GF LC

Makes: 5 servings   *Serving Size: 1/5 recipe*   *Prep Time: 10 minutes*

1 1/2	Tbsp lemon juice
1	Tbsp olive oil
2	Tbsp finely chopped fresh parsley
1/2	packet sugar substitute
6	large carrots, peeled and grated

1 In a medium bowl, whisk together all ingredients except carrots.

2 Add carrots and toss well to coat.

Exchanges/Choices
2 Vegetable   1/2 Fat

Calories	60
Calories from Fat	25
Total Fat	3.0 g
Saturated Fat	0.4 g
Trans Fat	0.0 g
Cholesterol	0 mg
Sodium	60 mg
Potassium	290 mg
Total Carbohydrate	9 g
Dietary Fiber	2 g
Sugars	4 g
Protein	1 g
Phosphorus	30 mg

Dietitian's Tip

Many people think carrots are in the starch exchange group, but they're not. They're in the vegetable group, which means you can eat more of them without your blood glucose going up!

Berry Crisp

Makes: 8 servings *Serving Size: 1/8 recipe* *Prep Time: 15 minutes*

nonstick cooking spray
1 pound strawberries, sliced
1 pint blueberries
1 tsp grated lemon zest
2 Tbsp lemon juice
2 Tbsp Splenda Sugar Blend
1 1/2 Tbsp cornstarch
1 tsp cinnamon

Topping
1 cup old-fashioned oats
1 Tbsp Splenda Sugar Blend
3 Tbsp Splenda Brown Sugar Blend
1/2 cup pecans, chopped
4 Tbsp trans-fat-free margarine, diced

1 Preheat oven to 350°F. Spray a 9-inch pie pan with cooking spray.

2 In a medium bowl, combine the berries, lemon zest, lemon juice, 2 Tbsp Splenda, cornstarch, and cinnamon. Mix well and pour into pie pan.

3 In another medium bowl, place all topping ingredients. Work the margarine into the dry ingredients with your hands until it is crumbly.

4 Sprinkle the crisp topping mixture evenly over the berries. Bake for 55 minutes or until the top is brown and the fruit is bubbly. Serve warm.

Exchanges/Choices
2 Carbohydrate 1 1/2 Fat

Calories	210
Calories from Fat	90
Total Fat	10.0 g
Saturated Fat	1.3 g
Trans Fat	0.0 g
Cholesterol	0 mg
Sodium	45 mg
Potassium	190 mg
Total Carbohydrate	28 g
Dietary Fiber	4 g
Sugars	13 g
Protein	3 g
Phosphorus	80 mg

Dietitian's Tip

This delicious and mouthwatering dessert is full of antioxidant-rich berries, vitamin C, and fiber from the oatmeal.

⚖.American Diabetes Association.
MyFoodAdvisor

This is an original recipe from the American Diabetes Association's online nutrition resource, **Recipes for Healthy Living**—your one-stop shop for diabetes-friendly recipes, meal plans, and other nutrition tips. Sign up today for the FREE *Recipes for Healthy Living* newsletter and to get access to the website by visiting **www.diabetes.org/recipes**.

OCTOBER

Great Veggie Fare

A healthy diabetes meal means filling half your plate with low-carb vegetables, such as broccoli, cauliflower, zucchini, tomatoes, spinach, and more! Most Americans say they like vegetables but admit that they aren't eating enough every day. Try a delicious veggie-packed meal this month, like the Veggie Chili, Eggplant Parmesan, or Roasted Butternut Squash Soup.

Veggie Chili (page 350)

If you're looking for a great vegetarian chili recipe, this is it. You won't miss the meat at all! Serve it with a crunchy salad and warm muffins or bread.

 gluten-free recipe, but always check ingredients for gluten.

 these recipes contain 15 grams of carbohydrate or less per serving.

 new recipe for the second edition.

OCTOBER RECIPES

OCTOBER

WEEK 1

GROCERY LIST

Fresh Produce
Bell pepper, green—1
Carrots, medium—2
Celery—4 stalks
Cilantro—1 bunch
Garlic—1 head
Mushrooms—2 pints
Onions, yellow or white,
    medium—3
Potatoes, Idaho, medium—2
Tarragon—1 bunch
Zucchini, medium—2

Meat, Poultry, & Fish
Chicken breasts, boneless,
    skinless—1 pound
Turkey kielbasa, 95% fat-
    free—1 pound

Grains, Bread, & Pasta
Pasta, farfalle, whole-
    wheat—16 ounces
Sandwich thins,
    whole-wheat—5

Dairy & Cheese
Buttermilk, low-fat—2/3 cup
Cheese, bleu—1/4 cup
Cheese, cheddar, reduced-fat,
    shredded—3/4 cup
Cheese, Parmesan—1 block
Cream cheese, fat-free—2
    ounces
Cream cheese, light—5 ounces
Eggs
Half-and-half, fat-free—
    1 1/2 cups
Milk, fat-free—1/2 cup
Yogurt, plain, fat-free—
    2 Tbsp

Canned Goods & Sauces
Beans, black, 16-ounce
    cans—3
Broth, chicken, fat-free, low-
    sodium, 14.5-ounce cans—3
Chickpeas (garbanzo beans),
    15-ounce can—1
Chilies, green, chopped,
    4-ounce can—1
Pumpkin, 15-ounce can—1
Tomatoes, diced, no-salt-
    added, 14.5-ounce cans—2

Frozen Foods
Spinach, 10-ounce package—1

Staples, Seasonings, & Baking Needs
Baking mix, reduced-fat—
    1 package
Bay leaf
Black pepper, ground
Cayenne pepper
Cornmeal
Cornstarch
Cumin
Mayonnaise, light
Nonstick cooking spray
Nutmeg, ground
Oil, canola
Oil, olive
Onion salt
Oregano
Paprika
Sage
Salt
Thyme

Miscellaneous
Almonds, slivered—1/4 cup
Wine, white

Black Bean Soup

Makes: 10 servings   *Serving Size: 1 cup*   *Prep Time: 15 minutes*

1 tsp olive oil
1 pound 95% fat-free turkey kielbasa, chopped
3 medium onions, coarsely chopped
2 medium celery stalks, diced
3 garlic cloves, minced
3 16-ounce cans black beans, rinsed and drained
4 cups water
1 15-ounce can no-salt-added diced tomatoes

1 4-ounce can chopped green chilies
1 tsp ground cumin
2 tsp dried oregano
1 bay leaf
1 green bell pepper, diced
1/2 tsp salt (optional)
1/4 tsp ground black pepper
1 Tbsp chopped fresh cilantro

1 Add oil to a large soup pot over high heat. Add kielbasa and sauté for 4–5 minutes or until beginning to brown.

2 Stir in onions, celery, and garlic. Sauté an additional 5 minutes or until onions turn clear.

3 Stir in remaining ingredients except cilantro and bring to a boil. Reduce heat and simmer 15 minutes.

4 Remove bay leaf and stir in cilantro.

Exchanges/Choices
1 Starch   2 Vegetable
2 Lean Meat

Calories 225
  Calories from Fat 30
Total Fat . . . . 3.5 g
  Saturated Fat . . . . 1.4 g
  Trans Fat . . . . 0.0 g
Cholesterol . . . . 30 mg
Sodium . . . . 605 mg
Potassium . . . . 595 mg
Total Carbohydrate . . . . . . 29 g
  Dietary Fiber . . . . 9 g
  Sugars . . . . 6 g
Protein . . . . 15 g
Phosphorus . . . . 225 mg

Chef's Tip

Serve a dollop of fat-free sour cream and a sprig of fresh cilantro on each serving of soup.

Cheese Muffins LC

Makes: 12 servings   *Serving Size: 1 muffin*   *Prep Time: 5 minutes*

nonstick cooking spray
2 cups reduced-fat baking mix
2/3 cup low-fat buttermilk
1 Tbsp canola oil
1 egg
3/4 cup reduced-fat shredded cheddar cheese
1/4 tsp ground black pepper

1 Preheat oven to 400°F. Coat a muffin pan with cooking spray.

2 In a medium bowl, mix together baking mix, buttermilk, oil, and egg with a fork. Stir vigorously.

3 Fold in remaining ingredients. Divide batter evenly among tins. Bake for 20 minutes until golden brown.

Exchanges/Choices
1 Starch   1/2 Fat

Calories 110
  Calories from Fat 40
Total Fat . . . . .4.5 g
  Saturated Fat . . . . .1.3 g
  Trans Fat . . . . .0.0 g
Cholesterol. . . . . 20 mg
Sodium . . . . 295 mg
Potassium. . . . . 55 mg
Total Carbohydrate . . . . . 14 g
  Dietary Fiber . . . . 1 g
  Sugars . . . . 2 g
Protein . . . . 4 g
Phosphorus . . . . 180 mg

Chef's Tip

To add some color to these muffins, stir in 1 Tbsp chopped fresh parsley when you add the cheese.

Pumpkin Pasta

Makes: 10 servings   *Serving Size: 1 cup*   *Prep Time: 15 minutes*

16	ounces whole-wheat farfalle pasta, uncooked
1	tsp olive oil
5	ounces light cream cheese, cubed
2	ounces fat-free cream cheese
1/4	cup freshly grated Parmesan cheese
1/2	cup fat-free milk
1	15-ounce can pumpkin
1/2	tsp cayenne pepper
1/4	tsp salt (optional)
1/4	tsp ground black pepper
1/4	tsp dried sage
	pinch ground nutmeg

1 Cook pasta according to package directions, omitting salt. Drain.

2 In a large saucepan, heat olive oil, cream cheeses, Parmesan cheese, and milk over low heat until cream cheese is melted, stirring frequently. Add remaining ingredients and cook until thoroughly heated.

3 Add cooked pasta to pan and toss gently to coat.

Exchanges/Choices

2 1/2 Starch   1 Fat

Calories	240
Calories from Fat	45
Total Fat	5.0 g
Saturated Fat	2.3 g
Trans Fat	0.0 g
Cholesterol	15 mg
Sodium	135 mg
Potassium	190 mg
Total Carbohydrate	38 g
Dietary Fiber	6 g
Sugars	3 g
Protein	11 g
Phosphorus	175 mg

Dietitian's Tip

This rare combination of flavors will have your guests coming back for more. This recipe is not only great in flavor, but an excellent source of vitamin A.

Mushroom and Bleu Cheese Polenta

Makes: 6 servings   *Serving Size: 1 cup*   *Prep Time: 10 minutes*

2	cups cornmeal
6	cups water
1	tsp olive oil
6	cups mushrooms, finely chopped
2	garlic cloves, minced
1/2	tsp dried thyme
1/2	cup white wine
1/2	cup fat-free half-and-half
1/2	tsp salt (optional)
1/4	tsp ground black pepper
1/4	cup bleu cheese
3	Tbsp freshly grated Parmesan cheese

1 In a large saucepan, combine cornmeal and water. While whisking, bring to a boil. Reduce to a simmer, whisking occasionally. Cook 20 minutes.

2 While polenta is cooking, heat oil in a medium nonstick skillet. Add mushrooms to skillet and sauté until all the liquid is evaporated (about 6–7 minutes). Add garlic and thyme and sauté for 30 seconds. Add wine and cook until liquid is evaporated.

3 Fold half-and-half into cooked polenta. Fold in salt (optional), pepper, bleu and Parmesan cheeses, and mushrooms until well mixed.

Exchanges/Choices
2 1/2 Starch   1 Vegetable
1/2 Fat

Calories	240
Calories from Fat	40
Total Fat	4.5 g
Saturated Fat	1.8 g
Trans Fat	0.1 g
Cholesterol	5 mg
Sodium	150 mg
Potassium	360 mg
Total Carbohydrate	41 g
Dietary Fiber	3 g
Sugars	3 g
Protein	8 g
Phosphorus	180 mg

Chef's Tip

Polenta is an Italian-style cornmeal that is served in different ways. This is a creamy version, but you can also cool it, slice it, and pan-fry it with a little cooking spray, salt (optional), pepper, and Parmesan cheese.

Creamed Spinach LC

Makes: 5 servings   *Serving Size: 1/4 cup*   *Prep Time: 10 minutes*

2 tsp olive oil
1 10-ounce package frozen spinach, thawed and drained
1 garlic clove, minced
1 Tbsp cornstarch
1 cup fat-free half-and-half
1/2 tsp salt (optional)
1/4 tsp ground black pepper

1 Add oil to a medium nonstick skillet over medium heat. Add spinach and cook 5–6 minutes or until liquid is evaporated. Stir in garlic and sauté an additional 30 seconds.

2 In a small bowl, whisk together remaining ingredients until all of the cornstarch is dissolved. Pour over spinach, stirring constantly. Bring to a boil, then reduce to a simmer for 5 minutes.

October is National Breast Cancer Awareness Month. Do self-checks every week and get a yearly mammogram!

Exchanges/Choices
1/2 Carbohydrate   1/2 Fat

Calories	65
Calories from Fat	20
Total Fat	2.5 g
Saturated Fat	0.7 g
Trans Fat	0.0 g
Cholesterol	0 mg
Sodium	90 mg
Potassium	230 mg
Total Carbohydrate	8 g
Dietary Fiber	2 g
Sugars	3 g
Protein	3 g
Phosphorus	95 mg

Dietitian's Tip

Although spinach is a nutritious food, creamed spinach is usually loaded with fat. We fixed that problem with some fat-free half-and-half.

Toasted Almond Chicken Salad Sandwich

Makes: 5 servings   *Serving Size: 1 sandwich*   *Prep Time: 20 minutes*

1   pound boneless, skinless chicken breasts
2   14.5-ounce cans fat-free, low-sodium chicken broth
1   Tbsp fresh tarragon, chopped
1/4 cup almond slivers, toasted
1/3 cup light mayonnaise
2   Tbsp fat-free plain yogurt
    dash ground black pepper
5   whole-wheat sandwich thins

1 Place chicken breasts in a large saucepan over medium heat. Pour chicken broth over the chicken breasts and bring to a low simmer for 20 minutes or until done. Shred chicken meat and set aside to cool.

2 In a medium bowl, combine remaining ingredients, except bread, and mix well.

3 Add chicken to mixture and toss well to coat. Divide the chicken salad into 5 equal portions. Top sandwich thin half with one portion of chicken salad. Top with another sandwich thin half. Repeat for remaining 4 sandwiches.

Exchanges/Choices
1 1/2 Starch   3 Lean Meat
1/2 Fat

Calories 285
  Calories from Fat 90
Total Fat . . . . 10.0 g
  Saturated Fat . . . . 1.4 g
  Trans Fat . . . . 0.0 g
Cholesterol . . . . 55 mg
Sodium . . . . 375 mg
Potassium . . . . 340 mg
Total Carbohydrate . . . . . . 25 g
  Dietary Fiber . . . . 6 g
  Sugars . . . . 4 g
Protein . . . . 26 g
Phosphorus . . . . 270 mg

Chef's Tip

How to make the ordinary more special: add a gourmet touch with fresh tarragon and toasted almonds.

Vegetarian Stew

Makes: 7 servings   *Serving Size: 1 cup*   *Prep Time: 15 minutes*

1/4	cup fat-free, low-sodium chicken broth
2	medium zucchini, diced
2	medium carrots, diced
2	celery stalks, diced
2	medium Idaho potatoes, peeled and finely diced
1	14.5-ounce can no-salt-added diced tomatoes
1	tsp paprika
1 1/2	tsp cumin
1	tsp onion salt
1	15-ounce can chickpeas (garbanzo beans)
1/4	tsp ground black pepper

1 In a large soup pot, add chicken broth, zucchini, carrots, celery, and potatoes over medium-high heat. Simmer for 5–6 minutes or until vegetables just begin to soften.

2 Add remaining ingredients and bring to a boil. Reduce heat and simmer, covered, for 30 minutes.

Exchanges/Choices
1 1/2 Starch   1 Vegetable

Calories	135
Calories from Fat	10
Total Fat	1.0 g
Saturated Fat	0.1 g
Trans Fat	0.0 g
Cholesterol	0 mg
Sodium	440 mg
Potassium	600 mg
Total Carbohydrate	28 g
Dietary Fiber	5 g
Sugars	6 g
Protein	5 g
Phosphorus	115 mg

Dietitian's Tip

This recipe is an excellent twist on a traditional stew—and packs in a lot of flavorful vegetables!

OCTOBER

WEEK 2

DAY 1
Cheese and Veggie
Pitas 336

DAY 2
Mostaccioli with Italian
Sausage 337

DAY 3
Blackened Tuna
Steaks 338
Roasted Acorn
Squash 339

DAY 4
Roasted Butternut
Squash Soup 340
Pumpkin Bread 341

DAY 5
Meatless Skillet
Lasagna 342

GROCERY LIST

Fresh Produce
Carrots, medium—3
Celery—3 stalks
Cucumber, medium—1
Garlic—3 cloves
Lettuce, romaine—1 head
Onion, red, medium—1
Onion, yellow or white,
    medium—1
Squash, acorn—4 pounds
Squash, butternut—2 pounds
Tomato—1

Meat, Poultry, & Fish
Tuna steaks, 4 ounces
    each—4
Turkey sausage, Italian,
    lean—5 (about
    14–15 ounces)

Grains, Bread, & Pasta
Pasta, farfalle—10 ounces
Pasta, mostaccioli, whole-
    wheat—16 ounces
Pita pockets, whole-wheat—4

Dairy & Cheese
Buttermilk, low-fat—1/3 cup
Cheese, mozzarella,
    part-skim, shredded—
    1 1/2 cups
Cheese, Parmesan—1 small
    block
Cheese, ricotta, fat-free—
    1 cup
Cheese, Swiss, reduced-
    fat—2 1/4 ounces
Eggs
Half-and-half, fat-free—1 cup

Canned Goods & Sauces
Broth, chicken, fat-free,
    low-sodium, 14.5-ounce
    cans—3
Pasta sauce, marinara,
    reduced-sodium (290 mg
    sodium per serving),
    24.5-ounce jars—3
Pumpkin, 15-ounce can—1

Frozen Foods

**Staples, Seasonings,
& Baking Needs**
Baking powder
Baking soda
Basil
Black pepper, ground
Cayenne pepper
Chili powder
Cinnamon
Flour, all-purpose
Garlic salt
Mayonnaise, light
Nonstick cooking spray
Nutmeg, ground
Oil, canola
Oil, olive
Paprika
Parsley
Salt
Splenda Sugar Blend for
    Baking
Thyme

Miscellaneous
Hummus—1/2 cup
Sunflower seeds—1/4 cup
Veggie burgers, 10-ounce
    package—1

Cheese and Veggie Pitas

Makes: 8 servings   *Serving Size: 1/2 pita*   *Prep Time: 15 minutes*

4	whole-wheat pita pockets
2	Tbsp light mayonnaise
2 1/4	ounces reduced-fat Swiss cheese
1/2	cup hummus
1/4	cup sunflower seeds
4	romaine lettuce leaves
1	medium red onion, thinly sliced
1	large tomato, cut into 4 equal slices
1	medium cucumber, thinly sliced

1 Slice one side of each pita to open pocket, but do not cut all the way through. Set aside.

2 Spread 1/2 Tbsp of mayonnaise in each pita.

3 Slice Swiss cheese into 4 even slices. Spread 2 Tbsp of hummus on each cheese slice and sprinkle 1 Tbsp sunflower seeds on top.

4 Layer lettuce leaf, onion slices, tomato slices, and cucumber slices on top of hummus.

5 Stuff each pita with sandwich filling and cut in half.

Exchanges/Choices
1 Starch   1 Vegetable
1 Med-Fat Meat

Calories	170
Calories from Fat	55
Total Fat	6.0 g
Saturated Fat	1.3 g
Trans Fat	0.0 g
Cholesterol	5 mg
Sodium	275 mg
Potassium	280 mg
Total Carbohydrate	23 g
Dietary Fiber	4 g
Sugars	4 g
Protein	8 g
Phosphorus	195 mg

Chef's Tip

You can often find different flavors of hummus at your grocery store. Experiment with roasted red pepper hummus, garlic hummus, or chili pepper hummus.

Mostaccioli with Italian Sausage

Makes: 10 servings *Serving Size: 1 cup* *Prep Time: 10 minutes*

16 ounces whole-wheat mostaccioli, uncooked

5 lean turkey Italian sausage links, sliced into 1/2-inch pieces (about 14–15 ounces)

3 garlic cloves, minced

2 24.5-ounce jars reduced-sodium marinara pasta sauce (290 mg sodium per serving)

1/2 Tbsp dried basil

1/2 cup shredded part-skim mozzarella cheese

1 Cook pasta according to package directions, omitting salt. Drain.

2 In a large saucepan, cook sausage over medium-high heat about 8 minutes or until sausage is no longer pink. Drain fat.

3 Add garlic and sauté 30 seconds. Add pasta sauce and basil. Bring to a boil; reduce heat and simmer about 10 minutes.

4 Add cooked pasta and mozzarella cheese to sauce and mix well.

Exchanges/Choices
3 Starch   1 Med-Fat Meat
1/2 Fat

Calories 325
  Calories from Fat 90
Total Fat . . . . .10.0 g
  Saturated Fat . . . . .2.2 g
  Trans Fat . . . . .0.1 g
Cholesterol. . . . . 25 mg
Sodium . . . . 620 mg
Potassium. . . . . 580 mg
Total Carbohydrate. . . . . . 44 g
  Dietary Fiber . . . . 6 g
  Sugars . . . . 7 g
Protein . . . . 16 g
Phosphorus . . . . 235 mg

Chef's Tip

The turkey Italian sausage in this recipe is a great substitute for regular sausage. The taste is superb without adding fat.

Blackened Tuna Steaks GF LC

Makes: 4 servings   *Serving Size: 1 steak*   *Prep Time: 10 minutes*

1	Tbsp paprika
1	tsp dried thyme
1/2	tsp ground black pepper
1/2	tsp garlic salt
1/2	tsp chili powder
1/4	tsp cayenne pepper
4	4-ounce tuna steaks
	nonstick cooking spray

1 In a small bowl, combine first 6 ingredients and mix well to incorporate.

2 Dredge one side of each tuna steak in blackening spice.

3 Coat a large nonstick skillet with cooking spray. Add tuna steaks spice side down to pan over medium-high heat. Cook on both sides for 4–5 minutes or until done.

Exchanges/Choices
4 Lean Meat

Calories	165
Calories from Fat	55
Total Fat	6.0 g
Saturated Fat	1.4 g
Trans Fat	0.0 g
Cholesterol	40 mg
Sodium	205 mg
Potassium	325 mg
Total Carbohydrate	1 g
Dietary Fiber	1 g
Sugars	0 g
Protein	26 g
Phosphorus	285 mg

Chef's Tip

Blackened meat or seafood dishes have great, bold flavor without added fat.

Roasted Acorn Squash GF

Makes: 8 servings   *Serving Size: 1/8 recipe*   *Prep Time: 5 minutes*

2 large acorn squash (4 pounds total)
   nonstick cooking spray
1/2 tsp salt (optional)
1/4 tsp ground black pepper
2 tsp olive oil

1 Preheat oven to 400°F.

2 Cut stem off each squash and cut in half lengthwise. Scoop out seeds; rinse and dry each squash half. Spray all sides of squash halves with cooking spray. Season inside of each half with salt (optional) and pepper. Place cut side down on a baking sheet coated with cooking spray. Bake for 45 minutes.

3 Scoop squash meat out into a medium bowl; discard skins. Add olive oil and beat with a sturdy whisk until fluffy.

Exchanges/Choices
1 Starch

Calories 85
  Calories from Fat 15
Total Fat . . . . 1.5 g
  Saturated Fat . . . . 0.2 g
  Trans Fat . . . . 0.0 g
Cholesterol . . . . 0 mg
Sodium . . . . 5 mg
Potassium . . . . 575 mg
Total Carbohydrate . . . . . . 19 g
  Dietary Fiber . . . . 6 g
  Sugars . . . . 6 g
Protein . . . . 1 g
Phosphorus . . . . 60 mg

Dietitian's Tip

Acorn squash is an excellent source of fiber, with about 8 grams per cup. Some people are unsure how to prepare squash, but this recipe proves it couldn't be easier.

Roasted Butternut Squash Soup LC

Makes: 12 servings   *Serving Size: 1 cup*   *Prep Time: 45 minutes*

1	large (or 2 medium) butternut squash (2 pounds total) nonstick cooking spray
1	tsp olive oil
3	medium carrots, finely diced
3	celery stalks, finely diced
1	medium onion, finely diced
3	14.5-ounce cans fat-free, low-sodium chicken broth
1	tsp dried thyme
1/2	tsp salt (optional)
1/4	tsp ground black pepper
1	cup fat-free half-and-half, heated

1 Preheat oven to 400°F.

2 Cut ends off of each squash and cut in half lengthwise. Scoop out seeds; rinse and dry each squash half. Spray all sides of squash halves with cooking spray. Place cut side down on a baking sheet coated with cooking spray. Bake for 45 minutes.

3 While squash is roasting, add oil and a generous amount of cooking spray to a large soup pot. Sauté carrots, celery, and onion over medium-high heat for 5–6 minutes or until onion is clear.

4 Add chicken broth, thyme, salt (optional), and pepper and bring to a boil. Reduce heat and simmer for 15 minutes.

5 Remove squash from oven and scoop out squash meat into soup pot; discard skins. Simmer for an additional 15 minutes, stirring occasionally.

6 Stir in heated half-and-half. Working in batches, purée soup in a blender until smooth. (You can also use an immersion blender right in the soup pot to purée soup.)

Exchanges/Choices

1/2 Starch   1 Vegetable

Calories	55
Calories from Fat	10
Total Fat	1.0 g
Saturated Fat	0.2 g
Trans Fat	0.0 g
Cholesterol	0 mg
Sodium	300 mg
Potassium	350 mg
Total Carbohydrate	10 g
Dietary Fiber	2 g
Sugars	4 g
Protein	2 g
Phosphorus	70 mg

Chef's Tip

Serve this delicious fall soup with Pumpkin Bread (page 341) and a green salad.

Pumpkin Bread

Makes: 12 servings   *Serving Size: 1 slice*   *Prep Time: 12 minutes*

nonstick cooking spray
1 15-ounce can pumpkin
1/3 cup low-fat buttermilk
1/4 cup canola oil
1 egg
2 egg whites
2 cups all-purpose flour
1/4 cup Splenda Sugar Blend for Baking
2 tsp baking powder
1 tsp baking soda
1/2 tsp salt
1 1/2 tsp ground cinnamon
1/4 tsp ground nutmeg

1 Preheat oven to 350°F. Coat a 9-inch loaf pan with cooking spray.

2 In a medium bowl, combine the pumpkin, buttermilk, oil, egg, and egg whites and mix well. Set aside.

3 In a large bowl, sift together the remaining ingredients.

4 Make a well in the center of the dry ingredients. Add pumpkin mixture all at once. Mix well.

5 Pour batter into loaf pan. Bake 50–60 minutes or until toothpick inserted in center comes out clean.

Exchanges/Choices
1 1/2 Carbohydrate   1 Fat

Calories 155
  Calories from Fat 45
Total Fat . . . . .5.0 g
  Saturated Fat . . . . .0.6 g
  Trans Fat . . . . .0.0 g
Cholesterol. . . . . 15 mg
Sodium . . . . 285 mg
Potassium. . . . . 120 mg
Total Carbohydrate . . . . . . 24 g
  Dietary Fiber . . . . 2 g
  Sugars . . . . 6 g
Protein . . . . 4 g
Phosphorus . . . . 125 mg

Dietitian's Tip

Pumpkin is a source of vitamin A, which helps your body's immune system and general repair and renewal.

Meatless Skillet Lasagna

Makes: 9 servings   *Serving Size: 1 cup*   *Prep Time: 5 minutes*

10 ounces farfalle pasta, uncooked

1 10-ounce package veggie burgers (4 burgers), crumbled

1 24.5-ounce jar reduced-sodium marinara pasta sauce (290 mg sodium per serving)

1 cup fat-free ricotta cheese

1 cup shredded, part-skim mozzarella cheese

1/4 cup freshly grated Parmesan cheese

1 Tbsp dried parsley

1 Cook pasta according to package directions, omitting salt; drain.

2 In a deep nonstick skillet or wok, cook crumbled veggie burgers for 3–4 minutes until done. Add pasta sauce and heat.

3 In a medium bowl, combine remaining ingredients and mix well. Add cheese mixture to sauce and mix well until thoroughly heated.

4 Add cooked pasta to sauce and toss to coat.

Mental Illness Awareness Week is in October. Be aware how your attitudes and beliefs are affecting your health.

Exchanges/Choices

2 1/2 Starch   2 Lean Meat

Calories	295
Calories from Fat	65
Total Fat	7.0 g
Saturated Fat	2.5 g
Trans Fat	0.0 g
Cholesterol	25 mg
Sodium	455 mg
Potassium	435 mg
Total Carbohydrate	38 g
Dietary Fiber	4 g
Sugars	7 g
Protein	19 g
Phosphorus	255 mg

Chef's Tip

Look for veggie burgers in interesting flavors, such as Italian-style or spicy.

OCTOBER

WEEK 3

GROCERY LIST

Fresh Produce

Basil—1 bunch
Beets, large—3 (18 ounces total)
Bell pepper, green—1
Broccoli—2 heads
Carrots—4
Garlic—1 head
Mushrooms, portobello, small—3
Onion, yellow or white—1
Oregano—1 bunch
Shallot—1
Squash, yellow, medium—1
Zucchini—2

Meat, Poultry, & Fish

Beef, ground, 95% lean—1 pound
Cod fillets, 4 ounces each—4
Scallops—1 pound
Shrimp, peeled and deveined—1 pound

Grains, Bread, & Pasta

Bread, whole-wheat—1 loaf
Oats, old-fashioned—1/4 cup
Rice, Arborio—1 small bag

Dairy & Cheese

Cheese, cheddar, sharp, reduced-fat, shredded—3 ounces
Cheese, Parmesan—1 small block
Eggs

Canned Goods & Sauces

Beans, black, 16-ounce can—1
Beans, kidney, 16-ounce can—1
Broth, chicken, fat-free, low-sodium, 14.5-ounce cans—2
Hot pepper sauce
Tomato sauce, 15-ounce can—1
Tomatoes, diced, no-salt-added, 14.5-ounce can—1

Staples, Seasonings, & Baking Needs

Black pepper, ground
Chili powder
Flour, all-purpose
Garlic powder
Mayonnaise, light
Nonstick cooking spray
Oil, canola
Oil, olive
Onion powder
Oregano
Parsley
Salt

Miscellaneous

Cereal, cornflakes—1 small box
Wine, white

Seafood Risotto

Makes: 9 servings   *Serving Size: 1 cup*   *Prep Time: 15 minutes*

nonstick cooking spray
1   shallot, minced
2 1/2   cups Arborio rice
2   14.5-ounce cans fat-free, low-sodium chicken broth
3 1/2   cups water
2   tsp olive oil
1   pound fresh scallops
1   pound peeled and deveined raw shrimp
1/2   cup white wine
1/4   tsp ground black pepper
1/4   cup freshly grated Parmesan cheese

1 Coat a large soup pot generously with cooking spray. Over medium-high heat, sauté shallots for 3–4 minutes or until they turn clear. Stir in rice and sauté for 1 more minute.

2 Stir in chicken broth and water and bring to a boil. Reduce heat to a simmer and stir constantly with a large wooden spoon for 20 minutes. Cover and remove from heat.

3 Add oil to a large nonstick skillet over medium-high heat. Add scallops and shrimp and sauté for 2 minutes. Add wine and cook until wine is reduced by half.

4 Fold seafood, pepper, and cheese gently into risotto.

Exchanges/Choices
2 1/2 Starch   2 Lean Meat

Calories 290
    Calories from Fat 20
Total Fat . . . . .2.5 g
    Saturated Fat . . . . .0.8 g
    Trans Fat . . . . .0.0 g
Cholesterol. . . . . 100 mg
Sodium . . . . 595 mg
Potassium. . . . . 345 mg
Total Carbohydrate . . . . . . 40 g
    Dietary Fiber . . . . 2 g
    Sugars . . . . 0 g
Protein . . . . 24 g
Phosphorus . . . . 345 mg

Chef's Tip

If you can't find Arborio rice, try pearl rice or any other small-grain rice in this recipe.

Roasted Veggie Panini

Makes: 5 servings   *Serving Size: 1 sandwich*   *Prep Time: 40 minutes*

1	medium zucchini
1	medium yellow squash
3	small portobello mushrooms
2	tsp olive oil
1	tsp garlic powder
2	tsp dried oregano
1/2	cup basil leaves, washed and dried
5	Tbsp light mayonnaise
	nonstick cooking spray
10	slices whole-wheat bread

1 Preheat oven to 400°F and prepare an indoor or outdoor grill.

2 Slice the zucchini and squash thinly lengthwise and then in half to make 3-inch strips. Pull the stem out of the portobello mushrooms and scrape out the scales with a spoon. Slice the mushrooms into 1-inch strips.

3 In a large bowl, combine the zucchini, squash, and mushrooms. Drizzle the olive oil over the vegetables and toss to coat. Sprinkle the garlic powder and oregano over the top and toss again to distribute.

4 Place the vegetable mixture in a 13 × 9-inch baking dish and roast in the oven for 30 minutes.

5 While the vegetables are roasting, finely chop basil leaves. In a small bowl, combine basil leaves with mayonnaise. Set aside in the refrigerator.

6 To assemble sandwiches, spread 1/2 Tbsp mayo on 5 slices of bread. Place 1/2 cup of the vegetable mixture on top of 1 slice of bread and top with other slice of bread. Repeat this process for remaining 4 sandwiches. Spray sandwiches with cooking spray and grill sandwiches on an indoor or outdoor grill over medium heat for 4 minutes on each side.

Chef's Tip

This sandwich can also be grilled in a nonstick skillet coated with cooking spray—cook for 4 minutes on each side over medium-high heat.

Exchanges/Choices
1 1/2 Starch   1 Vegetable
1 1/2 Fat

Calories	220
Calories from Fat	70
Total Fat	8.0 g
Saturated Fat	1.2 g
Trans Fat	0.0 g
Cholesterol	5 mg
Sodium	390 mg
Potassium	535 mg
Total Carbohydrate	30 g
Dietary Fiber	5 g
Sugars	6 g
Protein	9 g
Phosphorus	195 mg

Herbed Meatloaf LC

Makes: 6 servings   *Serving Size: 1 piece*   *Prep Time: 10 minutes*

	nonstick cooking spray
1	pound 95% lean ground beef
4	garlic cloves, minced
1/4	cup finely chopped fresh basil leaves
1/4	cup finely chopped fresh oregano leaves
1	Tbsp dried parsley
1	egg, slightly beaten
1/4	cup old-fashioned oats
1/2	tsp salt (optional)
1/4	tsp ground black pepper

1 Preheat oven to 400°F.

2 Coat a 5 × 9-inch loaf pan generously with cooking spray. In a medium bowl, combine all ingredients. Mix well.

3 Spread mixture evenly into loaf pan. Bake for 50–60 minutes or until no longer pink.

Exchanges/Choices
3 Lean Meat

Calories	130
Calories from Fat	45
Total Fat	5.0 g
Saturated Fat	2.1 g
Trans Fat	0.1 g
Cholesterol	75 mg
Sodium	55 mg
Potassium	295 mg
Total Carbohydrate	4 g
Dietary Fiber	1 g
Sugars	0 g
Protein	17 g
Phosphorus	170 mg

Chef's Tip

This recipe is a great example of what herbs can do for a meal! Ordinary meatloaf is transformed into a mouthwatering delight. Make meatloaf sandwiches with leftovers for lunch the next day.

Roasted Beets GF LC

Makes: 6 servings   *Serving Size: 1/6 recipe*   *Prep Time: 5 minutes*

nonstick cooking spray
- **3** large fresh beets (18 ounces total)
- **1** tsp olive oil
- **2** tsp chopped fresh basil
- **1/2** tsp salt (optional)

1 Preheat oven to 400°F.

2 Coat a 13 × 9-inch glass baking dish with cooking spray. Wash and dry beets; slice in half lengthwise. Place beets cut side down in the dish. Spray the beets generously with cooking spray. Roast in oven for 40 minutes. Remove beets from baking dish and let cool for 5 minutes.

3 Peel the skin off the roasted beets and slice into 1/4-inch-thick half moons. On a medium plate, arrange slices of beets in layers. Drizzle with olive oil and sprinkle with basil and salt (optional). Serve hot.

Exchanges/Choices
1 Vegetable

Calories	40
Calories from Fat	10
Total Fat	1.0 g
Saturated Fat	0.1 g
Trans Fat	0.0 g
Cholesterol	0 mg
Sodium	55 mg
Potassium	220 mg
Total Carbohydrate	7 g
Dietary Fiber	1 g
Sugars	6 g
Protein	1 g
Phosphorus	30 mg

Dietitian's Tip

Beets are low in carbohydrate and calories but high in nutrition.

Crispy Cod

Makes: 4 servings   *Serving Size: 1 fillet*   *Prep Time: 10 minutes*

	nonstick cooking spray
1 1/2	cups cornflake crumbs
1/2	tsp garlic powder
1/2	tsp onion powder
1	egg
2	egg whites
1	tsp hot pepper sauce (optional)
2	Tbsp all-purpose flour
4	4-ounce cod fillets

1 Preheat oven to 350°F. Coat a shallow baking pan with cooking spray.

2 In a medium bowl, combine cornflake crumbs, garlic powder, and onion powder.

3 In a separate bowl, lightly beat egg and egg whites. Add hot pepper sauce and mix well.

4 Place flour in a separate bowl.

5 Dip each cod fillet in flour, then egg mixture, then cornflake mixture, coating well.

6 Place fillets in baking pan. Spray fillets lightly with cooking spray and bake 18–20 minutes.

Exchanges/Choices
1 1/2 Starch   3 Lean Meat

Calories 225
  Calories from Fat 20
Total Fat . . . . 2.0 g
  Saturated Fat . . . . 0.5 g
  Trans Fat . . . . 0.0 g
Cholesterol . . . . 95 mg
Sodium . . . . 380 mg
Potassium . . . . 290 mg
Total Carbohydrate . . . . . . 25 g
  Dietary Fiber . . . . 1 g
  Sugars . . . . 3 g
Protein . . . . 26 g
Phosphorus . . . . 165 mg

Dietitian's Tip

This is a great-tasting replacement for traditionally high-fat fried fish.

Broccoli with Cheddar Cheese GF LC

Makes: 8 servings   *Serving Size: 1/2 cup*   *Prep Time: 10 minutes*

4	cups broccoli florets
1/2	tsp salt (optional)
1/4	tsp ground black pepper
3	ounces shredded, reduced-fat, sharp cheddar cheese

1 Steam broccoli until tender-crisp.

2 Sprinkle hot broccoli with salt (optional), pepper, and cheese.

Exchanges/Choices
1 Vegetable   1/2 Fat

Calories 40
  Calories from Fat 20
Total Fat . . . . .2.5 g
  Saturated Fat . . . . .1.3 g
  Trans Fat . . . . .0.0 g
Cholesterol. . . . . 5 mg
Sodium . . . . 95 mg
Potassium. . . . . 125 mg
Total Carbohydrate . . . . 2 g
  Dietary Fiber . . . . 1 g
  Sugars . . . . 1 g
Protein . . . . 4 g
Phosphorus . . . . 85 mg

Dietitian's Tip

Steaming vegetables in a small amount of water helps them retain their nutrients.

Veggie Chili

Makes: 8 servings   *Serving Size: 1 cup*   *Prep Time: 15 minutes*

1	Tbsp canola oil
1	medium onion, chopped
4	carrots, sliced
1	green bell pepper, chopped
1	zucchini, chopped
2	garlic cloves, minced
1	Tbsp chili powder
1	16-ounce can kidney beans, rinsed and drained
1	15.5-ounce can black beans, rinsed and drained
1	15-ounce can tomato sauce
2	14.5-ounce cans no-salt-added diced tomatoes with juice

1 Heat oil in a large soup pot over medium-high heat.

2 Add onion and carrots and sauté 5 minutes. Add green pepper and zucchini and sauté another 2 minutes.

3 Add garlic and sauté 30 seconds. Add all remaining ingredients; bring to a boil.

4 Cover, reduce heat, and simmer 30–35 minutes or until the vegetables are tender.

Exchanges/Choices

1 Starch   2 Vegetable
1/2 Fat

Calories	170
Calories from Fat	20
Total Fat	2.5 g
Saturated Fat	0.3 g
Trans Fat	0.0 g
Cholesterol	0 mg
Sodium	460 mg
Potassium	880 mg
Total Carbohydrate	30 g
Dietary Fiber	9 g
Sugars	9 g
Protein	9 g
Phosphorus	165 mg

Dietitian's Tip

The beans and veggies in this dish make it a great source of fiber, with 10 grams per serving. You should aim to get 20–35 grams of dietary fiber daily.

OCTOBER

WEEK 4

GROCERY LIST

Fresh Produce
Apples, red—5 (5 cups total)
Bananas—2–3
Bell pepper, green, large—1
Bell pepper, red, small—1
Broccoli—2 heads
Celery—2 stalks
Eggplant, medium—1 pound
Garlic—1 head
Mushrooms—1 pint
Onion, red, large—1
Onion, yellow or white,
    medium—1
Squash, butternut—2 pounds
Tomatoes, plum (Roma)—2
Zucchini—1

Meat, Poultry, & Fish
Pork chops, center-cut,
    bone-in—4 (20 ounces
    total)
Shrimp, medium, uncooked—
    1 pound

Grains, Bread, & Pasta
Bread crumbs, whole-
    wheat—1 cup
Oats, old-fashioned—1/2 cup
Pasta, penne, quinoa—
    12 ounces
Rice, brown—1 bag

Dairy & Cheese
Buttermilk, low-fat—
    1 1/4 cups
Cheese, cheddar,
    50% reduced-fat,
    shredded—1/2 cup
Cheese, mozzarella, part-
    skim, shredded—1/4 cup

Cheese, Parmesan—1 small
    block
Egg substitute—2 cups
Eggs—4
Margarine, trans-fat-free

Canned Goods & Sauces
Pasta sauce, marinara,
    reduced-sodium (290
    mg sodium per serving),
    24.5-ounce jar—1
Tomato paste, 4-ounce
    can—1
Tomatoes, diced, no-salt-
    added, 14.5-ounce cans—2

Staples, Seasonings,
& Baking Needs
Baking mix, reduced-fat—
    1 package
Basil
Black pepper, ground
Cajun seasoning
Cayenne pepper
Cinnamon
Cumin
Flour, all-purpose
Garlic salt
Nonstick cooking spray
Nutmeg
Oil, olive
Red pepper flakes
Salt
Splenda Brown Sugar Blend
Vanilla extract
Vinegar, balsamic

Miscellaneous
Cranberries, dried—1/3 cup
Pecans, chopped—1/4 cup

Pasta Primavera

Makes: 5 servings   *Serving Size: 2 cups*   *Prep Time: 15 minutes*

12	ounces quinoa penne pasta, uncooked
	nonstick cooking spray
2	Tbsp olive oil
1	large green bell pepper, cut into 2-inch strips
4	cups broccoli florets
1/4	tsp garlic salt (optional)
1/2	tsp ground black pepper
3	garlic cloves, minced
2	plum (Roma) tomatoes, cut into 1-inch chunks
3	Tbsp freshly grated Parmesan cheese

1 Cook pasta according to package directions, omitting salt. Drain.

2 Coat a large nonstick skillet with cooking spray and add olive oil over medium-high heat. Sauté green peppers for 5 minutes. Add broccoli, garlic salt (optional), and pepper and cook another 5–7 minutes; add garlic and sauté 30 seconds.

3 Add tomatoes and cook 2 more minutes.

4 In a large bowl, toss together the pasta and vegetable mixture. Sprinkle with Parmesan cheese and serve immediately.

Exchanges/Choices

3 1/2 Starch   1 Vegetable
1 Fat

Calories	335
Calories from Fat	70
Total Fat	8.0 g
Saturated Fat	1.3 g
Trans Fat	0.0 g
Cholesterol	0 mg
Sodium	65 mg
Potassium	705 mg
Total Carbohydrate	61 g
Dietary Fiber	7 g
Sugars	4 g
Protein	8 g
Phosphorus	385 mg

Dietitian's Tip

If you're not a vegetarian and want some added protein, try adding chicken breast or sun-dried tomato chicken sausage to this dish.

Shrimp Jambalaya

Makes: 8 servings　　　　*Serving Size: 1 cup*　　　　*Prep Time: 15 minutes*

1 1/2	tsp olive oil
1	medium onion, chopped
2	celery stalks, chopped
2	Tbsp tomato paste
1	tsp dried basil
1	Tbsp Cajun seasoning
	dash cayenne pepper (optional)
3	garlic cloves, minced
1/4	tsp cumin
2	14.5-ounce cans no-salt-added diced tomatoes, with juice
1 1/2	cups uncooked brown rice
1	pound uncooked medium shrimp, peeled and deveined

1 Add oil to a large, deep nonstick skillet or wok over medium-high heat. Add onions and celery and sauté for 5–7 minutes or until vegetables begin to caramelize. Stir in tomato paste and seasonings. Sauté for 1 minute.

2 Stir in tomatoes and rice. Bring to a boil, reduce heat and cover. Simmer for 10 minutes.

3 Add shrimp and cook for 4 minutes or until shrimp is done.

Exchanges/Choices

2 Starch　　　1 Vegetable
1 Lean Meat

Calories 210	
Calories from Fat 20	
Total Fat . . . . 2.5 g	
Saturated Fat . . . . 0.5 g	
Trans Fat . . . . 0.0 g	
Cholesterol . . . . 70 mg	
Sodium . . . . 490 mg	
Potassium . . . . 460 mg	
Total Carbohydrate . . . . . . 35 g	
Dietary Fiber . . . . 3 g	
Sugars . . . . 4 g	
Protein . . . . 12 g	
Phosphorus . . . . 250 mg	

Chef's Tip

Spice up this dish even more with a dash of Cajun hot sauce.

Eggplant Parmesan

Makes: 10 servings   *Serving Size: 1 slice eggplant*   *Prep Time: 15 minutes*

1/2 cup all-purpose flour
1/2 tsp salt (optional)
1/4 tsp ground black pepper
 1 cup whole-wheat bread crumbs
1/4 cup freshly grated Parmesan cheese
 2 eggs, beaten
 1 medium eggplant (1 pound), sliced into 10 1/2-inch-thick round slices
 2 tsp olive oil
   nonstick cooking spray
 1 24.5-ounce jar reduced-sodium marinara pasta sauce (290 mg sodium per serving)
1/4 cup shredded part-skim mozzarella cheese

1 Preheat oven to 375°F.

2 In a medium bowl, combine flour, salt (optional), and pepper. In another medium bowl, add bread crumbs and Parmesan cheese. In a third medium bowl, add eggs.

3 Dredge both sides of the eggplant slices in flour, then eggs, then bread crumbs, coating well. Set aside.

4 Add oil and a generous amount of cooking spray to a large nonstick skillet over medium-high heat. Cook eggplant in batches, recoating pan with cooking spray as necessary, for 2 minutes each side.

5 In a 13 × 9-inch baking dish, layer the eggplant slices along the bottom. Pour entire jar of sauce over the eggplant so all the slices are covered. Sprinkle mozzarella over the top and bake for 30 minutes.

Exchanges/Choices

1 Starch   1 Vegetable
1 Fat

Calories	155
Calories from Fat	55
Total Fat	6.0 g
Saturated Fat	1.4 g
Trans Fat	0.0 g
Cholesterol	40 mg
Sodium	245 mg
Potassium	315 mg
Total Carbohydrate	21 g
Dietary Fiber	4 g
Sugars	5 g
Protein	6 g
Phosphorus	95 mg

Chef's Tip

This dish, served with a big green salad, would be great for a dinner party.

Pork Chops with Cranberry Glaze GF LC

Makes: 4 servings   *Serving Size: 1 pork chop*   *Prep Time: 10 minutes*

4	bone-in, center-cut pork chops (20 ounces total)
1/4	tsp garlic salt
1/2	tsp ground black pepper
1	tsp olive oil
	nonstick cooking spray
1/4	large red onion, thinly sliced and separated into rings
1/2	cup balsamic vinegar
1/3	cup water
1/3	cup dried cranberries

1 Season pork chops well with garlic salt and pepper.

2 Add oil to a large nonstick skillet over medium-high heat. Sauté chops for 6–8 minutes or until browned, turning once. Remove from pan and keep chops warm.

3 Spray pan with cooking spray. Add onions and cook for 5–6 minutes or until they begin to caramelize. Stir in balsamic vinegar, water, and cranberries and simmer for 5–7 minutes or until cranberries are soft and sauce takes on a glaze consistency.

4 Pour cranberry sauce over pork chops.

Exchanges/Choices
1/2 Fruit   1/2 Carbohydrate
3 Lean Meat

Calories 215
    Calories from Fat 65
Total Fat . . . . .7.0 g
    Saturated Fat . . . . .2.3 g
    Trans Fat . . . . .0.0 g
Cholesterol. . . . . 60 mg
Sodium . . . . 130 mg
Potassium. . . . . 315 mg
Total Carbohydrate . . . . . . 15 g
    Dietary Fiber . . . . 1 g
    Sugars . . . . 12 g
Protein . . . . 21 g
Phosphorus . . . . 135 mg

Dietitian's Tip

Dried fruit contains more carbohydrate than fresh fruit, but adding just a few raisins, prunes, or cranberries is a great way to liven up a dish versus eating them alone for a snack.

Roasted Butternut Squash with Pecans GF LC

Makes: 6 servings   *Serving Size: 1/2 cup*   *Prep Time: 5 minutes*

1 large butternut squash (2 pounds), cut in half lengthwise, seeds discarded
  nonstick cooking spray
2 tsp trans-fat-free margarine, divided
1 Tbsp Splenda Brown Sugar Blend, divided
1/4 cup chopped pecans

1 Preheat oven to 400°F.

2 Spray both sides of squash with cooking spray and place face down in a glass baking dish. Bake for 45 minutes.

3 In a small bowl, mix 1 tsp margarine and 1 1/2 tsp brown sugar and microwave for 30 seconds to melt margarine. Add pecans and mix well. Spread mixture on a small baking sheet and bake for 3 minutes to toast nuts.

4 Remove squash from oven. Scoop squash meat into a large bowl; discard skins. Add remaining margarine and brown sugar and whip with a whisk until smooth. Fold in pecans.

Exchanges/Choices
1 Starch   1/2 Fat

Calories 85
  Calories from Fat 40
Total Fat . . . . .4.5 g
  Saturated Fat . . . . .0.6 g
  Trans Fat . . . . .0.0 g
Cholesterol. . . . . 0 mg
Sodium . . . . 15 mg
Potassium. . . . . 275 mg
Total Carbohydrate . . . . . . 12 g
  Dietary Fiber . . . . 3 g
  Sugars . . . . 3 g
Protein . . . . 1 g
Phosphorus . . . . 35 mg

Chef's Tip

Roasting vegetables really intensifies their flavors, as this dish shows. The brown sugar and pecans add sweet crunchiness.

Veggie Omelet GF LC

Makes: 4 servings   *Serving Size: 1 omelet*   *Prep Time: 10 minutes*

nonstick cooking spray
- 1/2 cup shredded zucchini
- 1/2 small red bell pepper, finely diced
- 1/2 cup sliced mushrooms
- 2 cups egg substitute
- 1/2 tsp salt (optional)
- 1/4 tsp ground black pepper
- 1/4 tsp crushed red pepper flakes
- 1/2 cup shredded 50% reduced-fat cheddar cheese

1 Add cooking spray to a large nonstick skillet over medium-high heat. Add zucchini, bell pepper, and mushrooms to pan and sauté for 5–6 minutes or until vegetables are soft.

2 Add cooking spray to a small nonstick pan (omelet pan) over medium heat. Pour 1/2 cup egg substitute in hot pan. Sprinkle with salt (optional), pepper, and red pepper flakes.

3 Once eggs set up and are still a little runny in the center, spread 1/4 cup of vegetable mixture on one side of eggs. Sprinkle the vegetable mixture with 2 Tbsp cheese.

4 Fold the other half of the eggs over the vegetables and gently flip the omelet using a wide spatula.

5 Repeat process for remaining three omelets.

Exchanges/Choices
2 Lean Meat

Calories	100
Calories from Fat	20
Total Fat	2.5 g
Saturated Fat	1.5 g
Trans Fat	0.0 g
Cholesterol	5 mg
Sodium	315 mg
Potassium	280 mg
Total Carbohydrate	4 g
Dietary Fiber	1 g
Sugars	2 g
Protein	17 g
Phosphorus	105 mg

Chef's Tip

Spoon a little salsa over each omelet for added flavor.

Banana-Oat Pancakes

Makes: 9 servings   *Serving Size: 1 pancake*   *Prep Time: 7 minutes*

1/2	cup old-fashioned oats
1 1/4	cups low-fat buttermilk
1	cup mashed bananas (about 2–3 bananas)
2	large eggs, beaten
1	tsp vanilla extract
1 1/2	cups reduced-fat baking mix nonstick cooking spray

1 In a large bowl, combine oats and buttermilk. Let stand until oats soften. Mix in mashed bananas, eggs, and vanilla extract. Gradually stir in baking mix.

2 Coat a griddle or nonstick skillet with cooking spray. Use 1/4 cup batter for each pancake and cook pancake until brown on bottom and some bubbles begin to break around edges. Turn pancake over. Cook until brown on bottom and firm to touch in center.

3 Repeat procedure until all batter is gone. Serve pancakes with sugar-free syrup.

Exchanges/Choices

1 Starch   1/2 Fruit
1/2 Fat

Calories	140
Calories from Fat	25
Total Fat	3.0 g
Saturated Fat	0.8 g
Trans Fat	0.0 g
Cholesterol	45 mg
Sodium	265 mg
Potassium	195 mg
Total Carbohydrate	24 g
Dietary Fiber	2 g
Sugars	6 g
Protein	5 g
Phosphorus	195 mg

Chef's Tip

If you like, serve sliced bananas on top of these pancakes.

Apple Crisp

Makes: 7 servings   *Serving Size: 1/2 cup*   *Prep Time: 15 minutes*

nonstick cooking spray
2   Tbsp Splenda Brown Sugar Blend
1/4   cup all-purpose flour
1/2   cup old-fashioned oats
2   Tbsp trans-fat-free margarine, softened
1   tsp ground cinnamon
1/2   tsp ground nutmeg
1   tsp vanilla extract
5   cups peeled, sliced red apples (about 5 apples)

1 Preheat oven to 375°F. Coat a 13 × 9-inch pan with cooking spray.

2 In a small bowl, combine all ingredients except apples. Blend with a fork until moistened (mixture should be crumbly).

3 Layer apples in pan and sprinkle brown sugar mixture evenly over top. Bake 30 minutes.

Exchanges/Choices
2 Carbohydrate

Calories 135
  Calories from Fat 25
Total Fat . . . . .3.0 g
  Saturated Fat . . . . .0.9 g
  Trans Fat . . . . .0.0 g
Cholesterol. . . . . 0 mg
Sodium . . . . 25 mg
Potassium. . . . . 140 mg
Total Carbohydrate . . . . . . 26 g
  Dietary Fiber . . . . 2 g
  Sugars . . . . 14 g
Protein . . . . 2 g
Phosphorus . . . . 40 mg

Chef's Tip

Top with light vanilla ice cream or frozen yogurt.

NOVEMBER

American Diabetes Month

Having diabetes doesn't mean the end of the world, food-wise. You can still eat a lot of your old favorites—just healthier versions of them, in moderation. Celebrate this month with delicious, low-fat, heart-healthy recipes.

Italian Sausage with Pepper Medley (page 389)
Spicy Sweet Potato Fries (page 158)

When the days grow shorter, you'll enjoy these hearty, slightly spicy foods! Sweet potato fries are a great alternative to the usual potato fries. Try them with this sausage medley or a tasty turkey burger.

 gluten-free recipe, but always check ingredients for gluten.

 these recipes contain 15 grams of carbohydrate or less per serving.

 new recipe for the second edition.

NOVEMBER

WEEK 1

DAY 1
Chili Lime Shrimp   364

DAY 2
Baked Potato
    Soup   365

DAY 3
Pesto Chicken Pita   366
Brussels Sprouts with
    Citrus Butter   367

DAY 4
10-Minute
    Tostadas   368
Tomato Salad
    with Cilantro
    Vinaigrette   369

DAY 5
Beef Stew   370

GROCERY LIST

Fresh Produce
Basil—1 bunch
Carrots, medium—2
Celery—2 stalks
Cilantro—1 bunch
Garlic—1 head
Lettuce, shredded—1 cup
Onions, yellow or white,
    medium—2
Potatoes, russet, medium—8
Scallions—1 bunch
Shallot, small—1
Tomatoes, medium—6

Meat, Poultry, & Fish
Beef round roast—1 pound
Chicken breasts, boneless,
    skinless—1 pound
Shrimp, medium, raw, peeled
    and deveined—9 ounces
Turkey bacon—5 slices

Grains, Bread, & Pasta
Pita pockets, whole-wheat—4
Tostada shells—4

Dairy & Cheese
Cheese, cheddar, 75%
    reduced-fat, shredded—
    1 1/4 cups
Cheese, Parmesan—1 small
    block
Half-and-half, fat-free—
    1 1/4 cups
Margarine, trans-fat-free

Canned Goods & Sauces
Beans, refried, with green
    chilies, 16-ounce can—1
Broth, beef, fat-free,
    low-sodium, 14.5-ounce
    cans—2
Broth, chicken, fat-free,
    low-sodium, 14.5-ounce
    cans—3
Chili-garlic sauce, Asian-
    style—1 small jar
Hot pepper sauce

Frozen Foods
Brussels sprouts, 1-pound
    bag—1

**Staples, Seasonings,
& Baking Needs**
Bay leaves
Black pepper, ground
Flour, all-purpose
Lemon juice
Lime juice
Mayonnaise, light
Nonstick cooking spray
Oil, olive
Parsley
Salt
Splenda Brown Sugar Blend
Vinegar, white wine

Miscellaneous
Pine nuts—2 Tbsp
Salsa

Chili Lime Shrimp LC NEW

Makes: 4 servings   *Serving Size: 4 ounces*   *Prep Time: 5 minutes*

1	tsp olive oil
	nonstick cooking spray
4	scallions (green and white parts), minced
1/4	cup lime juice
1	Tbsp minced garlic
1	Tbsp Splenda Brown Sugar Blend
1	tsp Asian-style chili-garlic sauce
9	ounces peeled and deveined raw medium shrimp

1 Add olive oil and a generous amount of cooking spray to a nonstick skillet over medium-high heat.

2 Add scallions and sauté for 3–4 minutes.

3 In a small bowl, whisk together lime juice, garlic, brown sugar, and chili-garlic sauce. Pour over scallions and simmer until reduced by half, about 3–4 minutes.

4 Add shrimp and sauté until shrimp is pink and just cooked through, about 4 minutes.

Exchanges/Choices
1/2 Carbohydrate   2 Lean Meat

Calories 100
  Calories from Fat 20
Total Fat . . . . .2.0 g
  Saturated Fat . . . . .0.4 g
  Trans Fat . . . . .0.0 g
Cholesterol. . . . . 105 mg
Sodium . . . . 570 mg
Potassium. . . . . 195 mg
Total Carbohydrate . . . . 6 g
  Dietary Fiber . . . . 0 g
  Sugars . . . . 2 g
Protein . . . . 14 g
Phosphorus . . . . 150 mg

Chef's Tip

You should be able to find the chili-garlic sauce in the ethnic foods aisle of the grocery store.

Baked Potato Soup

Makes: 9 servings   *Serving Size: 1 cup*   *Prep Time: 15 minutes*

nonstick cooking spray

1 medium onion, finely diced

5 slices turkey bacon, finely diced

6 medium russet potatoes, peeled and diced

3 14.5-ounce cans fat-free, low-sodium chicken broth

1 bay leaf

1/2 tsp salt (optional)

1/4 tsp ground black pepper

1 cup fat-free half-and-half

1/2 cup scallions, chopped

1/2 cup reduced-fat shredded cheddar cheese

1 Coat a large soup pot with cooking spray. Sauté onion for 3 minutes over medium heat. Add bacon and sauté for 3 minutes. Add potatoes, chicken broth, bay leaf, salt, and pepper. Turn heat to high and bring to a boil; then reduce heat to a low boil for 20 minutes.

2 Remove bay leaf.

3 Remove 4 cups of soup and purée in a blender or with a handheld immersion blender. Pour puréed soup back into pot and add half-and-half.

4 Garnish with scallions and cheddar cheese.

Exchanges/Choices

1 1/2 Starch   1/2 Fat

Calories 135
 Calories from Fat 25
Total Fat . . . . 3.0 g
 Saturated Fat . . . . 1.4 g
 Trans Fat . . . . 0.0 g
Cholesterol . . . . 10 mg
Sodium . . . . 525 mg
Potassium . . . . 485 mg
Total Carbohydrate . . . . . . 21 g
 Dietary Fiber . . . . 2 g
 Sugars . . . . 3 g
Protein . . . . 7 g
Phosphorus . . . . 155 mg

Chef's Tip

The immersion blender is a must-have kitchen tool for puréeing soups, sauces, smoothies, and desserts. It's easy to use and cleans up quickly!

Pesto Chicken Pita

Makes: 4 servings   *Serving Size: 1 pita*   *Prep Time: 10 minutes*

4	whole-wheat pita pockets
1/2	cup whole basil leaves
2	Tbsp pine nuts
2	Tbsp freshly grated Parmesan cheese
1/4	cup light mayonnaise
1/4	cup fat-free half-and-half
1	pound boneless, skinless chicken breasts

1 Slice one side of each pita to open pocket, but do not cut all the way through. Set aside.

2 In a blender or food processor, purée basil leaves, pine nuts, Parmesan cheese, and mayonnaise until a paste forms, about 2 minutes.

3 In a medium bowl, add basil mixture and half-and-half and whisk together. Reserve 4 Tbsp of basil sauce for later use.

4 Place each chicken breast between two pieces of plastic wrap and pound with a meat tenderizer or rolling pin until breasts are about 1/4 inch thick.

5 Place chicken breasts in a shallow dish and pour basil sauce over chicken.

6 Cook chicken breasts on an indoor or outdoor grill for 4 minutes on each side.

7 Toast pita pockets. Slice breast into strips and stuff inside pita. Add 1 Tbsp reserved basil sauce to each pita. Repeat procedure for remaining 3 pitas.

Exchanges/Choices
2 Starch	4 Lean Meat
1/2 Fat	

Calories	365
Calories from Fat	110
Total Fat	12.0 g
Saturated Fat	2.2 g
Trans Fat	0.0 g
Cholesterol	70 mg
Sodium	525 mg
Potassium	380 mg
Total Carbohydrate	35 g
Dietary Fiber	5 g
Sugars	2 g
Protein	31 g
Phosphorus	350 mg

Chef's Tip

You can also bake the chicken breasts in a 350°F oven for 20 minutes or until done instead of grilling them.

Brussels Sprouts with Citrus Butter GF LC

Makes: 5 servings   *Serving Size: 1/5 recipe*   *Prep Time: 8 minutes*

- **1**   1-pound bag frozen Brussels sprouts
- **2**   Tbsp trans-fat-free margarine
- **1**   Tbsp lemon juice
- **1/4**   tsp salt

1 Cook Brussels sprouts according to package directions.

2 Add remaining ingredients to a medium nonstick skillet over medium heat. Cook until margarine melts.

3 Add cooked Brussels sprouts and toss to coat.

Exchanges/Choices
1 Vegetable   1 Fat

Calories	70
Calories from Fat	35
Total Fat	4.0 g
Saturated Fat	1.1 g
Trans Fat	0.0 g
Cholesterol	0 mg
Sodium	165 mg
Potassium	255 mg
Total Carbohydrate	7 g
Dietary Fiber	4 g
Sugars	2 g
Protein	3 g
Phosphorus	50 mg

Dietitian's Tip

Brussels sprouts are also good topped with chopped, toasted nuts.

10-Minute Tostadas GF

Makes: 4 servings   *Serving Size: 1 tostada*   *Prep Time: 5 minutes*

4   tostada shells
1   16-ounce can fat-free refried beans with green chilies
3/4   cup shredded 75% reduced-fat cheddar cheese
1   cup shredded lettuce
1   cup tomatoes, seeded and chopped
       salsa and hot pepper sauce to taste

1 Preheat oven to 350°F.

2 Place tostada shells on a baking sheet. Spread 1/2 cup refried beans evenly on each tostada. Top each tostada with cheese. Bake in oven for 8–10 minutes or until cheese is melted.

3 Top with 1/4 cup lettuce and 1/4 cup tomatoes. Add salsa and hot pepper sauce as desired.

Exchanges/Choices
1 1/2 Starch   1 Med-Fat Meat

Calories 195
  Calories from Fat 40
Total Fat . . . . .4.5 g
  Saturated Fat . . . . .2.1 g
  Trans Fat . . . . .0.0 g
Cholesterol. . . . . 5 mg
Sodium . . . . 635 mg
Potassium. . . . . 560 mg
Total Carbohydrate . . . . . . 25 g
  Dietary Fiber . . . . 5 g
  Sugars . . . . 8 g
Protein . . . . 13 g
Phosphorus . . . . 275 mg

Dietitian's Tip

This tasty recipe works great when you're crunched for time. It's nutritious, with carbohydrate and fiber from the beans and protein and calcium from the cheese—all in just minutes!

Tomato Salad with Cilantro Vinaigrette GF LC

Makes: 8 servings   *Serving Size: 1/2 cup salad*   *Prep Time: 10 minutes*

- **2** Tbsp white wine vinegar
- **2** Tbsp olive oil
- **1** Tbsp chopped fresh cilantro
- **1** small shallot, minced
- **1/4** tsp salt
  dash ground black pepper
- **5** medium tomatoes, seeded and chopped

1 In a medium bowl, whisk together all ingredients except tomatoes.

2 Add tomatoes to bowl and toss gently to coat.

Exchanges/Choices
1 Vegetable   1/2 Fat

Calories 45
  Calories from Fat 30
Total Fat . . . . 3.5 g
  Saturated Fat . . . . 0.5 g
  Trans Fat . . . . 0.0 g
Cholesterol . . . . 0 mg
Sodium . . . . 75 mg
Potassium . . . . 195 mg
Total Carbohydrate . . . . 3 g
  Dietary Fiber . . . . 1 g
  Sugars . . . . 2 g
Protein . . . . 1 g
Phosphorus . . . . 20 mg

Chef's Tip

You can add some chopped cucumber to this salad if you like.

Beef Stew

Makes: 5 servings *Serving Size: 1 cup* *Prep Time: 20 minutes*

2   tsp olive oil
1   pound beef round roast, cut into 1/2-inch cubes
2   14.5-ounce cans fat-free, low-sodium beef broth
1/4 tsp ground black pepper
2   medium carrots, chopped
2   medium russet potatoes, peeled and chopped
2   medium celery stalks, chopped
1   medium onion, unevenly chopped
1   bay leaf
2   tsp dried parsley
1/4 cup cold water
2   Tbsp all-purpose flour

1 Add oil to a large soup pot over high heat. Add beef and cook for 15 minutes or until beef begins to brown. Add broth and pepper and bring to a boil. Reduce heat to a simmer, cover, and cook for 1 1/2 hours.

2 Add remaining ingredients except water and flour. Cover again and simmer 30 more minutes.

3 In a small bowl, whisk flour into cold water. Gradually stir the flour and water into the stew. Bring to a boil, stirring constantly, for 5 more minutes.

Exchanges/Choices
1 Starch   1 Vegetable
3 Lean Meat

Calories 225
  Calories from Fat 45
Total Fat . . . . .5.0 g
  Saturated Fat . . . . .1.3 g
  Trans Fat . . . . .0.0 g
Cholesterol. . . . . 40 mg
Sodium . . . . 475 mg
Potassium. . . . . 645 mg
Total Carbohydrate . . . . . . 19 g
  Dietary Fiber . . . . 3 g
  Sugars . . . . 4 g
Protein . . . . 25 g
Phosphorus . . . . 205 mg

Chef's Tip

This recipe takes a little longer to prepare, but it's well worth it—especially for the great-tasting leftovers.

NOVEMBER

WEEK 2

DAY 1
New England Clam
   Chowder   372

DAY 2
Creamy Shrimp
   and Mushroom
   Polenta   373
Green Beans
   Amandine   374

DAY 3
Beef and Cheese Skillet
   Casserole   375

DAY 4
Turkey Larb Lettuce
   Wraps   376
Fruit Salad with Yogurt
   Dressing   377

DAY 5
Tuna Spinach
   Bake   378

GROCERY LIST

Fresh Produce
Blueberries—1 cup
Chile, Serrano—1
Garlic—1 head
Grapes, green—2 cups
Lemon—1
Lettuce, butter (Bibb)—1 head
Mint—1 bunch
Mushrooms, baby bella,
   sliced—8 ounces
Onion, red, small—1
Onion, yellow or white,
   medium—1
Parsley—1 bunch
Potatoes, russet, medium—2
Spinach, 6-ounce bag—1
Strawberries—2 cups

Meat, Poultry, & Fish
Beef, ground, 95% lean—
   1 pound
Shrimp, raw—1 pound
Turkey, ground, 93% lean—
   1 1/2 pounds
Turkey bacon—4 slices

Grains, Bread, & Pasta
Pasta, farfalle, whole-
   wheat—8 ounces
Pasta, rotini, whole-wheat—
   8 ounces

Dairy & Cheese
Cheese, cheddar, 75%
   reduced-fat, shredded—
   1 1/2 cups
Cream cheese, light—2 Tbsp
Half-and-half, fat-free—
   1 1/2 cups

Margarine, trans-fat-free
Milk, fat-free—1 cup
Yogurt, plain, fat-free—
   1/2 cup

Canned Goods & Sauces
Clams, with juice, 10-ounce
   cans—2
Soup, cream of mushroom,
   condensed, reduced-fat,
   10.75-ounce can—1
Soy sauce, lite
Tomato sauce, 8-ounce
   can—1
Tomatoes, crushed,
   14.5-ounce can—1
Tuna, packed in water,
   6-ounce cans—2

Frozen Foods
Green beans, 1-pound
   bag—1

Staples, Seasonings,
& Baking Needs
Black pepper, ground
Cayenne pepper
Chili powder
Cornmeal
Garlic powder
Lemon juice
Lime juice
Nonstick cooking spray
Oil, olive
Salt
Splenda Sugar Blend
Vanilla extract

Miscellaneous
Almonds, slivered—1/4 cup

New England Clam Chowder

Makes: 5 servings   *Serving Size: 1 cup*   *Prep Time: 10 minutes*

nonstick cooking spray
4 slices turkey bacon, chopped
1 medium onion, finely diced
2 10-ounce cans chopped clams with juice
1/2 cup water
2 medium russet potatoes, finely diced
1 cup fat-free milk
1 cup fat-free half-and-half
1/2 tsp salt (optional)
1/4 tsp ground black pepper

1 Coat a medium soup pot with cooking spray. Add bacon and cook over medium-high heat for 4 minutes or until beginning to brown. Add onion and continue to cook another 3 minutes or until onion is clear.

2 Add clams with juice, water, and potatoes. Increase heat to high and bring to a boil. Boil for 20 minutes or until potatoes are soft.

3 Reduce heat to low and add milk and half-and-half. Simmer for 1 minute. Do not boil. Add salt and pepper.

Exchanges/Choices
1 Starch	1/2 Fat-Free Milk
1 Vegetable	2 Lean Meat

Calories 225
  Calories from Fat 35
Total Fat . . . . .4.0 g
  Saturated Fat . . . . .1.1 g
  Trans Fat . . . . .0.0 g
Cholesterol. . . . . 50 mg
Sodium . . . . 405 mg
Potassium. . . . . 920 mg
Total Carbohydrate . . . . . . 27 g
  Dietary Fiber . . . . 2 g
  Sugars . . . . 7 g
Protein . . . . 20 g
Phosphorus . . . . 455 mg

Chef's Tip

Serve this hearty chowder with a tossed salad.

Creamy Shrimp and Mushroom Polenta

Makes: 6 servings   *Serving Size: 1 cup*   *Prep Time: 15 minutes*

- **2** cups cornmeal (polenta)
- **6** cups water
- **1** Tbsp trans-fat-free margarine
  nonstick cooking spray
- **8** ounces sliced baby bella
  mushrooms
- **1** Tbsp minced garlic
- **2** Tbsp light cream cheese
- **1/2** cup fat-free half-and-half
- **1** pound medium raw shrimp,
  peeled and deveined
- **2** Tbsp chopped fresh parsley
- **1/2** tsp salt (optional)
- **1/2** tsp ground black pepper

1 In a large saucepan, combine cornmeal and water. While whisking, bring to a boil. Reduce to a simmer; whisking occasionally. Cook 20 minutes.

2 While polenta is cooking, heat margarine and a generous amount of cooking spray in a medium nonstick sauté pan. Add mushrooms to pan and sauté until all the liquid is evaporated (about 6–7 minutes). Add garlic and sauté for 30 seconds.

3 Stir in cream cheese and half-and-half and simmer until slightly thickened.

4 Add shrimp and cook for 3–4 minutes or until shrimp is pink and cooked through.

5 Fold the shrimp mixture into the cooked polenta and season with salt (optional), pepper, and fresh parsley.

Exchanges/Choices

2 1/2 Starch   2 Lean Meat

Calories	280
Calories from Fat	40
Total Fat	4.5 g
Saturated Fat	1.4 g
Trans Fat	0.0 g
Cholesterol	105 mg
Sodium	525 mg
Potassium	385 mg
Total Carbohydrate	41 g
Dietary Fiber	2 g
Sugars	3 g
Protein	16 g
Phosphorus	280 mg

Chef's Tip

You can save time by purchasing precooked shrimp. When adding precooked shrimp to the mushroom mixture in step 4, just reduce the cooking time to 1 minute so shrimp just gets warmed through but not overcooked.

Green Beans Amandine GF LC

Makes: 5 servings   *Serving Size: 1/2 cup*   *Prep Time: 2 minutes*

1 Tbsp trans-fat-free margarine
   nonstick cooking spray
1 1-pound bag frozen green beans,
   thawed
1/4 cup slivered almonds, toasted
1/2 tsp salt (optional)

1 Add margarine and a generous amount of cooking spray to a medium nonstick skillet over medium-high heat.

2 After margarine melts, add in remaining ingredients and sauté for 4–5 minutes.

Exchanges/Choices
1 Vegetable   1 Fat

Calories 70
  Calories from Fat 45
Total Fat . . . . 5.0 g
  Saturated Fat . . . . 0.8 g
  Trans Fat . . . . 0.0 g
Cholesterol . . . . 0 mg
Sodium . . . . 20 mg
Potassium . . . . 170 mg
Total Carbohydrate . . . . . . 6 g
  Dietary Fiber . . . . 3 g
  Sugars . . . . 1 g
Protein . . . . 2 g
Phosphorus . . . . 50 mg

Dietitian's Tip

Almonds provide taste and texture to this recipe, along with vitamin E.

Beef and Cheese Skillet Casserole

Makes: 7 servings   *Serving Size: 1 cup*   *Prep Time: 2 minutes*

2 cups whole-wheat rotini pasta, uncooked
1 pound 95% lean ground beef
1 14.5-ounce can crushed tomatoes
1 8-ounce can tomato sauce
2 tsp chili powder
1/8 tsp cayenne pepper
1 tsp garlic powder
1 tsp Splenda Sugar Blend
2/3 cup shredded 75% reduced-fat cheddar cheese

1 Cook pasta according to package directions, omitting salt. Drain.

2 In a large nonstick skillet, cook ground beef until beginning to brown, about 8–9 minutes. Drain any excess fat.

3 Add remaining ingredients except cheese and pasta and bring to a boil. Reduce heat and simmer for 6–7 minutes or until beginning to thicken. Fold in cheese and toss with pasta.

Exchanges/Choices
1 Starch   1 Vegetable
2 Lean Meat

Calories	215
Calories from Fat	45
Total Fat	5.0 g
Saturated Fat	2.2 g
Trans Fat	0.1 g
Cholesterol	45 mg
Sodium	370 mg
Potassium	535 mg
Total Carbohydrate	22 g
Dietary Fiber	4 g
Sugars	5 g
Protein	21 g
Phosphorus	245 mg

Chef's Tip

This is a quick and easy recipe the whole family will enjoy.

Turkey Larb Lettuce Wraps LC NEW

Makes: 4 servings   *Serving Size: 2 lettuce wraps*   *Prep Time: 10 minutes*

Dressing

1/4	cup lime juice
1	Tbsp lemon juice
2	Tbsp lite soy sauce
2	Tbsp Splenda Sugar Blend

Larb

1	Tbsp olive oil
	nonstick cooking spray
1	small red onion, minced
2	4-inch pieces lemon zest
1	Serrano chile, minced
1 1/2	pounds 93% lean ground turkey
1	tsp salt (optional)
1/2	tsp ground black pepper
1/2	cup chopped fresh mint leaves
8	leaves butter (Bibb) lettuce, washed and dried

1 In a small bowl, whisk together dressing ingredients. Set aside.

2 In a large skillet, add the olive oil and a generous amount of cooking spray over medium heat. Add the onion, lemon zest, and chile, and sauté until the vegetables begin to soften, about 5 minutes. Add the turkey, salt (optional), and pepper. Sauté until the turkey and vegetables are cooked through, about 7 minutes.

3 Add the dressing to the pan and simmer for 2 minutes. Remove the lemon zest and add the mint to the mixture. Stir well to incorporate and remove the pan from the heat.

4 Evenly divide the larb among the 8 lettuce leaves and fold over to make a wrap.

Exchanges/Choices

1 Vegetable   5 Lean Meat
2 Fat

Calories	330
Calories from Fat	160
Total Fat	18.0 g
Saturated Fat	4.2 g
Trans Fat	0.2 g
Cholesterol	130 mg
Sodium	395 mg
Potassium	525 mg
Total Carbohydrate	7 g
Dietary Fiber	1 g
Sugars	3 g
Protein	35 g
Phosphorus	350 mg

Chef's Tip

Use your potato peeler to gently peel the pieces of zest from the lemon. Be sure not to get the white part (pith), because it's bitter. Or you can use a zester (microplane) and use about 1 Tbsp of grated lemon zest (and omit the direction to remove the zest from the mixture).

Fruit Salad with Yogurt Dressing GF

Makes: 5 servings   *Serving Size: 1 cup*   *Prep Time: 15 minutes*

Fruit Salad
- **2** cups strawberries, sliced
- **1** cup blueberries
- **2** cups green grapes

Dressing
- **1/2** cup fat-free plain yogurt
- **1** Tbsp lemon juice
- **1/4** tsp vanilla extract

1 In a medium bowl, toss together strawberries, blueberries, and grapes.

2 In a small bowl, whisk together dressing ingredients. Pour dressing over fruit and gently toss.

World Diabetes Day is November 14. Celebrate by enjoying healthy food today!

Exchanges/Choices
1 1/2 Fruit

Calories	95
Calories from Fat	0
Total Fat	0.0 g
Saturated Fat	0.1 g
Trans Fat	0.0 g
Cholesterol	0 mg
Sodium	20 mg
Potassium	300 mg
Total Carbohydrate	22 g
Dietary Fiber	3 g
Sugars	17 g
Protein	2 g
Phosphorus	70 mg

Chef's Tip

This quick dressing really jazzes up plain fruit. Try it on more exotic fruits, too.

Tuna Spinach Bake

Makes: 6 servings *Serving Size: 1 cup* *Prep Time: 10 minutes*

nonstick cooking spray

4 cups whole-wheat farfalle pasta, uncooked

1 6-ounce bag fresh spinach (about 4 cups)

1/4 tsp ground black pepper

2 6-ounce cans tuna packed in water, drained

1 10.75-ounce can reduced-fat cream of mushroom condensed soup

1/2 cup reduced-fat shredded cheddar cheese

1 Preheat oven to 375°F. Coat a 9 × 9-inch baking dish with cooking spray. Set aside.

2 Cook pasta according to package directions, omitting salt. Drain.

3 Coat a medium nonstick skillet with cooking spray. Sauté spinach leaves over medium-high heat for 4 minutes.

4 In a medium bowl, mix pepper, tuna, soup, and cooked spinach. Pour pasta in bottom of baking dish. Pour tuna/spinach mixture over the pasta and spread evenly to coat.

5 Sprinkle cheese over the top and bake for 15 minutes.

Exchanges/Choices

2 Starch   2 Lean Meat

Calories 240
  Calories from Fat 35
Total Fat . . . . 4.0 g
  Saturated Fat . . . . 1.6 g
  Trans Fat . . . . 0.0 g
Cholesterol . . . . 30 mg
Sodium . . . . 525 mg
Potassium . . . . 475 mg
Total Carbohydrate . . . . . . 32 g
  Dietary Fiber . . . . 5 g
  Sugars . . . . 1 g
Protein . . . . 20 g
Phosphorus . . . . 255 mg

Chef's Tip

If you don't love tuna, try cooked, shredded chicken in this recipe.

NOVEMBER

WEEK 3

DAY 1
Pumpkin
    Pancakes   380

DAY 2
Pasta Fagioli   381

DAY 3
Mushroom Alfredo
    Halibut   382
Garlic Mashed
    Potatoes   383

DAY 4
Roasted Turkey   384
Cranberry Salad   385

DAY 5
Turkey Soup with
    White Beans   386

GROCERY LIST

Fresh Produce
Carrots, medium—4
Celery—1 head
Chives—1 bunch
Cranberries, 1-pound bag—1
Garlic—1 large head
Lemon—1
Mushrooms—1/2 pint
Onions, yellow or white—4
Orange, navel, medium—1
Potatoes, russet—2 pounds

Meat, Poultry, & Fish
Halibut fillets, 4 ounces
    each—4
Turkey—12 pounds
Turkey bacon—4 slices

Grains, Bread, & Pasta
Pasta, shell, quinoa—
    1 small box

Dairy & Cheese
Cheese, Parmesan—1 block
Eggs
Half-and-half, fat-free—
    2 cups
Margarine, trans-fat-free
Milk, fat-free—2 cups

Canned Goods & Sauces
Beans, cannellini, 16-ounce
    cans—3
Broth, chicken, fat-free,
    low-sodium, 14.5-ounce
    cans—5
Pumpkin, 15-ounce can—1
Tomatoes, diced, no-salt-
    added, 15-ounce cans—2

Staples, Seasonings, & Baking Needs
Baking powder
Basil
Black pepper, ground
Cinnamon
Flour, all-purpose
Garlic powder
Nonstick cooking spray
Nutmeg, ground
Oil, canola
Oil, olive
Oregano
Paprika
Parsley
Salt
Splenda Brown Sugar Blend
Splenda Sugar Blend

Pumpkin Pancakes

Makes: 7 servings   *Serving Size: 2 pancakes*   *Prep Time: 5 minutes*

1 1/2   cups all-purpose flour
2 1/4   tsp baking powder
    1   tsp ground cinnamon
  1/4   tsp ground nutmeg
  1/4   tsp salt
    2   cups fat-free milk
    3   tsp Splenda Brown Sugar Blend
    1   Tbsp canola oil
    2   eggs, lightly beaten
    1   15-ounce can pumpkin
        nonstick cooking spray

1 In a large bowl, sift together flour, baking powder, cinnamon, nutmeg, and salt.

2 In a medium bowl, whisk together milk, brown sugar, oil, eggs, and pumpkin. Make a well in the dry ingredients and pour in the wet ingredients. Stir mixture until liquid is incorporated and batter is smooth.

3 Coat a large nonstick skillet with cooking spray over medium heat. Once pan heats up, pour 1/3 cup batter to form pancakes. Cook pancakes until brown on bottom and some bubbles begin to break around edges. Turn pancake over. Cook until brown on bottom and firm to touch in center.

4 Repeat procedure until all batter is gone.

Exchanges/Choices
2 Starch   1/2 Fat

Calories 185
  Calories from Fat 30
Total Fat . . . . .3.5 g
  Saturated Fat . . . . .0.7 g
  Trans Fat . . . . .0.0 g
Cholesterol. . . . . 50 mg
Sodium . . . . 250 mg
Potassium. . . . . 285 mg
Total Carbohydrate . . . . . . 31 g
  Dietary Fiber . . . . 3 g
  Sugars . . . . 7 g
Protein . . . . 7 g
Phosphorus . . . . 295 mg

Chef's Tip

Serve these pancakes spread with trans-fat-free margarine and sprinkled with a mixture of sugar substitute, cinnamon, and nutmeg . . . or just top with a dusting of powdered sugar.

Pasta Fagioli

Makes: 6 servings　　　　*Serving Size: 1 cup*　　　　*Prep Time: 15 minutes*

nonstick cooking spray
4　slices turkey bacon, chopped
1　medium onion, minced
2　garlic cloves, minced
2　medium celery stalks, finely diced
2　medium carrots, finely diced
2　14.5-ounce cans fat-free, low-sodium chicken broth
2　16-ounce cans cannellini beans, rinsed and drained

1　15-ounce can no-salt-added diced tomatoes, drained
1　tsp dried parsley
1　tsp dried basil
1/4　tsp ground black pepper
1　cup small shell quinoa pasta, uncooked
1/4　cup freshly grated Parmesan cheese

1 Coat a large soup pot with cooking spray over high heat. Add bacon and sauté until crisp.

2 Reduce heat to medium and add onion, garlic, celery, and carrots. Sauté about 5–7 minutes or until vegetables begin to brown. Add broth and simmer for 5 minutes.

3 Stir in beans, tomatoes, parsley, basil, and pepper and simmer for 10 minutes. Add the pasta and continue to simmer for 10–15 minutes or until pasta is al dente.

4 Serve soup in a bowl sprinkled with Parmesan cheese.

Exchanges/Choices
1 1/2 Starch　　　2 Vegetable
1 Lean Meat

Calories 215	
Calories from Fat 25	
Total Fat . . . . .3.0 g	
Saturated Fat . . . . .1.2 g	
Trans Fat . . . . .0.0 g	
Cholesterol. . . . . 10 mg	
Sodium . . . . 355 mg	
Potassium. . . . . 770 mg	
Total Carbohydrate . . . . . . 35 g	
Dietary Fiber . . . . 8 g	
Sugars . . . . 4 g	
Protein . . . . 13 g	
Phosphorus . . . . 255 mg	

Chef's Tip

Al dente literally means "to the tooth" in Italian, meaning that the pasta should be soft but still have a little bit of a bite to it.

Mushroom Alfredo Halibut LC

Makes: 4 servings   *Serving Size: 1 fillet*   *Prep Time: 15 minutes*

1	tsp olive oil
	nonstick cooking spray
1/2	pint mushrooms, sliced
1/2	cup fat-free half-and-half
1/4	cup freshly grated Parmesan cheese
2	tsp garlic powder
4	4-ounce halibut fillets

1 Preheat oven to 350°F.

2 Add oil and a generous amount of cooking spray to a medium nonstick skillet over medium heat. Add sliced mushrooms and sauté for 5–7 minutes or until liquid is evaporated.

3 Heat half-and-half in the microwave for 1 minute. Turn off flame under mushrooms. Pour half-and-half over mushrooms. Add cheese and garlic powder and stir well.

4 Place each halibut fillet in a piece of aluminum foil. Pour 1/4 of mushroom sauce over fish and seal. Repeat procedure for remaining 3 fillets. Place foil packets on baking sheet and bake for 15 minutes or until fish flakes with a fork.

Exchanges/Choices
1/2 Carbohydrate   3 Lean Meat

Calories 175
　Calories from Fat 45
Total Fat . . . . 5.0 g
　Saturated Fat . . . . 1.5 g
　Trans Fat . . . . 0.0 g
Cholesterol . . . . 40 mg
Sodium . . . . 165 mg
Potassium . . . . 645 mg
Total Carbohydrate . . . . 4 g
　Dietary Fiber . . . . 0 g
　Sugars . . . . 2 g
Protein . . . . 27 g
Phosphorus . . . . 350 mg

Dietitian's Tip

Alfredo sauce is typically very high in fat, but the fat-free half-and-half solves that problem in this recipe.

Garlic Mashed Potatoes

Makes: 8 servings   *Serving Size: 1/2 cup*   *Prep Time: 15 minutes*

2 pounds russet potatoes, peeled and cut into chunks
8 garlic cloves, peeled
1 1/2 cups fat-free half-and-half, heated
2 Tbsp trans-fat-free margarine
1/4 cup fresh chives, chopped
1 tsp salt (optional)
1/4 tsp ground black pepper

1 Add potatoes and garlic cloves to a large soup pot and cover with cold water. Place on stove over high heat and bring to a boil. Boil for 20 minutes or until potatoes are softened. Drain and return to pot.

2 Add remaining ingredients and beat with an electric mixer until smooth.

Exchanges/Choices
1 1/2 Starch   1/2 Fat

Calories 125
  Calories from Fat 25
Total Fat . . . . .3.0 g
  Saturated Fat . . . . .1.0 g
  Trans Fat . . . . .0.0 g
Cholesterol. . . . . 0 mg
Sodium . . . . 70 mg
Potassium. . . . . 395 mg
Total Carbohydrate . . . . . . 23 g
  Dietary Fiber . . . . 2 g
  Sugars . . . . 3 g
Protein . . . . 3 g
Phosphorus . . . . 105 mg

Chef's Tip

This dish is a classic favorite and easy, too! Serve these potatoes with a wide variety of entrées.

Roasted Turkey GF LC

Makes: 20 servings   *Serving Size: 4–5 ounces turkey without skin*   *Prep Time: 15 minutes*

1   12-pound whole turkey
1   Tbsp salt
2   Tbsp trans-fat-free margarine, melted
1   lemon, cut in half
1   large onion, quartered

1 Preheat oven to 325°F.

2 Remove giblets from turkey. Rinse cavity. Rub cavity of bird lightly with salt.

3 Place turkey breast side up on rack in shallow roasting pan. Brush with melted margarine. Stuff the cavity with lemon halves and onion quarters.

4 When turkey begins to turn golden, place a tent of aluminum foil loosely over it.

5 Turkey will cook for about 3 1/2–4 1/2 hours, until internal temperature reaches 180°F. To ensure proper temperature readings, place the meat thermometer in the thigh muscle, so the thermometer does not touch bone.

6 Remove from oven and let stand about 15 minutes before slicing. Remove skin before serving.

Exchanges/Choices
5 Lean Meat

Calories 215
    Calories from Fat 65
Total Fat . . . . .7.0 g
    Saturated Fat . . . . .2.2 g
    Trans Fat . . . . .0.0 g
Cholesterol. . . . . 95 mg
Sodium . . . . 440 mg
Potassium. . . . . 370 mg
Total Carbohydrate . . . . 0 g
    Dietary Fiber . . . . 0 g
    Sugars . . . . 0 g
Protein . . . . 37 g
Phosphorus . . . . 265 mg

Chef's Tip

When roasting a bird this large, be sure to take the temperature in the thigh muscle to ensure the entire thing is cooked to 180°F. The thigh meat takes longer to cook than the breast meat, so you'll know the whole bird is done when the thigh meat is done.

Cranberry Salad GF LC

Makes: 8 servings　　　　*Serving Size: 1/8 recipe*　　　　*Prep Time: 10 minutes*

1　1-pound bag fresh cranberries
1　medium navel orange, peeled and cut into chunks
3/4　cup Splenda Sugar Blend

1 In a blender or food processor, pulse cranberries and orange chunks until finely ground. Pour into a medium bowl and stir in Splenda until incorporated.

2 Cover and refrigerate overnight.

Exchanges/Choices
1 Fruit

Calories	40
Calories from Fat	0
Total Fat	0.0 g
Saturated Fat	0.0 g
Trans Fat	0.0 g
Cholesterol	0 mg
Sodium	0 mg
Potassium	80 mg
Total Carbohydrate	11 g
Dietary Fiber	3 g
Sugars	6 g
Protein	0 g
Phosphorus	10 mg

Dietitian's Tip

Cranberries contain several antioxidants that may help fight against heart disease and some cancers.

Turkey Soup with White Beans LC

Makes: 10 servings   *Serving Size: 1 cup*   *Prep Time: 15 minutes*

1	Tbsp olive oil
2	small onions, finely diced
2	medium carrots, finely diced
2	medium celery stalks, finely diced
3	garlic cloves, minced
3	14.5-ounce cans fat-free, low-sodium chicken broth
1 1/2	tsp dried oregano
1/2	tsp paprika

2 1/2	cups cooked turkey meat, shredded (from Roasted Turkey recipe, page 384)
1	15-ounce can no-salt-added diced tomatoes with juice
1	16-ounce can cannellini beans, drained and rinsed
1/4	tsp salt (optional)
1/4	tsp ground black pepper

1 Add oil to a large soup pot over medium-high heat. Add onions, carrots, and celery and sauté for 5–7 minutes or until vegetables begin to soften. Stir in garlic and sauté an additional 30 seconds.

2 Add remaining ingredients and bring to a boil. Reduce heat and simmer for 20 minutes.

Exchanges/Choices

1/2 Starch   1 Vegetable
2 Lean Meat

Calories 145
  Calories from Fat 30
Total Fat . . . . 3.5 g
  Saturated Fat . . . . 0.8 g
  Trans Fat . . . . 0.0 g
Cholesterol . . . . 25 mg
Sodium . . . . 365 mg
Potassium . . . . 505 mg
Total Carbohydrate . . . . . . 13 g
  Dietary Fiber . . . . 3 g
  Sugars . . . . 4 g
Protein . . . . 15 g
Phosphorus . . . . 160 mg

Chef's Tip

Make use of that leftover turkey from Thanksgiving in this tasty soup.

NOVEMBER

WEEK 4

DAY 1
Unstuffed
Cabbage   388

DAY 2
Italian Sausage with
Pepper Medley   389

DAY 3
Cobb Salad   390
French Onion
Soup   391

DAY 4
Angel Hair with
Turkey Bacon and
Peas   392

DAY 5
Roasted Chicken   393
Sweet and Savory Baked
Apples   394

**DESSERT OF
THE MONTH**
Sweet Potato Pie   395

GROCERY LIST

Fresh Produce
Apples, Granny Smith,
    medium—2
Apples, honeycrisp,
    medium—2
Bell peppers, green—2
Bell pepper, red—1
Cabbage—1 head
Endive—1 head
Garlic—2 cloves
Lemons—2
Lettuce, romaine—1 head
Onions, yellow or white—6
Potatoes, sweet—1 1/2 pounds
Tomato, large—1

Meat, Poultry, & Fish
Beef, ground, 90% lean—
    1 pound
Chicken, fryer—3 pounds
Chicken breasts, boneless,
    skinless—1/2 pound
Turkey bacon—12 slices
Turkey sausage links, lean—5
    (14–15 ounces total)

Grains, Bread, & Pasta
Croutons, whole-grain—
    1/2 cup
Pasta, angel hair, whole-
    wheat—8 ounces
Rice, brown—1 bag

Dairy & Cheese
Cheese, Parmesan—1 small
    block
Cheese, Swiss, reduced-fat,
    shredded—1/2 cup
Cheese, wedges, spreadable,
    lite—6

Egg substitute—1/2 cup
Eggs
Half-and-half, fat-free—1 cup
Margarine, trans-fat-free

Canned Goods & Sauces
Broth, beef, fat-free, no-salt-
    added, 14.5-ounce cans—4
Milk, evaporated, fat-free—
    1 can
Tomatoes, diced, no-salt-
    added, 14.5-ounce cans—2

Frozen Foods
Peas—1 small bag

Staples, Seasonings,
& Baking Needs
Basil
Black pepper, ground
Cinnamon
Flour, all-purpose
Mustard, Dijon
Nonstick cooking spray
Nutmeg, ground
Oil, canola
Oil, olive
Oregano
Paprika
Red pepper flakes
Salt
Splenda Brown Sugar Blend
Splenda Sugar Blend
Vanilla extract
Vinegar, red wine
Vinegar, white wine

Miscellaneous
Almonds, slivered—6 Tbsp
Pie crust, unbaked, 9-inch—1

Unstuffed Cabbage

Makes: 5 servings   *Serving Size: 1/5 recipe*   *Prep Time: 20 minutes*

1   pound 90% lean ground beef
1   cup fat-free, low-sodium beef broth
8   cups cabbage, shredded
1   cup diced onion
2   14.5-ounce cans no-salt-added diced tomatoes with juice
4   Tbsp white wine vinegar
1   tsp Splenda Brown Sugar Blend
3/4 tsp salt
1/2 tsp ground black pepper
2 1/2 cups cooked brown rice

1 Sauté ground beef in a large, deep skillet until completely cooked. Drain off any excess fat.

2 Add beef broth and shredded cabbage and cook until cabbage begins to soften.

3 Add remaining ingredients except rice and simmer for 20 minutes or until cabbage is completely cooked.

4 Serve over rice.

Exchanges/Choices
1 1/2 Starch   3 Vegetable
2 Lean Meat   1 Fat

Calories	330
Calories from Fat	80
Total Fat	9.0 g
Saturated Fat	3.2 g
Trans Fat	0.5 g
Cholesterol	55 mg
Sodium	585 mg
Potassium	890 mg
Total Carbohydrate	40 g
Dietary Fiber	6 g
Sugars	10 g
Protein	24 g
Phosphorus	310 mg

Chef's Tip

This recipe tastes great and is a lot less time-intensive than your grandmother's stuffed cabbage. It's a one-skillet sensation that's sure to make you want more!

Italian Sausage with Pepper Medley GF LC

Makes: 5 servings   *Serving Size: 1/5 recipe*   *Prep Time: 10 minutes*

5	lean Italian turkey sausage links (14–15 ounces total)
1	tsp olive oil
2	green bell peppers, sliced into 1/2-inch strips
1	red bell pepper, sliced into 1/2-inch strips
1	medium onion, thinly sliced
1/2	tsp salt (optional)
1/8	tsp ground black pepper
1/2	tsp dried basil
1/2	tsp dried oregano
1/4	tsp crushed red pepper flakes
2	garlic cloves, minced
1	Tbsp water

1 Cook sausage in a large nonstick skillet over medium-high heat for 8–10 minutes or until done. Remove from pan and set aside.

2 Add oil to skillet. Add remaining ingredients and sauté for 4–5 minutes or until tender-crisp.

3 Serve peppers over sausage links.

Exchanges/Choices
1 Vegetable   2 Med-Fat Meat

Calories 160
 Calories from Fat 80
Total Fat . . . . .9.0 g
 Saturated Fat . . . . 2.0 g
 Trans Fat . . . . .0.2 g
Cholesterol. . . . . 45 mg
Sodium . . . . 500 mg
Potassium. . . . . 375 mg
Total Carbohydrate . . . . . . 8 g
 Dietary Fiber . . . . 2 g
 Sugars . . . . 4 g
Protein . . . . 14 g
Phosphorus . . . . 135 mg

Dietitian's Tip

This entrée features a terrific blend of flavors.

Cobb Salad GF LC

Makes: 8 servings   *Serving Size: 1/8 recipe*   *Prep Time: 15 minutes*

8	cups chopped romaine lettuce
2	cups chopped endive
6	slices turkey bacon, chopped
1/2	pound boneless, skinless chicken breasts, cooked and cubed
1	large tomato, seeded and diced
2	hard-boiled egg whites, sliced
1/4	cup red wine vinegar
2	Tbsp olive oil
2	tsp Dijon mustard

1 In a large salad bowl, toss together romaine and endive. Set aside.

2 Cook bacon in a large nonstick skillet until crisp. Arrange the chicken, tomato, egg whites, and cooled bacon over top of lettuce.

3 In a small bowl, whisk together remaining ingredients. Drizzle dressing over salad and toss to coat.

Exchanges/Choices

1 Vegetable   1 Lean Meat
1 Fat

Calories	105
Calories from Fat	55
Total Fat	6.0 g
Saturated Fat	1.2 g
Trans Fat	0.0 g
Cholesterol	20 mg
Sodium	205 mg
Potassium	300 mg
Total Carbohydrate	3 g
Dietary Fiber	2 g
Sugars	1 g
Protein	10 g
Phosphorus	100 mg

Chef's Tip

You can add almost anything to a Cobb salad— try cucumbers, avocado, bell peppers, or chopped ham.

French Onion Soup LC

Makes: 4 servings   *Serving Size: 1 cup*   *Prep Time: 10 minutes*

2	tsp canola oil
	nonstick cooking spray
5	small or 3 large onions, thinly sliced
3	14.5-ounce cans fat-free, no-salt-added beef broth
1/4	tsp salt (optional)
1/4	tsp ground black pepper
1/2	cup whole-grain croutons
1/2	cup shredded, reduced-fat Swiss cheese

1 Add oil and a generous amount of cooking spray to a medium soup pot over medium-high heat. Add onions and cook for 15–20 minutes until onions are deeply caramelized, stirring occasionally.

2 Add broth, salt, and pepper. Bring to a boil, then reduce heat and simmer for 25 minutes.

3 Pour soup into 4 soup bowls and top each with 2 Tbsp croutons and 2 Tbsp cheese.

Exchanges/Choices
3 Vegetable   1 Lean Meat
1/2 Fat

Calories 135
  Calories from Fat 40
Total Fat . . . . .4.5 g
  Saturated Fat . . . . .1.3 g
  Trans Fat . . . . .0.0 g
Cholesterol. . . . . 5 mg
Sodium . . . . 250 mg
Potassium. . . . . 375 mg
Total Carbohydrate. . . . . . 15 g
  Dietary Fiber . . . . 2 g
  Sugars . . . . 6 g
Protein . . . . 10 g
Phosphorus . . . . 165 mg

Chef's Tip

Caramelize means to cook until chocolate brown but not burned.

Angel Hair with Turkey Bacon and Peas

Makes: 4 servings   *Serving Size: 1 cup*   *Prep Time: 5 minutes*

8 ounces whole-wheat angel hair pasta, uncooked
1 cup fat-free half-and-half
1 tsp grated lemon peel
1 cup frozen peas
6 slices turkey bacon, cooked and chopped
2 tsp fresh lemon juice
1/4 cup freshly grated Parmesan cheese

1 Cook pasta according to package directions, omitting salt. Drain. Reserve 1/2 cup pasta cooking liquid.

2 In a large nonstick skillet, simmer half-and-half, pasta liquid, and lemon peel until slightly reduced, about 1 minute. Stir in peas, turkey bacon, and lemon juice. Simmer 2 minutes.

3 Add cooked pasta and cheese to skillet; toss to coat.

Exchanges/Choices
3 Starch   1 Med-Fat Meat

Calories 330
  Calories from Fat 55
Total Fat . . . . 6.0 g
  Saturated Fat . . . . 2.3 g
  Trans Fat . . . . 0.0 g
Cholesterol . . . . 20 mg
Sodium . . . . 430 mg
Potassium . . . . 330 mg
Total Carbohydrate . . . . . . 51 g
  Dietary Fiber . . . . 8 g
  Sugars . . . . 5 g
Protein . . . . 17 g
Phosphorus . . . . 345 mg

Chef's Tip

You'll love the flavor combination of sweet peas, tart lemon, and salty bacon in this dish.

Roasted Chicken GF LC

Makes: 6 servings   *Serving Size: 1 breast or 1 thigh or*   *Prep Time: 5 minutes*
                             1 drumstick and wing

nonstick cooking spray
1   3-pound fryer chicken, cut into
     8 pieces
1   Tbsp paprika
1/2 tsp salt
1/4 tsp ground black pepper

1 Preheat oven to 375°F.

2 Coat a 13 × 9-inch roasting pan with cooking spray. Arrange chicken pieces skin side up and spray generously with cooking spray. Season chicken with paprika, salt, and pepper.

3 Bake for 35 minutes or until juices run clear. Remove skin before serving.

Exchanges/Choices
3 Lean Meat

Calories 140
  Calories from Fat 45
Total Fat . . . . .5.0 g
  Saturated Fat . . . . .1.5 g
  Trans Fat . . . . .0.0 g
Cholesterol. . . . . 65 mg
Sodium . . . . 160 mg
Potassium. . . . . 190 mg
Total Carbohydrate . . . . 0 g
  Dietary Fiber . . . . 0 g
  Sugars . . . . 0 g
Protein . . . . 21 g
Phosphorus . . . . 145 mg

Dietitian's Tip

Taking the skin off poultry after cooking it is a good way to decrease the fat and extra calories.

Sweet and Savory Baked Apples GF NEW

Makes: 6 servings   *Serving Size: 1 apple*   *Prep Time: 10 minutes*

nonstick cooking spray

2 medium Granny Smith apples, peeled, seeded and diced

2 honeycrisp apples, peeled, seeded, and diced

2 1/2 tsp melted trans-fat-free margarine

2 Tbsp Splenda Brown Sugar Blend

1/8 tsp ground nutmeg

1/4 tsp salt (optional)

6 lite spreadable cheese wedges (Laughing Cow Lite Swiss Cheese Wedges)

6 Tbsp slivered almonds

1 Preheat oven to 350°F.

2 Place six 5-ounce ramekins on a baking sheet and coat each with cooking spray.

3 In a mixing bowl, combine apples, melted margarine, brown sugar, nutmeg, and salt (optional). Combine well.

4 Fill each ramekin about half full of apples. Place one cheese wedge on top of apples and press to spread over the apples. Fill the ramekins with the remaining apples, mounding them over the rim of the ramekin.

5 Bake in oven for 30 minutes. Remove from oven and top each ramekin with 1 Tbsp of slivered almonds. Return to the oven to finish baking.

6 Bake for 15 more minutes or until apples are bubbling and almonds are toasted. Remove from oven and let cool to just warmer than room temperature and serve. Can also be eaten cold or heated up in the microwave the next day.

Chef's Tip

Serve this as a side dish or as an appetizer with whole-grain crackers.

Exchanges/Choices
1/2 Fruit   1/2 Carbohydrate
1 Lean Meat   1 Fat

Calories	145
Calories from Fat	55
Total Fat	6.0 g
Saturated Fat	1.5 g
Trans Fat	0.0 g
Cholesterol	5 mg
Sodium	225 mg
Potassium	160 mg
Total Carbohydrate	18 g
Dietary Fiber	2 g
Sugars	12 g
Protein	4 g
Phosphorus	170 mg

American Diabetes Association.
MyFood**Advisor**

This is an original recipe from the American Diabetes Association's online nutrition resource, **Recipes for Healthy Living**—your one-stop shop for diabetes-friendly recipes, meal plans, and other nutrition tips. Sign up today for the FREE *Recipes for Healthy Living* newsletter and to get access to the website by visiting **www.diabetes.org/recipes**.

Sweet Potato Pie

Makes: 10 servings　　　　*Serving Size: 1 slice*　　　　*Prep Time: 10 minutes*

2	cups mashed cooked sweet potatoes
1	cup evaporated fat-free milk
1/4	cup + 2 Tbsp Splenda Sugar Blend
1	tsp vanilla extract
1	tsp ground cinnamon
1/4	tsp salt
1/2	tsp ground nutmeg
1/2	cup egg substitute
1	Tbsp trans-fat-free margarine
1	tsp lemon juice
1	9-inch unbaked pie crust

1 Preheat oven to 350°F.

2 In a medium bowl, combine all ingredients except pie crust and beat with an electric mixer on low-medium speed until smooth.

3 Spoon sweet potato mixture into pie crust. Bake for 45 minutes or until set.

4 Cool completely on wire rack. Serve with light whipped topping if desired.

The American Diabetes Association recommends eating only a small amount of saturated fat every day. This recipe is higher in saturated fat, so try to balance it by eating foods low in saturated fat at your other meals today.

Exchanges/Choices
2 Carbohydrate　　1 Fat

Calories	180
Calories from Fat	45
Total Fat	5.0 g
Saturated Fat	1.6 g
Trans Fat	0.0 g
Cholesterol	0 mg
Sodium	220 mg
Potassium	270 mg
Total Carbohydrate	28 g
Dietary Fiber	2 g
Sugars	14 g
Protein	5 g
Phosphorus	80 mg

Chef's Tip

We recommend roasting the sweet potatoes in the oven at 400°F for 1 hour. Remove the sweet potatoes from the oven and peel off the skin. Roasting is a great way to bring out the sweetness in the potato.

DECEMBER

Healthy Holiday Eating

As you relax and enjoy your friends and family over the holidays, try some of this month's recipes, such as the Pork Loin with Dried Plums, Asian Sesame Cornish Hens, and Green Salad with Raspberry Vinaigrette. These holiday dinner musts work great when serving large groups. This month proves that you can entertain your guests with healthy meals, and they won't even know the difference!

Raspberry Almond Layer Cake (page 431)

Make your holiday festivities extra special with this month's beautiful and tasty dessert. Your guests will love these fresh raspberries layered with almond cake and sprinkled with powdered sugar.

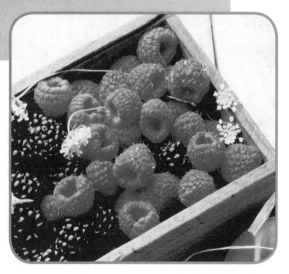

 gluten-free recipe, but always check ingredients for gluten.

 these recipes contain 15 grams of carbohydrate or less per serving.

 new recipe for the second edition.

DECEMBER RECIPES

DECEMBER

WEEK 1

DAY 1
Pepper Steak over
Rice   400

DAY 2
Spicy Chicken
Chili   401

DAY 3
Shrimp Marsala   402

DAY 4
Chicken
Drumsticks   403
Mashed Sweet
Potatoes   404

DAY 5
Roast with
Vegetables   405
Sage Apple
Stuffing   406

GROCERY LIST

Fresh Produce
Apple, Granny Smith—1
Bell peppers, green, large—2
Carrots—3
Celery—2 stalks
Garlic—2 cloves
Mushrooms, sliced—1 pint
Onions, yellow or white—3
Potatoes, sweet, large—7

Meat, Poultry, & Fish
Beef, bottom round roast—
3 pounds
Beef, top round steak,
boneless—1 pound
Chicken breasts, boneless,
skinless—1 pound
Chicken drumsticks—12
Shrimp, raw—1 pound

Grains, Bread, & Pasta
Bread crumbs, whole-
wheat—2 cups
Bread stuffing, whole-grain,
cubed—6 cups
Rice, brown—1 bag

Dairy & Cheese
Margarine, trans-fat-free

Canned Goods & Sauces
Beans, Great Northern,
16-ounce can—1
Beans, red kidney, 16-ounce
can—1

Broth, chicken, fat-free,
low-sodium, 14.5-ounce
cans—2
Chilies, green, chopped,
4-ounce can—1
Corn, 15-ounce can—1
Tomatoes, diced, no-salt-
added, 15-ounce cans—2

Staples, Seasonings, & Baking Needs
Black pepper, ground
Bouillon cubes, beef,
reduced-sodium—2
Cayenne pepper
Chili powder
Cinnamon
Cumin
Flour, all-purpose
Garlic powder
Mustard, Dijon
Nonstick cooking spray
Nutmeg, ground
Oil, olive
Sage
Salt
Vanilla extract
Vinegar, red wine

Miscellaneous
Wine, Marsala

Pepper Steak over Rice GF

Makes: 4 servings   *Serving Size: 3/4 cup beef and 1/2 cup rice*   *Prep Time: 10 minutes*

1   cup brown rice, uncooked
    nonstick cooking spray
1   pound boneless top round steak,
    cut into thin 1-inch slices
2   large green bell peppers, sliced
    into 1/2-inch-thick strips
1/4 tsp salt
1/4 tsp ground black pepper
1/4 cup water

1 Cook rice according to package directions, omitting salt.

2 Coat a large nonstick skillet with cooking spray over high heat. Add steak and sauté for about 4 minutes. Remove from pan and set aside.

3 Reduce heat to medium; add peppers to pan and sauté another 5 minutes. Add steak and any juices back to pan. Add salt, pepper, and water to pan. Sauté for 2 more minutes. Serve over rice.

World AIDS Day is December 1 every year. Are you aware of the scale of this terrible disease?

Exchanges/Choices
2 1/2 Starch   1 Vegetable
3 Lean Meat

Calories 345
  Calories from Fat 65
Total Fat . . . . .7.0 g
  Saturated Fat . . . . .2.3 g
  Trans Fat . . . . .0.1 g
Cholesterol. . . . . 75 mg
Sodium . . . . 185 mg
Potassium. . . . . 470 mg
Total Carbohydrate . . . . . . 40 g
  Dietary Fiber . . . . 4 g
  Sugars . . . . 3 g
Protein . . . . 29 g
Phosphorus . . . . 330 mg

Chef's Tip

Be sure not to overcook the meat in this recipe, or it will be too tough.

Spicy Chicken Chili

Makes: 7 servings   *Serving Size: 1 cup*   *Prep Time: 5 minutes*

nonstick cooking spray
1   pound boneless, skinless chicken breasts, cubed
1   Tbsp chili powder
1   tsp cumin
1/4 tsp cayenne pepper
1   16-ounce can Great Northern beans, rinsed and drained
1   16-ounce can red kidney beans, rinsed and drained

1   15-ounce can no-salt-added diced tomatoes
1   14.5-ounce can fat-free, low-sodium chicken broth
1/2 tsp salt (optional)
1/4 tsp ground black pepper
1   4-ounce can chopped green chilies
1   15-ounce can corn, drained (or 1 1/2 cups frozen corn, thawed)

1 Coat a large soup pot generously with cooking spray over high heat. Add chicken and sauté for 5 minutes.

2 Add remaining ingredients and bring to a boil. Reduce heat and simmer for 15 minutes.

Exchanges/Choices
1 1/2 Starch   1 Vegetable
2 Lean Meat

Calories	230
Calories from Fat	20
Total Fat	2.5 g
Saturated Fat	0.6 g
Trans Fat	0.0 g
Cholesterol	40 mg
Sodium	505 mg
Potassium	710 mg
Total Carbohydrate	30 g
Dietary Fiber	8 g
Sugars	4 g
Protein	23 g
Phosphorus	270 mg

Chef's Tip

This is a hearty winter dish that is easy to make.

Shrimp Marsala GF LC

Makes: 5 servings   *Serving Size: 1/5 recipe*   *Prep Time: 5 minutes*

2 tsp olive oil
1 pint sliced mushrooms
1 15-ounce can no-salt-added diced tomatoes, drained
1 cup Marsala wine
1 pound uncooked shrimp, peeled and deveined
1/2 tsp salt (optional)
1/4 tsp ground black pepper

1 Add oil to a large nonstick skillet over medium heat. Add mushrooms and sauté for 7–9 minutes. Add tomatoes and wine and simmer for 10 minutes.

2 Add shrimp, salt, and pepper. Sauté 4 more minutes or until shrimp are done.

Exchanges/Choices
1 Vegetable   2 Lean Meat

Calories 130
  Calories from Fat 25
Total Fat . . . . .3.0 g
  Saturated Fat . . . . .0.6 g
  Trans Fat . . . . .0.0 g
Cholesterol. . . . . 120 mg
Sodium . . . . 570 mg
Potassium. . . . . 300 mg
Total Carbohydrate . . . . 6 g
  Dietary Fiber . . . . 1 g
  Sugars . . . . 3 g
Protein . . . . 14 g
Phosphorus . . . . 210 mg

Chef's Tip

This dish is great over brown rice or linguine.

Chicken Drumsticks

Makes: 6 servings   *Serving Size: 2 drumsticks*   *Prep Time: 25 minutes*

1	small onion, chopped
2	garlic cloves, sliced
1/4	cup red wine vinegar
2	Tbsp Dijon mustard
1	Tbsp olive oil
1/2	tsp salt (optional)
1/4	tsp ground black pepper
12	chicken drumsticks, skin removed
2	cups whole-wheat bread crumbs

1 Preheat oven to 350°F.

2 In a blender or food processor, purée onion, garlic, vinegar, mustard, olive oil, salt, and pepper.

3 In a large bowl, add drumsticks and cover with marinade, turning to coat. Cover and refrigerate for 15 minutes.

4 Remove drumsticks from marinade and roll in bread crumbs, coating well.

5 Arrange drumsticks in the bottom of a shallow baking dish. Bake for 25–30 minutes or until done.

Exchanges/Choices
1 1/2 Starch   3 Lean Meat

Calories	285
Calories from Fat	70
Total Fat	8.0 g
Saturated Fat	1.7 g
Trans Fat	0.0 g
Cholesterol	80 mg
Sodium	235 mg
Potassium	310 mg
Total Carbohydrate	22 g
Dietary Fiber	4 g
Sugars	3 g
Protein	29 g
Phosphorus	215 mg

Dietitian's Tip

The dark meat in chicken drumsticks has more fat than white breast meat, but removing the skin helps, and they're delicious marinated.

Mashed Sweet Potatoes GF

Makes: 5 servings   *Serving Size: 1/5 recipe*   *Prep Time: 20 minutes*

3	large sweet potatoes
1 1/2	tsp vanilla extract
1/8	tsp ground cinnamon
1/8	tsp ground nutmeg
1	Tbsp trans-fat-free margarine

1 Wash and dry sweet potatoes and pierce on all sides with a fork. Microwave on high for about 15 minutes or until soft.

2 Cut potatoes in half lengthwise and scoop the meat out into a medium mixing bowl. Discard skins.

3 Mash the potato pulp with a potato masher or fork until smooth. Add remaining ingredients and mix well.

Exchanges/Choices
1 1/2 Starch

Calories	115
Calories from Fat	20
Total Fat	2.0 g
Saturated Fat	0.6 g
Trans Fat	0.0 g
Cholesterol	0 mg
Sodium	55 mg
Potassium	515 mg
Total Carbohydrate	23 g
Dietary Fiber	4 g
Sugars	7 g
Protein	2 g
Phosphorus	60 mg

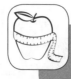

Dietitian's Tip

This is a much healthier version of a holiday favorite. Serve this dish any time of the year!

Roast with Vegetables

Makes: 8 servings   *Serving Size: 1/8 recipe*   *Prep Time: 15 minutes*

1   3-pound beef bottom round roast
     nonstick cooking spray
4   large sweet potatoes, cut in long
     wedges
1   medium onion, chopped
3   carrots, sliced
1   tsp ground black pepper
1   tsp garlic powder
1   cup water
2   reduced-sodium beef bouillon
     cubes

1 Preheat oven to 325°F. Place roast in a roasting pan coated with cooking spray.

2 Place potatoes, onion, and carrots around the roast in the pan. Sprinkle roast with pepper and garlic powder.

3 Add water and bouillon cubes to bottom of pan.

4 Bake for 1 1/2–2 hours, or until the meat is tender.

5 Slice and serve with vegetables and juice from pan.

Exchanges/Choices
1 Starch   1 Vegetable
5 Lean Meat

Calories 345
   Calories from Fat 80
Total Fat . . . . .9.0 g
   Saturated Fat . . . . .3.2 g
   Trans Fat . . . . .0.0 g
Cholesterol . . . . 105 mg
Sodium . . . . 230 mg
Potassium . . . . 880 mg
Total Carbohydrate . . . . . . 23 g
   Dietary Fiber . . . . 4 g
   Sugars . . . . 8 g
Protein . . . . 41 g
Phosphorus . . . . 310 mg

Chef's Tip

This roast makes great leftover sandwiches the next day.

Sage Apple Stuffing

Makes: 7 servings   *Serving Size: 1/2 cup*   *Prep Time: 10 minutes*

nonstick cooking spray
1   medium onion, diced
2   celery stalks, diced
1   Granny Smith apple, peeled and chopped coarsely
1   14.5-ounce can fat-free, low-sodium chicken broth
1/4   cup water
6   cups prepackaged whole-grain cubed bread stuffing
1   tsp dried sage
1/8   tsp salt (optional)
1/8   tsp ground black pepper

1 Preheat oven to 350°F.

2 Coat an 8-inch casserole dish with cooking spray.

3 Spray a large saucepan with cooking spray, and sauté onions and celery over medium-high heat until soft. Add chopped apple and sauté additional 3 minutes. Add broth and water and bring to a low boil.

4 In a medium bowl, toss stuffing, sage, salt, and pepper. Pour heated broth mixture over stuffing and let sit, covered, for 5 minutes.

5 Spread stuffing evenly in casserole dish and bake for 20–25 minutes or until golden brown on top.

Exchanges/Choices
2 Starch

Calories 145
  Calories from Fat 20
Total Fat . . . . .2.0 g
  Saturated Fat . . . . .0.4 g
  Trans Fat . . . . .0.0 g
Cholesterol. . . . . 0 mg
Sodium . . . . 575 mg
Potassium. . . . . 230 mg
Total Carbohydrate . . . . . . 30 g
  Dietary Fiber . . . . 5 g
  Sugars . . . . 6 g
Protein . . . . 5 g
Phosphorus . . . . 65 mg

Dietitian's Tip

You can buy prepackaged whole-wheat stuffing mix at the market.

DECEMBER
WEEK 2

DAY 1
20-Minute
   Chicken   408
Italian Veggies   409

DAY 2
Sweet and Sour Cabbage
   Skillet   410

DAY 3
Pork Tacos   411

DAY 4
Split Pea Soup   412

DAY 5
Roasted Red Pepper and
   Goat Cheese Stuffed
   Chicken   413
Mushroom Rice
   Pilaf   414

GROCERY LIST

Fresh Produce
Broccoli—1 head
Cabbage, green—1 head
Carrots, large—2
Celery—2 stalks
Garlic—1 head
Lemon—1
Lettuce—1 small head
Limes—2
Mushrooms—1 pint
Onions, yellow or white—2
Shallot—1
Tomatoes—2
Zucchini, small—2

Meat, Poultry, & Fish
Chicken breasts, boneless,
   skinless, 4 ounces each—8
Ham, chopped—1 cup
Pork tenderloins—2
   (1 1/4 pounds total)
Turkey, ground, 93% lean—
   1 1/4 pounds

Grains, Bread, & Pasta
Bread crumbs, whole-
   wheat—1/4 cup
Rice, brown—1 bag
Tortillas, whole-wheat,
   low-carb (10 grams of
   carb each)—12

Dairy & Cheese
Cheese, cheddar, 75%
   reduced-fat, shredded—
   1 1/2 cups
Cheese, goat, reduced-fat—
   3 1/2 Tbsp
Margarine, trans-fat-free

Canned Goods & Sauces
Broth, chicken, fat-free,
   low-sodium, 14.5-ounce
   cans—6
Red peppers, roasted
   (pimientos)—1 large jar

Staples, Seasonings, & Baking Needs
Basil
Bay leaf
Black pepper, ground
Chili powder
Cumin
Nonstick cooking spray
Oil, olive
Oregano
Paprika
Paprika, smoked
Sage
Salt
Splenda Brown Sugar Blend
Vinegar, white wine

Miscellaneous
Peas, split, green, 16-ounce
   package—1

20-Minute Chicken LC

Makes: 4 servings   *Serving Size: 1 chicken breast*   *Prep Time: 5 minutes*

1/4	cup whole-wheat bread crumbs
1	tsp dried basil
1/8	tsp ground black pepper
2	garlic cloves, minced
4	4-ounce boneless, skinless chicken breasts
	nonstick cooking spray
1	tsp trans-fat-free margarine
2	Tbsp lemon juice
1/2	cup fat-free, low-sodium chicken broth
1	Tbsp lemon zest

1 In a shallow dish, combine bread crumbs, basil, pepper, and garlic. Set aside.

2 Place each chicken breast between 2 sheets of plastic wrap; flatten to 1/4 inch thick using a meat tenderizer or rolling pin. Spray both sides of chicken with cooking spray. Dredge chicken in bread crumb mixture.

3 Coat a large nonstick skillet with cooking spray and melt margarine over medium-high heat. Add chicken and cook 4 minutes on each side or until done. Remove chicken from pan and set aside.

4 Add lemon juice, broth, and lemon zest to skillet and cook 1 minute. Spoon sauce over chicken breasts.

Exchanges/Choices
1/2 Starch   3 Lean Meat

Calories 160
  Calories from Fat 30
Total Fat . . . . .3.5 g
  Saturated Fat . . . . .1.0 g
  Trans Fat . . . . .0.0 g
Cholesterol. . . . . 65 mg
Sodium . . . . 135 mg
Potassium. . . . . 250 mg
Total Carbohydrate. . . . . . . 6 g
  Dietary Fiber . . . . 1 g
  Sugars . . . . 1 g
Protein . . . . 25 g
Phosphorus . . . . 195 mg

Chef's Tip

Pounding the chicken breasts flat makes them cook more quickly, so they're more tender. If your chicken is too dry, it's overcooked!

Italian Veggies GF LC

Makes: 8 servings   *Serving Size: 1/2 cup*   *Prep Time: 10 minutes*

nonstick cooking spray
1   Tbsp olive oil
3   garlic cloves, minced
2   cups carrots, sliced (about
    2 medium or 1 large carrot)
2   cups broccoli florets
    (1 medium head)
2   cups zucchini, thinly sliced
    (2 small zucchini)
1/2 tsp salt
1   Tbsp water

1 Add oil and a generous amount of cooking spray to a large nonstick skillet over medium-high heat. Add all ingredients except water and sauté for 5–6 minutes.

2 Turn heat to high, add water, and cover vegetables. Steam for 3–4 minutes or until tender-crisp.

Exchanges/Choices
1 Vegetable   1/2 Fat

Calories 40
  Calories from Fat 20
Total Fat . . . . .2.0 g
  Saturated Fat . . . . .0.3 g
  Trans Fat . . . . .0.0 g
Cholesterol. . . . . 0 mg
Sodium . . . . 175 mg
Potassium. . . . . 235 mg
Total Carbohydrate . . . . 5 g
  Dietary Fiber . . . . 2 g
  Sugars . . . . 2 g
Protein . . . . 1 g
Phosphorus . . . . 35 mg

Chef's Tip

Sautéing these veggies with garlic before steaming them adds great flavor.

Sweet and Sour Cabbage Skillet NEW

Makes: 4 servings   *Serving Size: 1 1/2 cups*   *Prep Time: 10 minutes*

1	tsp olive oil
	nonstick cooking spray
6	cups shredded green cabbage
1	medium onion, thinly sliced
1 1/4	pounds 93% lean ground turkey
1/4	cup white wine vinegar
2	Tbsp Splenda Brown Sugar Blend
1	tsp salt (optional)
1/2	tsp ground black pepper
1	cup fat-free, low-sodium chicken broth
1/2	tsp smoked paprika

1 Add olive oil and a generous amount of cooking spray to a large skillet over medium-high heat.

2 Add cabbage and onions and sauté until beginning to caramelize, about 10–12 minutes.

3 Add ground turkey to the cabbage mixture and sauté another 5–7 minutes or until turkey is just cooked through.

4 Add remaining ingredients and simmer for 5–7 minutes.

Exchanges/Choices

1/2 Carbohydrate	2 Vegetable
4 Lean Meat	1 Fat

Calories 310
  Calories from Fat 125
Total Fat . . . . 14.0 g
  Saturated Fat . . . . 3.4 g
  Trans Fat . . . . 0.2 g
Cholesterol . . . . 110 mg
Sodium . . . . 140 mg
Potassium . . . . 625 mg
Total Carbohydrate . . . . . 16 g
  Dietary Fiber . . . . 3 g
  Sugars . . . . 8 g
Protein . . . . 31 g
Phosphorus . . . . 320 mg

Chef's Tip

This recipe is a great substitution for sauerkraut and sausage, which is traditionally a high-fat and very-high-sodium dish. If you don't have smoked paprika, you can use regular paprika or omit that ingredient. The smoked paprika mimics the flavor you get from kielbasa and is a great substitute for the fatty sausage.

Pork Tacos LC NEW

Makes: 12 servings   *Serving Size: 1 taco*   *Prep Time: 45 minutes*
(includes marinating time)

2 limes, juiced
2 garlic cloves, minced
1 1/2 Tbsp chili powder
1 tsp cumin
1 tsp dried oregano
1/2 tsp salt
1/2 tsp ground black pepper
2 pork tenderloins (1 1/4 pounds total)
12 whole-wheat, low-carb tortillas (10 grams of carb per tortilla), warmed
2 tomatoes, diced
1 1/2 cups shredded lettuce
1 1/2 cups shredded 75% reduced-fat cheddar cheese

1 In a large bowl, combine lime juice, garlic, chili powder, cumin, oregano, salt, and pepper. Add pork and coat well. Marinate in refrigerator for 30 minutes or up to 4 hours.

2 Preheat oven to 375°F. Place tenderloins in a shallow baking dish and bake for 30 minutes or until pork is done.

3 Remove pork from oven and let rest for 10 minutes. Cut pork into 1-inch chunks.

4 Serve pork in warm tortillas topped with tomatoes, 2 Tbsp lettuce, and 2 Tbsp cheese.

Exchanges/Choices
1/2 Starch   2 Lean Meat

Calories	140
Calories from Fat	40
Total Fat	4.5 g
Saturated Fat	1.2 g
Trans Fat	0.0 g
Cholesterol	30 mg
Sodium	435 mg
Potassium	280 mg
Total Carbohydrate	13 g
Dietary Fiber	8 g
Sugars	1 g
Protein	19 g
Phosphorus	200 mg

Chef's Tip

You can also top these tacos with avocado and fresh salsa.

American Diabetes Association.
My Food**Advisor**

This is an original recipe from the American Diabetes Association's online nutrition resource, **Recipes for Healthy Living**—your one-stop shop for diabetes-friendly recipes, meal plans, and other nutrition tips. Sign up today for the FREE *Recipes for Healthy Living* newsletter and to get access to the website by visiting **www.diabetes.org/recipes**.

Split Pea Soup

Makes: 8 servings   *Serving Size: 1/8 recipe*   *Prep Time: 15 minutes*

1   Tbsp olive oil
1   large carrot, finely diced
2   celery stalks, finely diced
1   shallot, minced
1   garlic clove, minced
1   tsp salt (optional)
1/4   tsp ground black pepper
1   16-ounce package green split peas
3   14.5-ounce cans fat-free, low-sodium chicken broth
1   cup chopped ham

1 Add oil to a large soup pot over medium-high heat. Sauté carrots, celery, and shallots for 3–4 minutes or until shallots begin to turn clear. Add garlic and sauté 1 more minute.

2 Add remaining ingredients except ham and bring to a boil. Simmer uncovered for 25–30 minutes.

3 Purée soup in a blender or with an immersion blender until smooth. Stir in ham and bring back to a simmer over medium heat for 2–3 minutes.

Exchanges/Choices
2 Starch   2 Lean Meat

Calories 220
   Calories from Fat 20
Total Fat . . . . .2.5 g
   Saturated Fat . . . . .0.4 g
   Trans Fat . . . . .0.0 g
Cholesterol. . . . . 10 mg
Sodium . . . . 545 mg
Potassium. . . . . 750 mg
Total Carbohydrate . . . . . . 33 g
   Dietary Fiber . . . . 12 g
   Sugars . . . . 6 g
Protein . . . . 17 g
Phosphorus . . . . 205 mg

Chef's Tip

This soup freezes well and tastes great when reheated.

Roasted Red Pepper and Goat Cheese Stuffed Chicken GF LC

Makes: 4 servings   *Serving Size: 1 chicken breast*   *Prep Time: 15 minutes*

4 4-ounce boneless, skinless chicken breasts
1 cup jarred roasted red peppers, finely chopped
3 1/2 Tbsp reduced-fat goat cheese
2 garlic cloves, minced
1/2 tsp salt (optional)
1/2 tsp ground black pepper
1 tsp paprika
nonstick cooking spray

1 Preheat oven to 350°F.

2 Place each chicken breast between 2 sheets of plastic wrap; flatten to 1/4 inch thick using a meat tenderizer or rolling pin. Set aside.

3 In a medium bowl, combine red peppers, goat cheese, and garlic. Spread 3 Tbsp of this mixture on one side of the pounded chicken breast. Roll breast and secure the seam with a toothpick. Repeat procedure for remaining 3 chicken breasts.

4 Sprinkle all sides of rolled chicken breasts with salt, pepper, and paprika.

5 Coat a medium glass or metal baking dish with cooking spray and place chicken in dish seam side down. Spray chicken breasts generously with cooking spray. Bake for 30 minutes or until chicken is done.

6 To serve, remove toothpicks and slice each piece into 5 rounds. Serve over Mushroom Rice Pilaf (page 414).

Exchanges/Choices
1 Vegetable   3 Lean Meat

Calories	165
Calories from Fat	35
Total Fat	4.0 g
Saturated Fat	1.5 g
Trans Fat	0.0 g
Cholesterol	70 mg
Sodium	220 mg
Potassium	320 mg
Total Carbohydrate	5 g
Dietary Fiber	1 g
Sugars	2 g
Protein	26 g
Phosphorus	210 mg

Chef's Tip

Impress your foodie friends with this easy and healthy meal!

Mushroom Rice Pilaf

Makes: 5 servings   *Serving Size: 2/3 cup*   *Prep Time: 10 minutes*

1 tsp olive oil	**1** Add oil to a medium saucepan over medium-high heat. Sauté mushrooms and onion for 6–7 minutes or until liquid is evaporated.
1 pint mushrooms, finely chopped	
1 medium onion, finely diced	
1 cup uncooked brown rice	**2** Add rice and stir constantly over heat for 2 minutes. Pour broth, sage, and bay leaf over mixture and stir. Bring to a boil.
3 cups fat-free, low-sodium chicken broth	
1/4 tsp dried sage	
1 bay leaf	**3** Reduce heat and simmer, covered, for 40 minutes (or according to package directions).
1/2 tsp salt (optional)	
1/4 tsp ground black pepper	**4** Remove bay leaf. Season with salt and pepper and fluff rice with a fork.

Exchanges/Choices
2 Starch   1 Vegetable

Calories 170
  Calories from Fat 20
Total Fat . . . . 2.0 g
  Saturated Fat . . . . 0.4 g
  Trans Fat . . . . 0.0 g
Cholesterol . . . . 0 mg
Sodium . . . . 310 mg
Potassium . . . . 315 mg
Total Carbohydrate . . . . . . 33 g
  Dietary Fiber . . . . 2 g
  Sugars . . . . 2 g
Protein . . . . 6 g
Phosphorus . . . . 175 mg

Chef's Tip

It's important to brown the rice after cooking the mushrooms and before adding the liquid. This imparts great toasted flavor to the rice and elevates this dish from the ordinary to the extraordinary.

DECEMBER

WEEK 3

DAY 1

Noodle-less Spinach and Eggplant Lasagna   416

DAY 2

Salmon with Citrus Sauce   417

Artichoke Salad   418

DAY 3

Asian Sesame Cornish Game Hens   419

DAY 4

Pork Loin with Dried Plums   420

Garlic Olive Oil Potatoes   421

DAY 5

Italian Soup   422

GROCERY LIST

Fresh Produce

Eggplant, large—1
Garlic—1 head
Lemons—2
Onions, yellow or white—2
Potatoes, red, new—1 pound
Spinach, baby—6 ounces
Tomato, medium—1

Meat, Poultry, & Fish

Cornish game hens,
   1 1/4 pounds each—4
Pork tenderloin—1 pound
Salmon fillets, 4 ounces
   each—4
Turkey sausage links,
   Italian—3

Dairy & Cheese

Cheese, mozzarella, reduced-
   fat, shredded—1 cup
Cheese, Parmesan—1 block
Cheese, ricotta, fat-free—
   15 ounces
Eggs
Yogurt, Greek, plain,
   fat-free—1 cup

Canned Goods & Sauces

Artichoke hearts, 14-ounce
   cans—2
Beans, Great Norther,
   16-ounce can—1
Broth, chicken, fat-free,
   low-sodium, 14.5-ounce
   cans—3
Hot pepper sauce
Jam, raspberry, seedless,
   sugar-free—1 jar
Olives, black, 2-ounce can—1

Pasta sauce, tomato basil,
   reduced-sodium,
   24-ounce jar—1
Preserves, apricot, sugar-
   free—1 jar
Soy sauce, lite
Tomatoes, crushed, 32-ounce
   can—1

Frozen Foods

Spinach, 9-ounce package—1

**Staples, Seasonings,
& Baking Needs**

Basil
Black pepper, ground
Flour, all-purpose
Honey
Nonstick cooking spray
Oil, olive
Oil, sesame
Oregano
Parsley
Red pepper flakes
Salt
Sesame seeds
Vinegar, balsamic
Vinegar, red wine
Vinegar, rice wine

Miscellaneous

Orange juice—1 cup
Prunes (dried plums),
   pitted—8

Noodle-less Spinach and Eggplant Lasagna NEW

Makes: 10 servings   *Serving Size: 1 slice*   *Prep Time: 20 minutes*

nonstick cooking spray

1   large eggplant, peeled and sliced lengthwise into 10 thin strips

9   ounces frozen chopped spinach, thawed and drained well

15   ounces fat-free ricotta cheese

1   cup fat-free plain Greek yogurt

1   Tbsp minced garlic

1   Tbsp dried parsley

1   egg

1/4   cup freshly grated Parmesan cheese

1/2   tsp ground black pepper

1   24-ounce jar reduced-sodium tomato basil pasta sauce

1   cup shredded reduced-fat mozzarella cheese

1   Preheat oven to 350°F. Coat two baking sheets with cooking spray. Lay eggplant slices, without overlapping, on the baking sheets and spray with cooking spray. Bake for 10 minutes or until eggplant begins to soften. Remove from oven and set aside to cool.

2   In a medium bowl, combine spinach, ricotta, yogurt, garlic, parsley, egg, Parmesan cheese, and black pepper. Stir to combine.

3   Coat a 9 × 13-inch baking dish with cooking spray. Pour 1 1/2 cups of pasta sauce into the pan and spread to coat. Layer 5 pieces of eggplant in the bottom of the pan and top with the entire ricotta and spinach mixture. Gently spread the ricotta and spinach mixture evenly over the first layer of eggplant.

4   Layer 5 more pieces of eggplant on top of the ricotta and spinach mixture and top with remaining pasta sauce. Spread evenly. Top with 1 cup shredded mozzarella and bake for 25 minutes or until cheese is melted and beginning to brown.

Chef's Tip

Make this the day before and slice it cold. Then, portion it into individual servings and put into airtight containers and freeze. No more need to purchase frozen meals at the grocery store! You just made your own!

Exchanges/Choices

1/2 Starch   1 Vegetable
2 Lean Meat

Calories	165
Calories from Fat	55
Total Fat	6.0 g
Saturated Fat	2.0 g
Trans Fat	0.0 g
Cholesterol	40 mg
Sodium	345 mg
Potassium	505 mg
Total Carbohydrate	16 g
Dietary Fiber	4 g
Sugars	8 g
Protein	14 g
Phosphorus	235 mg

Salmon with Citrus Sauce LC

Makes: 4 servings   *Serving Size: 1 salmon fillet*   *Prep Time: 10 minutes*

nonstick cooking spray
4   4-ounce salmon fillets
1/4   tsp ground black pepper
1   cup orange juice
1/4   cup lemon juice
3   Tbsp lite soy sauce
1   Tbsp rice wine vinegar
2   tsp sesame oil
1/4   tsp crushed red pepper flakes

1 Preheat oven to 350°F. Coat a shallow baking dish with cooking spray.

2 Season both sides of salmon fillets with pepper and arrange in bottom of the baking dish. Bake for 18–20 minutes or until done.

3 While salmon is baking, add remaining ingredients to a medium saucepan over high heat. Bring to a boil, stirring constantly. Reduce heat and simmer for 15 minutes.

4 Remove salmon from pan and serve with sauce.

Exchanges/Choices
1/2 Fruit   4 Lean Meat
1 Fat

Calories 260
  Calories from Fat 115
Total Fat . . . . 13.0 g
  Saturated Fat . . . . 2.1 g
  Trans Fat . . . . 0.0 g
Cholesterol . . . . 80 mg
Sodium . . . . 475 mg
Potassium . . . . 510 mg
Total Carbohydrate . . . . . . 9 g
  Dietary Fiber . . . . 0 g
  Sugars . . . . 6 g
Protein . . . . 27 g
Phosphorus . . . . 280 mg

Chef's Tip

This is an easy way to cook salmon steaks.

Artichoke Salad GF LC

Makes: 8 servings   *Serving Size: 1/2 cup*   *Prep Time: 10 minutes*

Dressing

1/2	tsp dried oregano
1/4	cup red wine vinegar
2	Tbsp olive oil
1/8	tsp salt
1/8	tsp ground black pepper

Salad

2	14-ounce cans artichoke hearts, drained and quartered
1	2-ounce can sliced black olives, drained
1	medium tomato, seeded and finely diced
1	small onion, thinly sliced

1 In a small bowl, whisk together all dressing ingredients; set aside.

2 In a large bowl, combine all salad ingredients. Pour dressing over salad and toss to coat.

Exchanges/Choices

2 Vegetable	1/2 Fat

Calories	80
Calories from Fat	35
Total Fat	4.0 g
Saturated Fat	0.6 g
Trans Fat	0.0 g
Cholesterol	0 mg
Sodium	240 mg
Potassium	215 mg
Total Carbohydrate	9 g
Dietary Fiber	4 g
Sugars	1 g
Protein	3 g
Phosphorus	50 mg

Dietitian's Tip

This is another great luncheon salad—it's so easy and elegant!

Asian Sesame Cornish Game Hens LC

Makes: 8 servings   *Serving Size: 1/2 Cornish hen*   *Prep Time: 5 minutes*

nonstick cooking spray
1/4   cup sugar-free apricot preserves
1   tsp lite soy sauce
1   tsp rice wine vinegar
1   tsp sesame oil
1/4   tsp hot pepper sauce
2   Tbsp sesame seeds
4   Cornish game hens (about 1 1/4 pounds each)

1 Preheat oven to 350°F. Coat a large glass or metal baking dish with cooking spray.

2 In a small saucepan, combine preserves, soy sauce, vinegar, sesame oil, and hot pepper sauce over medium heat. Bring to a simmer, stirring occasionally. Simmer about 10 minutes or until the sauce becomes glaze-like.

3 Wash and pat dry Cornish game hens. Arrange hens breast side up in the baking dish. Brush each hen generously with glaze. Sprinkle with sesame seeds and bake for 30–35 minutes or until done. Remove the skins before eating.

Exchanges/Choices
4 Lean Meat

Calories 180
Calories from Fat 55
Total Fat . . . . 6.0 g
Saturated Fat . . . . 1.4 g
Trans Fat . . . . 0.0 g
Cholesterol . . . . 130 mg
Sodium . . . . 90 mg
Potassium . . . . 320 mg
Total Carbohydrate . . . . 2 g
Dietary Fiber . . . . 0 g
Sugars . . . . 0 g
Protein . . . . 29 g
Phosphorus . . . . 195 mg

Dietitian's Tip

Be sure to remove the skins of these moist hens before eating them, to reduce saturated fat and calories!

Pork Loin with Dried Plums `GF`

Makes: 4 servings   Serving Size: 1/4 recipe   Prep Time: 15 minutes

Pork

1	pound pork tenderloin
8	pitted prunes (dried plums)
1/2	tsp salt (optional)
1/4	tsp ground black pepper
	nonstick cooking spray

Glaze

1	cup balsamic vinegar
1/4	cup sugar-free seedless raspberry jam
1	Tbsp honey

1 Preheat oven to 375°F.

2 Using a small sharp knife, make 6–8 slits in the side of the tenderloin to form several small pockets in a row. Do not cut all the way through. Stuff 1–2 prunes into each pocket. Season the tenderloin well with salt and pepper.

3 Coat a large sauté pan with cooking spray and heat over high heat. Add whole pork tenderloin and sear on each side for 3 minutes. Remove from pan and set aside.

4 Add vinegar, jam, and honey to pan over high heat. Bring to a boil for 5 minutes. Purée mixture in blender and set aside.

5 Spread 2 Tbsp glaze on all sides of the tenderloin and transfer to a baking sheet. Bake for 25–30 minutes or until done.

6 Reheat the remaining glaze, if necessary, and pour over cooked tenderloin. Slice thinly and serve.

Exchanges/Choices

1/2 Fruit   1 1/2 Carbohydrate
3 Lean Meat

Calories	235
Calories from Fat	25
Total Fat	3.0 g
Saturated Fat	1.0 g
Trans Fat	0.0 g
Cholesterol	60 mg
Sodium	55 mg
Potassium	555 mg
Total Carbohydrate	30 g
Dietary Fiber	1 g
Sugars	20 g
Protein	22 g
Phosphorus	220 mg

Dietitian's Tip

Prunes (dried plums) are a good source of fiber and potassium.

Garlic Olive Oil Potatoes GF

Makes: 4 servings   *Serving Size: 1/2 cup*   *Prep Time: 10 minutes*

1   pound red new potatoes, quartered
1 1/2   tsp olive oil
1/2   tsp salt (optional)
1/2   tsp ground black pepper
2   garlic cloves, minced

1 Preheat oven to 400°F.

2 In a large bowl, toss all ingredients together and spread evenly on a baking sheet. Bake 30 minutes or until golden brown.

Exchanges/Choices
1 Starch   1/2 Fat

Calories 100
   Calories from Fat 20
Total Fat . . . . .2.0 g
   Saturated Fat . . . . .0.3 g
   Trans Fat . . . . .0.0 g
Cholesterol. . . . . 0 mg
Sodium . . . . 5 mg
Potassium. . . . . 445 mg
Total Carbohydrate. . . . . . 19 g
   Dietary Fiber . . . . 2 g
   Sugars . . . . 1 g
Protein . . . . 2 g
Phosphorus . . . . 60 mg

Chef's Tip

Another classic recipe with wonderful flavor—this can be a side dish for any meat or poultry entrée.

Italian Soup NEW LC

Makes: 10 servings   *Serving Size: 1 cup*   *Prep Time: 15 minutes*

nonstick cooking spray
1 medium onion, finely diced
3 Italian turkey sausage links
32 ounces fat-free, low-sodium chicken broth
1 1/2 cups water
1 1/2 cups canned, crushed tomatoes
1 16-ounce cans Great Northern beans, rinsed and drained
1/2 Tbsp dried basil
1/4 tsp dried oregano
1/4 tsp ground black pepper
6 ounces fresh baby spinach

1 Spray a large soup pot with cooking spray. Add onion and sauté over medium-high heat for 3 minutes or until clear.

2 Squeeze sausage meat from casing and discard casing. Add sausage to pot and break up into pieces with a spoon. Cook until brown, about 7–8 minutes.

3 Add remaining ingredients except baby spinach. Reduce heat and simmer for 15 minutes.

4 Add baby spinach and cook for an additional 1–2 minutes.

Exchanges/Choices
1/2 Starch   1 Vegetable
1 Lean Meat

Calories 110
   Calories from Fat 30
Total Fat . . . . .3.5 g
   Saturated Fat . . . . .0.8 g
   Trans Fat . . . . .0.1 g
Cholesterol. . . . . 20 mg
Sodium . . . . 505 mg
Potassium. . . . . 460 mg
Total Carbohydrate . . . . . . 11 g
   Dietary Fiber . . . . 3 g
   Sugars . . . . 3 g
Protein . . . . 10 g
Phosphorus . . . . 125 mg

Dietitian's Tip

This one-pot meal provides healthy carbs from the beans, protein from the turkey sausage, and veggies from the spinach and tomatoes. Healthy eating and cooking can be easy and delicious!

American Diabetes Association.
MyFoodAdvisor

This is an original recipe from the American Diabetes Association's online nutrition resource, **Recipes for Healthy Living**—your one-stop shop for diabetes-friendly recipes, meal plans, and other nutrition tips. Sign up today for the FREE *Recipes for Healthy Living* newsletter and to get access to the website by visiting **www.diabetes.org/recipes**.

DECEMBER
WEEK 4

GROCERY LIST

Fresh Produce
Asparagus—1 pound
Basil—1 bunch
Cilantro—1 bunch
Garlic—2 large cloves
Limes—3
Onion, red, large—1
Onion, yellow or white,
    small—1
Pepper, jalapeño—1
Raspberries—1 1/2 pints
Salad greens, mixed, baby
    field—4 cups

Meat, Poultry, & Fish
Halibut fillets—4 (about
    1 1/2 pounds total)
Pork chops, center-cut, boneless,
    4 ounces each—4
Turkey, ground, 93% lean—
    3/4 pound

Grains, Bread, & Pasta
Bread crumbs, whole-
    wheat—1/2 cup
Pasta, penne, whole-wheat—
    8 ounces
Tortillas, corn, 6-inch—10
Tortillas, whole-wheat, low-carb
    (10 grams carb and
    7 grams fiber)—16

Dairy & Cheese
Cheese, cheddar, 75% reduced-
    fat, shredded—1 1/2 cups
Cheese, Mexican-style, reduced-
    fat, shredded—1/3 cup
Eggs
Egg substitute—1/2 cup
Yogurt, Greek, plain, fat-
    free—1/2 cup

Canned Goods & Sauces
Applesauce, unsweetened—
    1 small jar
Beans, black, 15.5-ounce can—1
Beans, refried, fat-free,
    16-ounce can—1
Broth, chicken, fat-free, low-
    sodium, 14.5-ounce can—1
Hot pepper sauce
Preserves, raspberry, seedless,
    sugar-free, 10-ounce jar—1
Tomato paste, no-salt-added,
    4-ounce can—1
Tomato sauce, no-salt-added,
    8-ounce cans—2

Staples, Seasonings,
& Baking Needs
Almond extract
Black pepper, ground
Cake mix, yellow, 18.25-ounce
    package (3 grams fat per
    serving)—1
Cayenne pepper
Chili powder
Cumin
Flour, all-purpose
Honey
Nonstick cooking spray
Oil, canola
Oil, olive
Oregano
Red pepper flakes
Salt
Sugar, powdered
Vinegar, red wine
Vinegar, white wine

Miscellaneous
Pine nuts—1 Tbsp
Salsa
Tomatoes, sun-dried, not
    packed in oil—1 small
    package

Enchiladas

Makes: 5 servings   *Serving Size: 2 enchiladas*   *Prep Time: 15 minutes*

nonstick cooking spray
3/4   pound 93% lean ground turkey
1   16-ounce can fat-free refried beans
1/3   cup shredded, reduced-fat Mexican-style cheese, divided
1/4   tsp crushed red pepper flakes
1/2   tsp salt (optional)
1/4   tsp ground black pepper
10   6-inch corn tortillas, steamed
2   8-ounce cans no-salt-added tomato sauce
2   tsp chili powder
1   tsp cumin
1/4   tsp cayenne pepper

1 Preheat oven to 375°F. Coat a large glass or metal baking dish with cooking spray.

2 In a large nonstick skillet, cook turkey for 7–9 minutes or until beginning to brown; drain excess fat. Stir in beans, half the cheese, and the red pepper flakes, salt, and pepper. Reduce heat and cook for 3 minutes.

3 Fill one tortilla with about 1/4 cup of meat and bean mixture and roll tortilla. Repeat for remaining tortillas.

4 Line baking dish with enchiladas, seam side down.

5 In a small bowl, combine remaining ingredients except the cheese. Pour tomato sauce over enchiladas and sprinkle with remaining cheese. Bake for 20–25 minutes or until cheese is bubbly.

Exchanges/Choices

2 Starch   1 Vegetable
2 Lean Meat   1 Fat

Calories 335
  Calories from Fat 90
Total Fat . . . . .10.0 g
  Saturated Fat . . . . .2.6 g
  Trans Fat . . . . .0.1 g
Cholesterol. . . . . 55 mg
Sodium . . . . 555 mg
Potassium. . . . . 890 mg
Total Carbohydrate . . . . . . 42 g
  Dietary Fiber . . . . 11 g
  Sugars . . . . 5 g
Protein . . . . 24 g
Phosphorus . . . . 445 mg

Chef's Tip

To steam tortillas, layer them between sheets of damp paper towels and microwave on high for 1 minute.

Breaded Pork Cutlets

Makes: 4 servings   *Serving Size: 1 cutlet*   *Prep Time: 15 minutes*

1/3 cup all-purpose flour
1/2 cup egg substitute
1/2 tsp salt (optional)
1/4 tsp ground black pepper
1/2 cup whole-wheat bread crumbs
4   4-ounce boneless, center-cut
     pork chops
     nonstick cooking spray

1 Preheat oven to 350°F.

2 Place flour in a shallow dish. Place egg substitute in a shallow dish. Add salt and pepper to bread crumbs and place in a shallow dish.

3 Place 1 pork chop between two sheets of plastic wrap. Using a meat tenderizer or rolling pin, pound chops to 1/4-inch thickness. Repeat for remaining 3 chops.

4 Dredge each chop in flour, coating all sides, then dip into egg substitute and roll in bread crumb mixture, coating well.

5 Coat a baking dish with cooking spray and line the bottom of the pan with chops. Spray each chop with more cooking spray. Bake for 20–25 minutes.

Exchanges/Choices
1 Starch   4 Lean Meat

Calories 250
  Calories from Fat 65
Total Fat . . . . .7.0 g
  Saturated Fat . . . . .2.6 g
  Trans Fat . . . . .0.0 g
Cholesterol. . . . . 60 mg
Sodium . . . . 115 mg
Potassium. . . . . 375 mg
Total Carbohydrate . . . . . . 17 g
  Dietary Fiber . . . . 2 g
  Sugars . . . . 1 g
Protein . . . . 27 g
Phosphorus . . . . 210 mg

Chef's Tip

Add herbs to the bread crumbs for an extra kick. Try 1 tsp each of dried oregano, thyme, and basil.

Red Onion Marmalade GF LC

Makes: 4 servings   *Serving Size: 1/4 recipe*   *Prep Time: 10 minutes*

1	Tbsp olive oil
1	large red onion, thinly sliced (about 1 1/2 cups)
1/3	cup red wine vinegar
1 1/2	Tbsp honey
1/4	tsp salt
	dash ground black pepper

1 Add oil to a medium saucepan over high heat. Add onion and sauté for 7–10 minutes or until beginning to caramelize.

2 Add remaining ingredients and bring to a boil. Reduce heat and simmer for 15–20 minutes or until thickened.

Exchanges/Choices
1/2 Carbohydrate   1 Vegetable
1/2 Fat

Calories	80
Calories from Fat	30
Total Fat	3.5 g
Saturated Fat	0.5 g
Trans Fat	0.0 g
Cholesterol	0 mg
Sodium	150 mg
Potassium	95 mg
Total Carbohydrate	12 g
Dietary Fiber	1 g
Sugars	9 g
Protein	1 g
Phosphorus	15 mg

Chef's Tip
Be sure to cook this tasty meat accompaniment until the onions are nice and soft.

Halibut Fish Tacos LC NEW

Makes: 8 servings *Serving Size: 1 taco* *Prep Time: 20 minutes*

3 limes, juiced
1/2 tsp crushed red pepper flakes
1 Tbsp cilantro, chopped
4 halibut fillets (about 1 1/2 pounds)
1/4 tsp salt (optional)
1/4 tsp ground black pepper
   nonstick cooking spray
1 jalapeño pepper, minced
8 small whole-wheat, low-carb tortillas (10 grams carb and more than 7 grams fiber), warmed

Sauce
1/2 cup fat-free plain Greek yogurt
1 tsp hot pepper sauce

1 In a medium bowl, combine lime juice, red pepper flakes, and cilantro. Add fish to marinade and marinate in the refrigerator for 15 minutes.

2 Remove fish from marinade and season with salt (optional) and pepper.

3 Coat a large sauté pan with cooking spray. Sauté jalapeño pepper over medium heat for 2 minutes; then add halibut and sauté for an additional 2–3 minutes on each side.

4 Remove fish and peppers from pan and shred fish into large pieces, mixing the pepper while shredding.

5 In a small bowl, combine sauce ingredients.

6 Evenly divide fish among 8 tortillas. Top each taco with a dollop of yogurt sauce.

Exchanges/Choices
1/2 Starch   3 Lean Meat

Calories	155
Calories from Fat	35
Total Fat	4.0 g
Saturated Fat	0.3 g
Trans Fat	0.0 g
Cholesterol	25 mg
Sodium	270 mg
Potassium	470 mg
Total Carbohydrate	12 g
Dietary Fiber	7 g
Sugars	1 g
Protein	24 g
Phosphorus	255 mg

Chef's Tip

If jalapeño peppers are too spicy for you, substitute with a green bell pepper.

Green Salad with Raspberry Vinaigrette GF LC

Makes: 5 servings   *Serving Size: 1 cup*   *Prep Time: 5 minutes*

Dressing

1/4	cup white wine vinegar
1/2	cup fresh raspberries, puréed
1 1/2	Tbsp olive oil
1/4	tsp salt
	pinch ground black pepper

Salad

4	cups mixed baby field greens
1	cup fresh raspberries
1	Tbsp pine nuts

1 In a small bowl, whisk dressing ingredients.

2 In a medium salad bowl, toss together salad ingredients. Drizzle dressing over salad and toss gently to coat.

Exchanges/Choices
1/2 Carbohydrate   1 Fat

Calories	75
Calories from Fat	55
Total Fat	6.0 g
Saturated Fat	0.7 g
Trans Fat	0.0 g
Cholesterol	0 mg
Sodium	125 mg
Potassium	145 mg
Total Carbohydrate	6 g
Dietary Fiber	3 g
Sugars	2 g
Protein	1 g
Phosphorus	30 mg

Chef's Tip

Serve this beautiful, tasty salad to your holiday party guests.

Pasta with Asparagus and Sun-Dried Tomatoes

Makes: 4 servings   *Serving Size: 1/4 recipe*   *Prep Time: 5 minutes*

8	ounces whole-wheat penne pasta, uncooked
1	Tbsp olive oil, divided
1	pound asparagus, trimmed, cut into 1/2-inch pieces
1/2	cup chopped sun-dried tomatoes
1/2	cup chopped fresh basil
2	large garlic cloves, minced
1/2	tsp dried oregano
1/4	tsp crushed red pepper flakes
1	14.5-ounce can fat-free, low-sodium chicken broth
2	Tbsp tomato paste

1 Cook pasta according to package directions, omitting salt; drain.

2 Heat 2 tsp oil in a large nonstick skillet over medium-high heat. Add asparagus and sauté about 5 minutes. Remove asparagus from pan and set aside.

3 Add 1 tsp oil to skillet over medium-high heat. Add sun-dried tomatoes, basil, garlic, oregano, and red pepper flakes, and sauté about 3 minutes.

4 Add broth and tomato paste to skillet and bring to a low boil. Stir occasionally and cook for 5–7 minutes or until sauce thickens.

5 Add sauce and cooked asparagus to cooked pasta and toss to coat.

Exchanges/Choices
2 1/2 Starch   2 Vegetable
1 Fat

Calories	290
Calories from Fat	45
Total Fat	5.0 g
Saturated Fat	0.7 g
Trans Fat	0.0 g
Cholesterol	0 mg
Sodium	465 mg
Potassium	675 mg
Total Carbohydrate	54 g
Dietary Fiber	9 g
Sugars	7 g
Protein	11 g
Phosphorus	230 mg

Chef's Tip
If you want, sprinkle some Parmesan cheese on this pasta before serving.

Black Bean Quesadillas [NEW]

Makes: 8 servings   *Serving Size: 1 quesadilla*   *Prep Time: 5 minutes*

nonstick cooking spray
1/4   small onion, finely diced
1   15.5-ounce can black beans, rinsed and drained
1/4   tsp cumin
1/2   cup salsa
8   whole-wheat, low-carb tortillas (10 grams carb and 7 grams fiber),
1 1/2   cups shredded 75% reduced-fat cheddar cheese

1 Spray a large nonstick skillet with cooking spray. Add onions and sauté until clear. Add beans, cumin, and salsa; cook about 3 more minutes. Remove from pan.

2 Spray skillet with cooking spray and add 1 tortilla to pan.

3 Top tortilla with 3 Tbsp cheese and about 3 Tbsp bean mixture. Fold tortilla in half. Cook tortilla until golden; about 2 minutes each side.

4 Repeat procedure for remaining 7 quesadillas.

Exchanges/Choices
1 Starch   1 Med-Fat Meat

Calories 140
  Calories from Fat 35
Total Fat . . . . 4.0 g
  Saturated Fat . . . . 1.2 g
  Trans Fat . . . . 0.0 g
Cholesterol . . . . 5 mg
Sodium . . . . 495 mg
Potassium . . . . 210 mg
Total Carbohydrate . . . . . 19 g
  Dietary Fiber . . . . 10 g
  Sugars . . . . 1 g
Protein . . . . 15 g
Phosphorus . . . . 190 mg

Chef's Tip

You can top the tortilla with additional salsa or guacamole.

Raspberry Almond Layer Cake

Makes: 14 servings *Serving Size: 1 slice* *Prep Time: 15 minutes*

Cake

nonstick cooking spray
1 18.25-ounce package yellow cake mix (3 grams of fat per serving)
1 1/4 cups water
1 egg
3 egg whites
1/4 cup canola oil
3 Tbsp unsweetened applesauce
1 tsp almond extract

Filling

1 10-ounce jar sugar-free seedless raspberry preserves

Topping

1/4 cup powdered sugar
1 cup fresh raspberries

Exchanges/Choices

2 1/2 Carbohydrate 1 Fat

Calories	225
Calories from Fat	70
Total Fat	8.0 g
Saturated Fat	1.7 g
Trans Fat	0.0 g
Cholesterol	10 mg
Sodium	250 mg
Potassium	80 mg
Total Carbohydrate	41 g
Dietary Fiber	1 g
Sugars	22 g
Protein	3 g
Phosphorus	125 mg

---

1 Preheat oven to 350°F. Coat two 8-inch cake pans with cooking spray.

2 In a large bowl, mix together cake ingredients and beat with an electric mixer on low speed for 30 seconds. Increase speed to medium and beat for 2 minutes.

3 Divide batter evenly between cake pans and bake for 30–35 minutes or until a toothpick inserted in the center comes out clean. Cool 10 minutes in pan. Run knife around side of pan before removing. Cool completely.

4 To prepare filling, heat preserves in a small saucepan over low heat for 3–4 minutes or until they just begin to thin. Do not simmer or boil.

5 To assemble cake, using a long, sharp knife, slice cakes in half lengthwise to create 4 cake halves. Place one of the bottom cake halves on a large plate or cake plate, cut side up. Spoon 1/3 of the raspberry preserves on top and spread evenly over entire cake within 1/4 inch of the sides. Top with one of the top cake halves, cut side up. Spoon another 1/3 of the raspberry preserves on top and spread over entire cake within 1/4 inch of the sides. Top with the other bottom half, cut side up. Spoon the remaining raspberry preserves on top and spread over entire cake within 1/4 inch of the sides. Top with the last top cake half, cut side down.

6 To top cake, sift 1/4 cup powdered sugar over entire cake, letting some sprinkle down onto the plate. Line the fresh raspberries along the bottom edge of the cake and pile 3 of them on the top center of the cake to garnish.

Chef's Tip

Use mint leaves in your garnish for added color.

INDEX

blackened catfish, 12
broccoli scallop pasta, 213
catfish, breaded, 141
chimichurri salmon, grilled, 124
cod, crispy, 348
cod, peanut-crusted, 9
crab cakes, 153
crab tostadas, 259
halibut (*see* halibut)
linguine with red clam sauce, 92
Mediterranean shrimp wrap, 136
New England clam chowder, 372
orange roughy with citrus cream sauce, 239
oysters Rockefeller, 50
perch, baked, 309
salmon (*see* salmon)
seafood risotto, 344
seafood stew, 105
shrimp (*see* shrimp)
tilapia, lemon herb with zucchini, 56
tuna (*see* tuna)
flank steak
grilled with onion rings, 236
marinated, 60
French onion soup, 391
fried rice, 258
frittata
Italian garden, 196
zucchini and green pepper, 318
fruits
apples (*see* apples)
berry compote, 149
Brussels sprouts with citrus butter, 367
cherry tarts, 251
with dip, 203
grilled, 221
Mandarin orange chicken salad, 308
pear pecan salad, 242
pear salad with almonds, 70
pork chops, apple and raisin stuffed, 225
pork chops, grilled with peach compote, 187
pork chops with cranberry glaze, 355
pork loin with dried plums, 420
pretzel and strawberry delight, 180
salad, 87
salad with yogurt dressing, 377
shrimp skewers with pineapple and peppers, 208

smoothies, 132
turkey and apple grilled cheese, 168
turkey and avocado wraps, 42

G

garbanzos. *see* chickpeas (garbanzos)
garlic
butter mushrooms, 140
parsnips, garlic and herb-mashed, 61
potatoes, mashed, 383
potatoes, olive oil, 421
glazes
chicken breasts with raspberry balsamic glaze, 23
orange-glazed pork loin medallions, 233
pork chops with cranberry glaze, 355
tuna steaks with balsamic glaze, 46
gluten-free
acorn squash, roasted, 339
apples, sweet and savory baked, 394
artichoke salad, 418
asparagus, roasted, 33
asparagus with scallions, 117
beef kabobs, 197
beef tenderloin, 40
beef tenderloin, blackened, 100
beets, roasted, 347
berry compote, 149
black bean salsa chicken, 165
blackened catfish, 12
broccoli Amandine, 294
broccoli salad with raisins, 193
broccoli with cheddar cheese, 349
Brussels sprouts, roasted, 296
Brussels sprouts with citrus butter, 367
butterfly steak, 148
butternut squash soup, roasted with pecans, 356
Cajun French fries, 68
candied walnut salad, 24
caprese salad, 214
carrots, honey tarragon, 169
carrot salad, 322
cauliflower florets with lemon mustard butter, 125
cauliflower "potato" salad, 310